ADULT-GERONTOLOGY PRIMARY CARE NURSE PRACTITIONER REVIEW & RESOURCE MANUAL

Sharon Stark, PhD, RN, AGPCNP-BC, CFN, CPG

Lynda Stoodley, DNP, NP-C, AGACNP-BC, AGPCNP-BC

NURSING KNOWLEDGE CENTER

Library of Congress Cataloging-in-Publication Data

Names: Stoodley, Lynda, author. | Stark, Sharon W., author. | Nursing Knowledge Center, issuing
    body.
Title: Adult-gerontology primary care nurse practitioner review and resource manual / by Lynda
    Stoodley and Sharon Stark.
Description: Silver Spring, MD : Nursing Knowledge Center, American Nurses Association,
    [2017] | Includes bibliographical references.
Identifiers: LCCN 2017047885| ISBN 9780976821335 (pbk.) | ISBN 9780976821342 (epub) |
    ISBN 9780976821359 (epdf) | ISBN 9780976821366 (mobi)
Subjects: | MESH: Geriatric Nursing | Nurse Practitioners | Test Taking Skills | United States |
    Study Guide | Outlines
Classification: LCC RC954 | NLM WY 18.2 | DDC 618.97/0231--dc23 LC record available at
    https://lccn.loc.gov/2017047885

The American Nurses Association (ANA) is the only full-service professional organization
representing the interests of the nation's 3.4 million registered nurses through its constituent/
state nurses associations and its organizational affiliates. The ANA advances the nursing
profession by fostering high standards of nursing practice, promoting the rights of nurses in the
workplace, projecting a positive and realistic view of nursing, and lobbying the Congress and
regulatory agencies on healthcare issues affecting nurses and the public.

ISBN print   978-0-9768213-3-5
ISBN ePDF   978-0-9768213-5-9
ISBN ePub   978-0-9768213-4-2
ISBN mobi   978-0-9768213-6-6

First printing, December 2017

ADULT-GERONTOLOGY PRIMARY CARE NURSE PRACTITIONER REVIEW AND RESOURCE MANUAL

December 2017

Please direct your comments and queries to: revmanuals@ana.org

The healthcare services delivery system is a volatile marketplace demanding superior knowledge, clinical skills, and competencies from all registered nurses. Nursing autonomy of practice and nurse career marketability and mobility in the new century hinge on affirming the profession's formative philosophy, which places a priority on a lifelong commitment to the principles of education and professional development. The knowledge base of nursing theory and practice is expanding, and while care has been taken to ensure the accuracy and timeliness of the information presented in the *Adult-Gerontology Primary Care Nurse Practioner Review and Resource Manual*, clinicians are advised to always verify the most current national guidelines and recommendations and to practice in accordance with professional standards of care used with regard to the unique circumstances that apply in each practice situation. In addition, the editors wish to note that provision of information in this text does not imply an endorsement of any particular products, procedures, or services.

Therefore, the authors, editors, American Nurses Association (ANA), American Nurses Association's Publishing (ANP), and the Nursing Knowledge Center (NKC) cannot accept responsibility for errors or omissions, or for any consequences or liability, injury, and/or damages to persons or property from application of the information in this manual and make no warranty, express or implied, with respect to the contents of the *Adult-Gerontology Primary Care Nurse Practioner Review and Resource Manual*. Completion of this manual does not guarantee that the reader will pass the certification exam. The practice examination questions are not a requirement to take a certification examination. The practice examination questions cannot be used as an indicator of results on the actual certification.

Published by

Nursing Knowledge Center
8515 Georgia Avenue, Suite 400
Silver Spring, MD 20910-3402
www.nursecredentialing.org

INSTRUCTIONS FOR OBTAINING CONTINUING EDUCATION CREDIT FOR STUDY OF THE *ADULT-GERONTOLOGY PRIMARY CARE NURSE PRACTITIONER REVIEW AND RESOURCE MANUAL*

The Nursing Knowledge Center offers continuing nursing education contact hours (CE) to those who review and study this manual and successfully complete an online module. To obtain CE credit you must purchase and review the manual, pay required fees to enroll in the online module, and complete all module components by the published CE expiration date including disclosures, pre- and post-tests, and the course evaluation. The continuing nursing education contact hours online module can be completed at any time prior to the published CE expiration date and a certificate can be printed from the online learning management system immediately after successful completion of the online module. To purchase the online module for this manual visit the Nursing Knowledge Center's online catalog at https://learn.ana-nursingknowledge.org/. Please contact online support with any questions about the CE or module.

INQUIRIES OR COMMENTS

If you have any questions about the content of the manual please e-mail revmanuals@ana.org. You may also mail any comments to Editorial Project Manager at the address listed below.

Nursing Knowledge Center
Attn: Editorial Project Manager
8515 Georgia Avenue, Suite 400
Silver Spring, MD 20910-3492
Fax: (301) 628-5342

CE PROVIDER INFORMATION

ANA's Center for Continuing Education and Professional Development is accredited as a provider of continuing nursing education by the American Nurses Credentialing Center's Commission on Accreditation.

ANCC Provider Number 0023.

ANA is approved by the California Board of Registered Nursing, Provider Number CEP6178.

DISCLAIMER

Review and study of this manual and successful completion of the online module do not guarantee success on a certification examination. Purchase of this manual and completion of the online module are not required to obtain certification.

CONTENTS

CHAPTER 1

PREPARING FOR THE CERTIFICATION EXAMINATION

BEFORE YOU BEGIN STUDYING

Confirm the eligibility criteria. The eligibility criteria will vary for each exam, but may include things like clinical practice hours, degree and license required, etc. Please check the American Nurses Credentialing Center (ANCC) website for details on the particular eligibility criteria for your exam.

Review the general testing handbook. The general testing handbook can be found on ANCC's website (http://nursecredentialing.org/GeneralTestingandRenewalHandbook). It provides information on how the exam is scored, policies, etc.

TAKE ADVANTAGE OF ALL OF ANCC'S RESOURCES

1. Test Content Outline. The test content outline includes the number of questions for each domain of practice and identifies the areas that are included on the examination.

2. Test Reference List. Review the test reference list for review resources. While the list is not all-inclusive, it will act as a guide to help you prepare.

3. Sample Questions. In addition to the review questions at the back of this book, you can find sample questions that are similar to those on the actual examination on ANCC's website. For many exams there are also banks of practice questions available from the Nursing Knowledge Center's website: https://learn.ana-nursingknowledge.org/. Make sure to look at practice tests designed for the exam.

Develop a personal study plan approximately 3 months before you plan to take your exam. This could include self-study, finding a study buddy or group, taking a review course, taking an online narrated review course, reviewing current textbooks and articles, or other methods. The key is to have a study plan that works for you and follow through on it.

Arrange for special testing accommodations. The American Nurses Credentialing Center and its testing vendor make every effort to reasonably accommodate candidates with documented disabilities as defined by the Americans with Disabilities Act (ADA). If you have a disability as de-fined under the ADA, you must notify ANCC by submitting a report regarding your request from your physician or a qualified healthcare professional. The information must be on the physician's or other qualified healthcare professional's letterhead, typed, dated, and signed by the healthcare professional. Refer to the General Test Handbook for more details.

TIPS FOR PREPARING FOR THE EXAM

Step 1: Assess Current Knowledge

General Content

Examine the table of contents of this book and the test content outline, available at http://nurse-credentialing.org/Exam61-AdultGeroPrimaryCareNP-TCO.

- ▶ What content do you need to know?
- ▶ How well do you know these subjects?

Take a Review Course

- ▶ Taking a review course is an excellent way to assess your knowledge of the content that will be included in the exam.
- ▶ If you plan to take a review course, take it well before the exam so you will have plenty of time to master any areas of weakness the course uncovers.
- ▶ If some topics in the review course are new to you, concentrate on these in your studies.

Step Two: Develop Your Study Plan

- ▶ Write up a formal plan of study.
  - ▷ Include topics for study, timetable, resources, and methods of study that work for you.
  - ▷ Decide whether you want to organize a study group or work alone.
  - ▷ Schedule regular times to study.
  - ▷ Avoid cramming; it is counterproductive. Try to schedule your study periods in 1-hour increments.
  - ▷ Gather your study resources (general test handbook, Test Content Outline, Test Reference List, sample questions, etc.).
- ▶ You will need to know facts and be able to interpret and analyze this information utilizing critical thinking.

Personalize Your Study Plan

- ▶ How do you learn best? Choose study methods that fit your learning style.
- ▶ Have a specific place with good lighting set aside for studying. Find a place with no distractions. Assemble your study materials.
- ▶ Make sure to focus on the areas you are weakest and reassess periodically.

Step Three: Implement Your Study Plan

▶ Refer to your study plan regularly. Write it up or type it out and put it someplace you will see it regularly. Post it at your desk or even put it into your calendar.

▶ Stick to your schedule.

▶ Take breaks when you get tired.

▶ If you start procrastinating, get help from a friend or reorganize your study plan.

▶ It is not necessary to follow your plan rigidly. Adjust as you learn where you need to spend more time.

▶ Make sure you reference the Test Reference List and Test Content Outline on ANCC's website for the latest updates and information about the exam.

Pace Your Studying

▶ Stop studying for the examination when you start to feel overwhelmed and take a break. If you need to, adjust your study plan:

▷ Break overwhelming tasks into smaller tasks that you know you can do.

▷ Try a new study method.

Work with Others

▶ Put together a study group.

▷ Study groups can provide practice in analyzing cases, interpreting questions, and critical thinking.

▷ You can discuss a topic and take turns presenting cases for the group to analyze.

▷ Study groups can also provide moral support and help you stay on track.

Step Four: Final Preparation

Use practice exams when studying to get accustomed to the exam format and time restrictions. The Nursing Knowledge Center has a bank of sample questions available online in many specialty areas.

Practice tests can help you learn to judge the time it should take you to complete the exam and are useful for gaining experience in analyzing questions. However, keep in mind that books of questions may not uncover the gaps in your knowledge that a more systematic content review text will reveal. If you feel that you don't know enough about a topic, refer to a text from the reference list to learn more. After you feel that you have learned the topic, practice questions are a wonderful tool to help improve your test-taking skills.

Know your test-taking style and be aware of your potential pitfalls. Do you rush through the exam without reading the questions thoroughly? Practice reading the question completely, including all four choices. Choice "a" may sound good at first glance, but "d" is actually correct. Do you get stuck and dwell on a question for a long time? Remember that computer-based exams allow you to mark questions you are unsure about and go back to them later. You should spend about 45 to 60 seconds per question and finish with time to review the questions you marked. There is also no penalty for guessing; you are encouraged to respond to every examination question.

THE NIGHT BEFORE THE EXAM

▶ Be prepared to get to the exam on time.

   ▷ Know the test site location and how long it takes to get there.

   ▷ Take a "dry run" beforehand to make sure you know how to get to the testing site, if necessary.

▶ Get a good night's sleep.

▶ Eat sensibly.

▶ Avoid alcohol the night before.

▶ Assemble the required material to be admitted to the exam. Make sure you have the required form of ID. Reference the general test handbook for information about what you'll need.

▶ Read over the exam room rules. Know what you can and cannot bring with you.

THE DAY OF THE EXAM

▶ Get there early. You must arrive to the test center at least 15 minutes before your scheduled appointment time. If you are late, you may not be admitted.

▶ You will be given a dry erase board, which will be collected at the end of the exam.

▶ Nothing else is allowed in the exam room. You will be required to put all personal items in a designated area such as a locker.

▶ Items such as eye-wear, jewelry, etc. are subject to visual inspection

▶ No water or food will be allowed. You may leave the testing room to use the restroom or get a drink of water, but you will need to sign out according to the instructions that will be explained at the test site. Your testing time will not be increased to accommodate a break.

▶ Think positively. You have studied hard and are well-prepared.

▶ Remember your anxiety reduction strategies.

TIPS FOR DEALING WITH ANXIETY

Leading up to the Exam

Everyone experiences anxiety when faced with taking the certification exam.

▶ Taking a review course or setting up your own study plan will help you feel more confident about taking the exam. There is no substitute for being well-prepared.

▶ Take practice tests and time yourself to get used to feeling of working on a timer. Remember that the total time for each test is usually 4 hours. Time is not meant to be a factor in the examination.

▶ Brush up on test-taking skills.

▶ Practice relaxation techniques. A few minutes of deep breathing, meditation, or even just listening to soothing music can help you calm down and focus.

▶ Don't put too much stock in what others tell you about their exam experience. Remember that everything they can tell you is based on their memory of a stressful situation; it may not be very accurate. People tend to remember those items with which they are less comfortable; for instance, those with a limited background in women's health may say that the exam was "all women's health." In fact, the test content outline ensures that the exam covers multiple content areas without over-emphasizing any one.

Exam Day Anxiety

Test anxiety is a specific type of anxiety. Symptoms include upset stomach, sweaty palms, tachycardia, trouble concentrating, and a feeling of dread. But there are ways to cope with test anxiety.

▶ Avoid alcohol, excess coffee, caffeine, and any new medications that might sedate you, dull your senses, or make you feel agitated.

▶ Take a few deep breaths and concentrate on the task at hand.

▶ Use relaxation techniques such as breathing exercises, progressive muscle relaxation, or imagery and visualization.

▶ Go into the exam with a strategy in mind. Plan to take water and bathroom breaks at specific intervals and take that opportunity to stretch. Mark questions you're unsure of to come back to them later rather than spending too much time on one question.

INTERNET RESOURCES

▶ ANCC website: www.nursecredentialing.org

　▷ Test Content Outline: http://nursecredentialing.org/Exam61-AdultGeroPrimaryCareNP-TCO

　▷ Test Reference List: http://nursecredentialing.org/Exam61-AGPCNP-TRL

　▷ Sample Questions: http://nursecredentialing.org/AdultGeroPrimaryCareNP-SampleQuestions

▶ General Testing and Renewal Handbook: http://nursecredentialing.org/GeneralTestingandRenewalHandbook

▶ ANA Bookstore: www.nursesbooks.org.

　▷ ANA Nursing: Scope and Standards of Practice

　▷ ANA specialty scope and standards

　▷ Code of Ethics for Nurses

　▷ Other titles that may be listed on your Test Reference List

▶ Nursing Knowledge Center website: https://learn.ana-nursingknowledge.org/

　▷ Practice questions

　▷ Webinars and review courses

　▷ Certification Exam Test-Taking Strategies Web Course

CHAPTER 2

FOUNDATIONS OF ADVANCED PRACTICE NURSING

▶ Discuss role and scope of practice for adult-gerontology primary care nurse practitioners (AGPCNPs)

▶ Identify credentialing issues related to AGPCNP practice

DIMENSIONS OF THE NURSE PRACTITIONER (NP) ROLE

Important Factors Influencing the NP Role

AGPCNP Role

▶ Collaborate with health, social, political, cultural, and spiritual systems to eliminate barriers

▶ Assist patients to minimize health risks

　▷ Assume responsibility for their own health

　▷ Modify risk factors to prevent complications

▶ Practice holistically

▶ Recognize and address frequent and atypical responses to disease and treatment

▶ Serve as advocate and change agent

▶ Provide information, education, and resources

State Nurse Practice Acts

▶ Authority for nurse practitioner (NP) practice is found in state legislative statutes and in rules and regulations. The role of state boards of nursing is to protect the public. State boards of nursing grant authority for NP practice via nurse practice acts and promulgate rules and regulations passed by state legislatures. The Nurse Practice Act defines who can use the NP title, scope of practice, restrictions on practice, requirements that must be met to be credentialed within a state for practice, and rules and regulations for NP practice. Some states require a collaborative agreement with a physician, specify the types of drugs that might be prescribed, or define some type of oversight board on NP practice.

▶ Statutory law is implemented in regulatory language. Rules and regulations may vary with each state. Each state may further define scope of practice and practice requirements and restrictions.

▶ Beginning in 1999, the National Council for State Boards of Nursing (NCSBN) began implementing an interstate compact for nursing practice requirements to reduce state-to-state discrepancies in nursing requirements for practice. The Advanced Practice Registered Nurse (APRN) Compact addresses the need to promote consistent access to high-quality advanced practice nursing care within states and across state lines. The Uniform APRN Licensure/Authority to Practice Requirements, developed by the NCSBN with APRN stakeholders in 2000, establishes the foundation for this APRN Compact. Similar to the existing Nurse License Compact for recognition of registered nurse (RN) and licensed practical nurse (LPN) licenses, the APRN compact offers states the mechanism for mutually recognizing APRN license and authority to practice. A state must either be a member of the current nurse compact for RN and LPN, or enter into both compacts simultaneously to be eligible for the APRN Compact. To determine which states participate, view the state compact map at https://www.ncsbn.org/nurse-licensure-compact.htm.

▶ The APRN Joint Dialogue Group, consisting of an APRN Consensus Work Group and the NCSBN Advanced Practice Advisory Committee, forwarded a consensus model for APRN regulation in 2008. The model identifies APRN roles and population foci for licensure and specialty practice areas. The model identifies adult and gerontology as one population, with older adults as a potential specialty. A copy of the consensus statement and regulatory model can be found at http://www.aacn.nche.edu/education/pdf/APRNReport.pdf.

LEGAL AND FINANCIAL ISSUES

Nurse Practitioner Professional Practice

Licensure

▶ "The process by which boards of nursing grant permission to an individual to engage in nursing practice after determining that the applicant has attained the competency necessary to perform a unique scope of practice" (NCSBN 2017).

▶ "The purpose of a professional license is to protect the public from harm by setting minimal qualifications and competencies for safe entry-level practitioners" (NCSBN 2011).

▶ "Licensure is necessary when the regulated activities are complex and require specialized knowledge and skill and independent decision making. The licensure process determines if the applicant has the necessary skills to safely perform a specified scope of practice by predetermining the criteria needed and evaluating licensure applicants to determine if they meet the criteria" (NCSBN 2017).

▶ "Licensure benefits both the public and the individual nurse because essential qualifications for nursing practice are identified; a determination is made as to whether or not an individual meets those qualifications; and an objective forum is provided for review of concerns regarding a nurse's practice when needed. Licensure benefits nurses because clear legal authorization for the scope of practice of the profession is established. Licensure also protects the use of titles. Only a licensed nurse is authorized to use certain titles (i.e., registered nurses [RNs], licensed practical/vocational nurses [LPN/VNs], advanced practice registered nurses [APRNs], etc.) or to represent themselves as a licensed nurse" (NCSBN 2011).

Certification

▶ "A process by which a non-governmental agency or association certifies that an individual licensed to practice a profession has met certain predetermined standards specified by that profession for specialty practice. Its purpose is to assure various publics that an individual has mastered a body of knowledge and acquired skills in a particular specialty" (American Nurses Credentialing Center [ANCC] 2017).

Accreditation

▶ "A process of review that healthcare organizations participate in to demonstrate the ability to meet predetermined criteria and standards of accreditation established by a professional accrediting agency (Accreditation Commission for Health Care [ACHC], n.d.).

▶ Accreditation represents agencies as credible and reputable organizations dedicated to ongoing and continuous compliance with the highest standard of quality (ACHC, n.d.).

Scope of Practice

▶ Describes the who, what, where, when, why, and how of nursing practice, practice boundaries, and membership of a profession.

▶ Defines a specific legal scope determined by state statutes, boards of nursing, educational preparation, and common practice within a community. For example, adult nurse practitioners are not legally authorized to care for children. A state might require an NP to have formal educational preparation in pediatrics. Broad variation exists from state to state.

▶ General scope of practice is specified in many published professional documents (e.g., *Nursing: Scope and Standards of Practice,* American Nurses Association [ANA] 2015b; *Nursing's Social Policy Statement,* ANA 2010). In addition, many organizations have completed role-delineation studies that attempt to qualify the core behaviors that all APRNs must possess, as well as core knowledge and behaviors required of practitioners in a particular specialty. For example, core knowledge for a pediatric nurse practitioner will be inherently different from that of an adult-gerontology primary care nurse practitioner. It is critical that these statements about specific scope and standards exist so that everyone—including nurses—will have access to materials that they can refer to when there are specific questions related to role. This is especially important when the traditional role of nurses is being changed or "advanced" at an uneven rate through changes in state law. As the nurse practitioner role has expanded into new practice settings, including hospice, acute care, and home care, it is important that core knowledge, as well as state law protecting NPs in their practice settings, also expand, providing the legal authorization and title protections necessary for these practice settings.

▶ Prescriptive authority is recognized as within the scope of practice for nurse practitioners in all fifty states, though there is significant variability from state to state. This has created inherent difficulty in collecting data related to NP prescribing practices. The *Nurse Practitioner* journal publishes a comprehensive update of legislative requirements and recent changes in its January issue each year. Data collected by Nurse Practitioner Alternatives, Inc., since 1996 has documented stability within prescribing patterns by NPs. Data from 2004 document that the majority (72 percent) of NPs possess their own Drug Enforcement Administration (DEA) number, write between six and twenty-five prescriptions in an average clinical day (79 percent), recommend between one and twenty over-the-counter preparations in an average clinical day (90 percent), and manage between 25 percent and 100 percent of their patient encounters independently (97 percent; Scudder 2006).

Standards of Practice

▶ Authoritative statements by which quality of practice, service, or education can be judged (e.g., *Nursing: Scope and Standards of Practice*).

▶ Professional standards focus on the minimum levels of acceptable performance as a way of providing consumers with a means of measuring the quality of care they receive. They may be written at the generic level to apply to all nurses (e.g., following universal precautions), as well as to define practice by specialty.

▶ The presence of acceptable standards of practice may be used to legally describe the standard of care that must be met by a provider. These standards may be precise protocols that must be followed or recommendations for more general guidelines.

▶ Healthy People 2020 Objectives (https://www.healthypeople.gov/2020/topics-objectives) and the World Health Organization's (WHO) "Health for All" (Morrison 1985) are, respectively, national and international policy statements that describe objectives to be met to help all persons to obtain a level of health that will permit them to lead socially and economically productive lives. It is expected that over time, these objectives will form the basis for international standards of practice.

Patient Rights

Patient Self-Determination Act of 1990

Federal law requires healthcare agencies to have written policies on advance directives. The right to refuse care extends to life-prolonging care (including nutrition and hydration). Patients must have the mental capacity to refuse care. Failure to respect and comply with patient requests may result in lawsuits against providers (Patient Self-Determination Act of 1990).

Confidentiality

▶ Patients and families have a right to assume that personal health information will be kept private and will not be disclosed unless they consent to release the information. Patient confidentiality has several dimensions:

▷ Oral information: Information shared will not be disclosed to others who are not directly involved in the care of the patient.

    ▷ Written information: Confidentiality of any healthcare encounter is protected under federal statute through the Health Insurance Portability and Accountability Act (HIPAA) of 1996.

    ▷ Individual right to privacy is respected when requesting or responding to a request for a patient's medical record.

    ▷ The statute requires that the provider discuss confidentiality issues with patients, establish consent, and clarify any questions about disclosure of information.

    ▷ The provider is required to obtain a signed medical authorization and consent form to release medical records and information.

▶ Exceptions to guaranteed confidentiality occur when society determines that the need for information outweighs the principle of confidentiality. Examples might be when records are released to insurance companies; to attorneys involved in litigation; in answering court orders, subpoenas, or summonses; in cases of suspected child abuse; or if a patient reveals an intent to harm someone.

Health Insurance Portability and Accountability Act (HIPAA)

▶ Patients must be given detailed, written information on privacy rights and how their information may be used.

▶ Covers all forms of information including paper, verbal, and electronic.

▶ Provides civil and criminal penalties for violations ranging up to $250,000 and 10 years in prison.

NP Responsibilities

▶ Keep all patient information confidential.

▶ Never leave information on computer screens where unauthorized persons can gain access. Locate and position screens so they are not visible to passersby.

▶ Never share computer access codes with unauthorized persons.

▶ Do not leave telephone messages with confidential information unless granted permission.

▶ Do not discuss patient information with anyone not directly involved in patient care.

▶ Do not post any information on social media that may identify a patient.

Informed Consent

▶ Informed consent is the right of all competent adults and emancipated minors to accept or reject treatment recommended by a healthcare provider.

▶ Informed consent must be provided in terms the patient can understand.

▶ The clinician has the duty to explain relevant information to the patient and family so that they can make an appropriate decision.

▶ Relevant information usually includes diagnosis and nature and purpose of proposed treatment or description of procedure.

▶ Benefits and risks of proposed treatment or procedure, with an explanation of the possibility for death or serious harm or side effects, must be given.

▶ Discuss alternative methods of treatment and the possible effects of not having the treatment or procedure.

▶ It must be documented in medical records that this information has been provided (Dunphy et al. 2015).

Decisional Capacity

▶ Decision-making capability is the ability to cognitively process information and render a decision.

▶ The clinician must determine the patient's ability to cognitively process information provided.

▶ Competence is a legal term referring to the determination by a court that a person possesses sufficient cognitive function to make decisions regarding their health care and legal matters. If a person is declared incompetent, a legal guardian is appointed and the incompetent person's ability to exercise basic rights is limited.

Advance Directives

▶ When a person is not capable of making decisions, a person's preferences may be expressed by way of a written living will or healthcare durable power of attorney (DPOA) created when the patient was still competent.

▶ A living will is a written document prepared in advance of a terminal illness or irreversible loss of consciousness or competence.

▶ These provisions go into effect when

▷ The patient has become incompetent,

▷ The patient is determined to be terminally ill, and

▷ No further interventions will alter the patient's course to a reasonable degree of medical certainty.

Durable Power of Attorney

▶ Competent persons can identify in writing an agent to act on their behalf, should they become mentally incapacitated. Decisions made by the designated agent are

▷ Binding,

▷ Not limited to circumstances of terminal illness,

▷ Flexible enough to carry out the patient's wishes throughout the course of illness, and

▷ Often accompanied by a DPOA over financial issues as well.

▶ Legislation in most states enables family members to make medical decisions when no DPOA exists.

Guardianship

▶ Usually granted in response to a petition filed by family or caregiver

▶ Court decision transfers decision-making power from the patient ("ward") to a proxy ("guardian")

▶ Usually a "limited" guardianship—gives proxy power to make certain decisions that the patient is incapable of making

▶ Often necessary when a person has no family and lacks decision-making capacity

ETHICS

▶ Ethics is a discipline in which one attempts to identify, organize, analyze, and justify human acts by applying certain principles to determine the right thing to do in a given situation.

▶ Ethical dilemmas result when two or more choices exist and two or more of the outcomes are unfavorable.

Code of Ethics for Nurses

▶ The ethical behavior for nurses is defined in the *Code of Ethics for Nurses with Interpretive Statements* (ANA 2015a). Ethical codes are statements based on beliefs about individuals, nursing, health, and society.

▶ Nursing code statements deal with nursing behavior and attitudes about patients.

▶ In addition to courts, other bodies and agencies can use codes and standards to evaluate nursing practice.

TABLE 2–1.
IMPORTANT ETHICAL PRINCIPLES

Justice	Treat patients fairly and ensure they receive the services they deserve.
Veracity	Be truthful to patients.
Fidelity	Keep commitments and honor word to patients.
Confidence	Respect patients' right to privacy and protect information given confidentially.
Autonomy	Competent decision-making by individuals; self-determination; right to choose for oneself. Balance protection and limiting personal freedom.
Informed Consent	Protects a person's autonomy.
Beneficence	Doing good (finding alternatives) for patients to provide greatest good and do no harm.
Nonmaleficence	Nurses should avoid harming patients.

Ethical Decision-Making

▶ Moral concepts such as advocacy, accountability, loyalty, caring, compassion, and human dignity are the foundation for ethical behavior.

▶ Ethical behavior incorporates respect for the person and his or her autonomy. Thus, no decision is truly ethical if the caregiver does not involve the patient in decision-making to the full extent of the patient's capacity.

▶ Duty to help others (beneficence), avoidance of harmful behavior (nonmaleficence), and fairness are foundational components of ethical behavior.

Managing Ethical Dilemmas

▶ Dilemmas occur when the needs and obligations of some conflict with needs of others.

▶ Ethical dilemmas are common; often there is no right or wrong answer to an ethical issue.

Ethical Issues Affecting Older Patients

▶ Refusing procedures that could be life-saving

▶ Discontinuing life-extending medications and treatments

▶ Care of incapacitated patients without advance directives

▶ Unnecessary treatments or procedures

ADVOCACY

▶ An advocate is one who pleads for, supports, or recommends on behalf of another.

▶ Nurse advocacy is promoted by the Code of Ethics for Nurses, which supports patients as free agents with rights of self-determination.

Mandatory Advocacy

▶ **Abuse**: Physical or mental maltreatment

▷ Financial: Theft, fraud, undue influence

▷ Psychological: Name-calling, threats of violence or neglect

▷ Sexual: Forced or exploitative sexual conduct

▶ **Neglect:** Passive abuse, withholding needed care

▶ **Self-neglect:** Usually because of diminished physical or mental ability, but can be intentional

▶ Mandatory abuse and neglect reporting for certain populations (e.g., children, older adults, disabled adults) by healthcare personnel is required by almost every state (Buppert and Klein 2017).

QUALITY ASSURANCE

▶ Quality assurance is a system designed to evaluate and monitor the quality of patient care and facility management.

▶ Formal programs provide a framework for systematic, deliberate, continuous evaluation and monitoring of individual clinical practice. Programs promote responsibility and accountability to deliver high-quality care, and provide for an organized means of problem-solving. Thus, a good program identifies educational needs, improves the documentation of care, and reduces the clinician's overall exposure to liability.

▶ Programs identify components of structure, process, and outcomes of care. They also look at the organizational effectiveness, efficiency, and patient and provider interactions.

▶ ◆ May be implemented through audits, utilization review, peer review, outcome studies, and measurements of patient satisfaction.

Quality Improvement (QI)

▶ "Consists of systematic and continuous actions that lead to measurable improvement in healthcare services and the health status of targeted patient groups" (Health Resources and Services Administration 2011, 1).

▶ QI plan: Identify and prioritize areas for improvement by assessing quality of care congruent with mission of organization.

▷ Identify goals, objectives, and timeframe.

▷ Determine performance measures and indicators of performance.

▷ Define measurement population.

▷ Describe data collection plan and method, and analysis plan.

▶ ◆ Implementation of quality improvement initiatives can include peer review, safety, error reduction, self-monitoring, and use of technology.

Total Quality Management (TQM)

▶ Quality management includes quality monitoring, retrospective review, and quality committee activities (Hashmi, n.d.). TQM entails continuous, systematic actions, and ongoing evaluation of work that lead to measurable improvement in healthcare services, patient health status, and satisfaction of targeted groups. TQM includes

▷ Establishing long-term best care goals and problem-solving;

▷ Seeking, soliciting, and responding to suggestions;

▷ Monitoring, recording, and resolving complaints of patients, staff, professionals, and health entities immediately;

▷ Involving all staff in development and review of mission statement;

▷ Sharing responsibility for setting quality goals;

▷ Measuring daily operation outcomes in light of stated commitment to quality;

▷ Proactive and preventive quality improvement programs; and

▷ Support systems for staff having difficulties.

RISK MANAGEMENT

▶ Risk management is a process by which a business or other party reduces financial loss. Healthcare institutions' risk of financial loss exists in relation to patient care; employee, patient, and visitor injury; system failure; and functions of the organization. Institutional quality management programs are closely related to risk management. Quality management programs in health care are concerned with assessing and improving patient care. Risk management, although it has a preventative function, is most active after a problem incident.

▶ Risk management includes

▷ Evaluating risk of loss by identifying potential risks,

▷ Analyzing chance of potential risk becoming actual, and

▷ Acting to reduce occurrence of risk or loss.

Institutional Risks for Financial Loss

▶ Inadequate patient care

▶ Visitor accidents

▶ System breakage and equipment failure or loss

▶ Employee injury and personnel problems

▶ Corporate liability for malpractice actions of employees and others

▶ Issues related to any function undertaken by the organization

NURSE PRACTITIONER LEGAL AND FINANCIAL ISSUES

Accountability and Competence

▶ Level of conduct for which a nurse is held accountable. Standard of care is what a reasonably prudent nurse would do in the same or similar circumstance. Standards of care are flexible and constantly changing as knowledge and technology expands. Institutions can develop standards, which employees are expected to follow (e.g., policies and procedures). If an institution's standards are higher than those of a professional organization, a nurse is held to the higher standard while in that institution.

▶ **Accountability** is being responsible or answerable to another or to some authority. Accountability is to patients, employers, peers, the profession of nursing, and the public. Nurses are accountable for

▷ Safe and appropriate patient care,

▷ Documentation of care provided,

▷ Appropriate and timely communication with other practitioners, and

▷ Maintaining adequate level and currency of knowledge and skill to practice.

▶ **Competence** is possessing the needed knowledge, ability, skills, and intent to perform certain activities:

▷ Appropriate education

▷   Experience

▷   Specific knowledge

Liability

▶   Sources of legal risk

▷   Patients, procedures

▷   Quality of medical records

▶   Risk reduction or management

▷   Activities or systems are designed to recognize and intervene to reduce the risk of injury to patients and subsequent claims against healthcare providers.

▷   Malpractice insurance does not protect clinicians from charges of practicing outside their scope of practice. All clinicians should carry their own liability insurance coverage to ensure their own legal representation by an attorney to advocate for them.

Negligence and Malpractice

▶   Negligence is the failure to use care and judgment that a reasonably prudent and careful nurse would use in the same or similar circumstance that causes or results in harm to a patient. Negligence is any conduct that falls below an established standard. Negligence is not intentional. Standards are widely interpreted. Negligence needs to be established to pursue a malpractice case. Accepted standards of comparison are most likely to be national standards. To prove negligence in a malpractice claim, each of four elements listed below must be established by a preponderance of evidence.

▶   Malpractice

▷   Negligent professional acts of individuals engaged in professions requiring highly technical or professional skills

▷   The plaintiff has the burden of proving the four elements of negligence:

1.   Duty: The clinician has the duty to exercise reasonable care when undertaking and providing treatment when a patient-clinician relationship exists.

2.   Breach of duty: The clinician violates the applicable standard of care in treating the patient's condition.

3.   Proximate cause: There is a causal relationship between the breach in the standard of care and the patient's injuries.

4.   Damages: The patient suffers permanent and substantial damages as a result of the malpractice.

▷   High-risk areas for malpractice:

▶   Safety issues

▶   Medication errors

▶   Nursing assessment

▶   Competent knowledge of medical procedures

▶ Use of equipment

▶ Communication

▶ Documentation

▶ Failure to follow established policies, procedures, or standards of care

TABLE 2–2.
MALPRACTICE INSURANCE

TYPES	COVERAGE
Occurrence-based	Policy continues for claims occurring while policy is in effect, even after policy is terminated.
	Limits available to pay a claim are limits that were in place during policy term.
Claims made	Policy coverage as long as the insured pays premiums for initial policy and renewals
	Coverage ceases for cases that company did not accept during the policy term.

Reimbursement

▶ NPs are reimbursed as primary care providers in some form for their services under Medicare, Medicaid, Federal Employee Benefit Plan, Tricare (formerly Champus), veterans' and military programs, and federally funded school-based clinics.

▶ Private insurance plans may elect to reimburse for NP services even if not mandated to do so by state law. In some states, the insurance code may be interpreted rigidly to exclude reimbursement of NPs.

▶ Managed care organizations (MCOs) have frequently excluded NPs from being designated as primary care providers and carrying their own caseload. Thus, in many MCOs the only employment arrangement left open to NPs is that of a salaried employee. The NPs' contributions as salaried employees are often not visible and may be credited to their collaborating physicians, giving them "ghost" provider status. Without a legitimate method to document services provided and revenue generated, NP job security is often at risk. A recent focus of legislative activity by many state NP organizations has been to enact state laws that allow NPs to be impaneled as primary care providers in both health maintenance organizations (HMOs) and preferred provider organizations (PPOs). These efforts have led to opposition from state medical organizations.

▶ The concept of the medical home is a new model for patient care. Efforts are underway by professional nursing organizations to include nurse practitioners as primary care providers in the medical home model.

▶ State and national policy are in considerable flux regarding what services and procedures NPs may bill for and whether they will be paid directly. Incorrect billing places the healthcare provider at risk for fraud and abuse charges whether they knowingly violate the law or are just ignorant of the regulations.

▶ NPs must be aware of specific regulations and policies for patient care services. Resources include the Centers for Medicare and Medicaid Services (CMS) at www. cms.hhs.gov.

▶ Coding and billing is the responsibility of NP providers.

▶ Knowledge of regulations for payers is a requisite competency.

Healthcare Payment Systems

▶ Per diem payment

▶ Diagnosis-related groups (DRGs) and prospective payment (PP)

▶ Medicare (1965), Parts A, B, and D; Medicaid (1965) Title XIX (see table 2–3)

▶ Managed care; capitation

▶ HMOs, PPOs, independent practice associations (IPAs)

▶ Case management

TABLE 2–3.
COMPARING MEDICARE AND MEDICAID ⊙

MEDICARE	MEDICAID
• Federally administered.	• Administered by individual states, which make rules.
• Direct reimbursement to NPs is 85 percent of physician fee.	• States follow CMS rules and regulations for directing Medicaid program.
• "Incident to" reimbursement.	• Covers NP services.
• Services furnished incidental to physician's care.	• If a state has applied to CMS for a Medicaid waiver, it is important that NPs be allowed to act as primary care providers.
• Physicians must provide initial service and regular subsequent visits.	
• Physician must be present in office but not in exam room in some states.	• NPs apply to state Medicaid for Medicaid provider number.
• Services billed under physician's provider number at 100 percent of physician rate.	

Specific rules and regulations for Medicare and Medicaid can be found at www.cms.hhs.gov.

Performance Assessment

▶ "The Healthcare Integrity and Protection Data Bank (HIPDB) was established by the Health Insurance Portability and Accountability Act of 1996, Public Law 104-191, (HIPDB's authorizing statute is also referred to as Section 1128E of the Social Security Act). The purpose of the HIPDB was to help combat healthcare fraud and abuse. The HIPDB is no longer operational; however, information previously collected and disclosed by the HIPDB is now collected and disclosed by the National Practitioner Data Bank (NPDB)" (https://www.npdb.hrsa.gov/resources/hipdbArchive.jsp).

▶ The NPDB is maintained by the Department of Health and Human Services (HHS), Health Resources and Services Administration (HRSA), Bureau of Health Professions (BHP), Division of Practitioner Data Banks (DPDB). Developed as a result of the Health Care Quality and Improvement Act of 1986 (American Health Lawyers Association, n.d.), and amended in 1998, the NPDB and HIPDB are flagging systems intended to facilitate a comprehensive review of healthcare practitioners' professional credentials, with a goal of improving the quality of health care. The information contained in the NPDB includes a practitioner's licensure, professional society memberships, malpractice payment history, and record of clinical privileges. Online access is available to providers, agencies, and NPs to perform queries at http://www.npdb.hrsa.gov/pract/selfQueryBasics.jsp.

▶ Other programs monitoring and comparing healthcare quality include the Health Plan Employer Data and Information Set (HEDIS) developed by the National Committee on Quality Assurance (NCQA). HEDIS is a set of standardized performance measures designed to ensure that purchasers and consumers have the information they need to reliably compare the performance of managed healthcare plans (www.ncqa.org/).

CURRENT TRENDS

Fiscal Issues

▶ Growing competition in the job market for NPs as the numbers of NPs have increased and NPs have begun to directly compete with physicians and physician assistants.

▶ Reimbursement struggles with Medicare and private insurance.

▶ Increasing costs for malpractice insurance; many states have launched legislative initiatives on medical tort reform in an attempt to hold down malpractice premiums.

▶ Growing concerns over reimbursement fraud and abuse, as well as coding issues leading to overbilling and underbilling, particularly for Medicare patients, prompted the Centers for Medicare and Medicaid Services in 2007 to require all providers to obtain a National Provider Identifier (NPI). Information may be obtained at https://www.cms.gov/Medicare/CMS-Forms/CMS-Forms/downloads/CMS10114.PDF.

▶ Information on how to apply for an NPI can be found at https://nppes.cms.hhs.gov/NPPES/StaticForward.do?forward=static.instructions.

NP Education

▶ Recognition of the need to ensure the quality of NP education, faculty, and curricula has led to efforts by the National Organization of Nurse Practitioner Faculties (NONPF) and the American Association of Colleges of Nursing (AACN) to promulgate core competency statements (APRN Consensus Work Group and NCSBN APRN Advisory Committee 2008).

▶ In addition, NONPF, AACN, numerous NP professional organizations, NP accrediting bodies, and educational organizations have jointly promulgated criteria for evaluating nurse practitioner programs. In combination with accreditation standards for graduate programs and specialty areas, the criteria provide a basis for evaluating the quality of nurse practitioner programs (National Task Force on Quality Nurse Practitioner Education 2016).

▶ AACN, working with NONPF (with input from other groups), has developed a practice doctorate in nursing. In the future, the practice doctorate is expected to be the graduate degree for advanced practice nursing preparation, including but not limited to the four current APRN roles: clinical nurse specialist, nurse-anesthetist, nurse-midwife, and nurse practitioner.

▶ The board of NONPF regards the practice doctorate of nursing as an important evolutionary step in the preparation of nurse practitioners. They anticipate that the practice doctorate degree will become the standard for entry into nurse practitioner practice; however, much like the movement of educational preparation of NPs from the post–basic certification to master's degree, this evolution will be gradual. NONPF does not support any finite deadline for NP programs to be at doctoral-level preparation, but instead encourages NP educators to continue to sustain the highest quality programs to prepare NPs for clinical practice (NONPF 2015). In 2006, NONPF published *Practice Doctorate Nurse Practitioner Entry-Level Competencies*.

Practice Environment

▶ Health disparities: There is growing recognition of disparities in the health services and outcomes of different populations in the United States. The National Institute on Minority Health and Health Disparities (NIMHD) at the National Institutes for Health (NIH) is a government organization with a mission to promote minority health and to lead, coordinate, support, and assess the NIH effort to reduce and ultimately eliminate health disparities (https://www.nimhd.nih.gov).

▶ Health literacy: Now recognized as one of the largest contributors to health outcomes is the ability of a patient and family to understand and act on health information. Both the Health and Medicine Division (HMD; formerly the Institute of Medicine [IOM]) and the Agency for Healthcare Research and Quality (AHRQ) have launched efforts to quantify and offer solutions to the problems that result from inadequate health literacy. The IOM report on health literacy (Nielsen-Bohlman, Panzer, and Kindig 2004) may be viewed at https://www.nap.edu/catalog/10883/health-literacy-a-prescription-to-end-confusion and the AHRQ study (AHRQ 2015) can be viewed at https://www.ahrq.gov/sites/default/files/wysiwyg/research/findings/nhqrdr/nhqdr14/2014nhqdr.pdf.

▶ Patient Bill of Rights: In 2010, after President Obama signed the Affordable Care Act, a new updated Patient's Bill of Rights went into effect, which included patient protections. Children with preexisting conditions were often denied coverage and with the updated bill, denial of coverage for children with preexisting conditions was no longer allowed. As of 2014, this extended to adults. Other changes included the disallowance of lifetime limits on coverage and of cutting off insurance coverage because of an unintentional mistake on an application. Other components included the ability for the insured to choose which doctor to see and the ban on charging more for using emergency room services outside of the insurer's network. Young adults can stay on their parents' insurance until their twenty-sixth birthday and recommended preventative health care must be provided with no out-of-pocket costs. Lastly, new insurance holders are allowed to appeal insurance company decisions (Centers for Medicare and Medicaid Services, n.d.). With the most recent change in government, these may change.

▶ Disaster preparation: Increasing attention is being paid to preparing registered nurses to assume emergency roles during disaster with mass casualties. Potential disasters may be natural, accidental, or intentional (ANA 2016):

▷ Natural environmental (severe weather or earthquakes)

▷ Chemical

▷ Biological (pandemic influenza)

▷ Radiological or nuclear

▷ Terror attacks

▷ Explosive

▷ "ANA encourages nurses to strengthen the capacity of the health services in emergencies by joining a volunteer registry, knowing and understanding their employer's disaster response plan, and being personally prepared for emergencies" (http://www.nursingworld.org/MainMenuCategories/WorkplaceSafety/Healthy-Work-Environment/DPR/ANAAction). "The type of response and the level of response needed often depend on the type and severity of disaster" (ANA 2016). More information can be found at http://www.nursingworld.org/disasterpreparedness.

▶ Direct-to-consumer advertising: Patients frequently present to the office already having formed their diagnosis and wanting specific treatments. NPs must be knowledgeable about the newest products on the market to appropriately counsel and treat patients.

▶ Complementary and alternative modalities and medicines (CAM): There is a greater recognition of patient use of complementary and alternative modalities and medicines. Research suggests that 40–50 percent of patients are currently using a form of complementary or alternative therapy, despite the dearth of research on which to base treatment regimens. NPs as providers need to learn about common CAM treatments, and particularly about how some herbal products interact with prescription drugs. The National Center for Complementary and Integrative Health (NCCIH) is the federal government's lead agency for scientific research on complementary and alternative medicine (https://nccih.nih.gov).

▶ Since the 2000 release of the IOM report, *To Err Is Human: Building a Safer Health System* (Kohn, Corrigan, and Donaldson 2000), attention has increased on changes all healthcare providers should make to reduce medical errors. In response, The Joint Commission (formerly the Joint Commission on Accreditation of Healthcare Organizations [JCAHO], www.jointcommission.org) issued a list of abbreviations that should not be used in health care (https://www.jointcommission.org/facts_about_do_not_use_list/). In addition, the Institute for Safe Medication Practices has published a list of dangerous abbreviations related to medication use that it recommends be explicitly prohibited (https://www.ismp.org/tools/errorproneabbreviations.pdf). The list of banned abbreviations includes many symbols traditionally used in patient charts and writing prescriptions.

Health Policy and Delivery Issues

Health disparities are "differences in health outcomes between groups that reflect social inequalities" (Frieden 2011, 1).

- Access to care: Availability of care for all, including disadvantaged, underserved, and minority populations

  ▷ Barriers to access

    ▶ Decline related to decreased employer insurance coverage

    ▶ Financial inability to pay for services

    ▶ Impediments to care because of decreased providers and/or healthcare facilities

    ▶ Personal and cultural beliefs that block seeking care or compliance with care

Legislative Regulations

- Social policy determines what services citizens will pay for because of moral commitment to provide for the less fortunate.

- Economics determine program availability, eligibility, modifications to services, and services to control expenses.

- Legislative regulations (Health Care Financing Administration [HCFA]) provided choice for Medicare recipients for managed care or fee for service.

- Congressional Office of Technology Assessment has called for improved public information about healthcare providers' quality and treatment effectiveness.

- The Patient Self-Determination Act of 1990 provides information for advance directives.

- The Older Americans Act attempts to meet needs for social services, mental and physical health services, nutritional services, training, research to disseminate knowledge about aging, long-term care ombudsman, and more (National Council on Aging 2016).

Professional Organizations

- Participation in professional organizations is important because nurse practitioners, acting as a unified group, can influence the direction of the profession and of healthcare policy in the United States. All NPs should be involved and active in their professional organizations at the national, state, and local levels.

- State organizations work diligently to monitor and enforce laws and regulations affecting NP practice and health policy. In addition, these associations provide a group of peers for discussion and continuing education. Many state NP organizations have local chapters.

- National organizations

  ▷ The American Association of Nurse Practitioners (AANP) is focused on advocacy and keeping NPs current on legislative, regulatory, and clinical practice issues that affect NPs in the rapidly changing healthcare arena). "On January 1, 2013, the American Academy of Nurse Practitioners (founded in 1985) and the American College of Nurse Practitioners (founded in 1995) came together to form the American Association of Nurse Practitioners™ (AANP), the largest full-service national professional membership organization for NPs of all specialties" (https://www.aanp.org/about-aanp).

▷ The American Academy of Nurse Practitioners Certification Board (AANPCB; formerly American Academy of Nurse Practitioners Certification Program [AANPCP]) has a mission to promote excellence in NP practice, education, and research; shape the future of health care through advancing health policy; serve as the source of information for NPs, the healthcare community, and patients; and build a positive image of the NP role as a leader in the national and global healthcare community (https://www.aanpcert.org/ptistore/control/index).

▷ The Gerontological Advanced Practice Nurses Association (GAPNA) represents the interests of all advanced practice nurses who work with older adults. These APNs are active in a variety of settings across the continuum, including primary, acute, postacute, and long-term care (https://www.gapna.org).

▷ NONPF is an organization of nurse practitioner educators who are instrumental in setting standards for nurse practitioner education. NONPF developed core competencies describing domains of practice with critical behaviors that should be exhibited by all entry-level NPs (www.nonpf.org).

Health Models and Theories

▶ ˢ **Health Belief Model** (Janz and Becker 1984): A framework originally developed in the 1950s by Godfrey Hochbaum, Irwin Rosenstock, and Stephen Kegels to explain why people did not participate in health prevention and screening initiatives. Becker extended the model to include people's compliance with treatment for illness. It is based on people's perceived threat of susceptibility, seriousness, benefits action, and barriers for making changes to reduce the threat of disease, and is used for motivating people to take positive health actions to avoid negative health consequences.

▶ ˖ **Maslow's Hierarchy of Needs** (Maslow 1954): Posits a hierarchy of needs from basic to complex. Basic needs must be met before complex needs are met. From basic to complex, Maslow's hierarchy of needs is as follows:

▷ Survival/physiologic needs: Food, water, air, sleep, shelter

▷ Safety and security: Prevention of and protection from harm

▷ Love/belonging: Affection, friendship and family, trust and acceptance, and belonging

▷ Esteem: Self-esteem, personal worth, recognition, and accomplishment

▷ Self-actualization: Self-aware, personal growth, less concerned with opinions of others, and fulfilling self-potential

▶ ˗ **Transtheoretical Model of Change** (Prochaska and Velicer 1997): Conceptual model of intentional behavior change. Changes in health behavior involve six stages of change:

1. Precontemplation: No intention to take action to change in foreseeable future but person may be aware of the problem behavior

2. Contemplation: Intention to start the healthy behavior in foreseeable future

3. Preparation: Ready to take action within 30 days

4. Action: Recently changed behavior (within last 6 months) with intention to keep moving forward

5. Maintenance: Sustained change in behavior (more than 6 months) with intention to maintain change going forward

6. Termination: No desire to return to unhealthy behaviors and confident of no relapse

▶◣ **Social Cognitive and Self-Efficacy Theory** (Bandura 1986): Based on a persons' belief in their ability to perform behaviors to accomplish specific goals, and personal confidence in the ability to exert control over self-motivation, behavior, and social environment.

▶ • **Wellness Model** (National Wellness Institute 2017): Encompasses multiple dimensions—physical, emotional, mental, and spiritual. Every person has an optimal level of function, even with chronic illness or during the dying process.

▶ • **Family Systems Theory** (Kerr 2000): Grounded in general systems theory, in which there are interacting parts within and outside of families. Families interact in patterns in which predictable interaction patterns emerge. Boundaries can be viewed on a continuum from open to closed boundaries. Open boundaries permit outside influence. Closed boundaries create isolation.

▶ Aging theories

  ▷ Biological

    ▶ Wear and tear; cellular aging; immunological; free radicals

  ▷ Sociological

    ▶ Continuity; disengagement; activity; age-stratification

  ▷ Geriatric or Age-Related Stressors

    ▶ Physical disability

    ▶ Lost youthful appearance, beauty

    ▶ Interpersonal and social support loss or change

    ▶ Forced reliance on caregivers, confrontation

    ▶ Loss and grief

    ▶ Role loss

▶ • **Systems Theory in Practice Settings** (Walonick 1993): A collection of parts are the components of a system that are needed to make the system work in an interconnecting network to meet system goals. Systems theory attempts to explain system parts.

  ▷ **Input**

    ▶ Connections between the parts

      ▷ Staff-patients

      ▷ Materials–financial resources

  ▷ **Process**: Throughput; process of the work

  ▶ Processes to meet system goals

   ▷ Daily operations

  ▷ **Output:** Product of the work

  ▶ Success in meeting system goals and the ability of a system to change in response to feedback about meeting those goals

▶ ◦**Learning Theory (**Graduate Student Instructor Teaching and Resource Center 2017)

  ▷ Behaviorist: Associationist/Associationism School of Learning (Skinner, Pavlov)

  ▶ Learning results through reinforced associated behavior

  ▷ Cognitive School of Learning (Piaget, Perry)

  ▶ Mental thought processing or information processing

  ▷ Humanist (Knowles)

  ▶ Self-actualization is the prime objective to assist adult learners to develop and achieve full emotional, psychological, and intellectual potential

   ▷ Premise of this theory is that adults learn best by doing

Learning and Adult Education

▶ Learning should be continuous (lifelong), be related to information already mastered, be purposeful, make sense to the learner, and involve as many senses as possible.

▶ Adult education

  ▷ Best when the learner is involved and learning is relevant

  ▷ Uses multisensory approach

  ▶ Auditory, visual, and kinesthetic

  ▷ Should be repetitious

  ▷ Uses appropriate educational material

  ▶ Consider age, gender, culture, language

  ▷ Assesses reading level

  ▶ Can be done in most word processing programs

Adult Learner Accommodations

▶ Increase time allowed.

▶ Help learner identify association between items.

▶ Promote physical comfort.

▶ Set realistic, mutual goals.

▶ Eliminate distractions.

▶ Ensure glasses and/or hearing aids are on and working.

▶ Encourage verbal response and allow time.

► Incorporate techniques for good communication.

► Reinforce correct responses and provide immediate feedback.

► Use examples relating to learner's life and experience.

► Use simple, black-on-white, large-letter visuals.

► Include a family member when possible and appropriate.

► Provide new information in writing (at appropriate reading level).

► Always treat adult learners with respect and dignity.

Older Adult Learning Considerations

► • Learn best by pacing selves to incoming stimuli

► - Do not learn "unnecessary" or "irrelevant" tasks

► - Solve problems differently than younger adults

► - Tend to refer back to previous experience

► - Approach to problems literal, not hypothetical

► - Use fewer organizational skills

► ¹ More cautious and take fewer risks

► ⁻ Less likely to change strategies

► - More affected by information overload

Factors Affecting Teaching and Learning

► Educational level

▷ • Keep written material at a 6th- to 7th-grade reading level.

► Socioeconomic status

▷ Assist with accessing resources.

► Support systems

▷ Identify and include them.

► Age

▷ Affects information processing

► Culture

▷ Incorporate beliefs, language needs, and health practices.

Health Literacy

Health literacy is the capacity to obtain, process, and understand basic health information and services and requires appropriate communication techniques.

► Use opened-ended questions to ensure understanding.

► Make incremental goals for information mastery.

► Have patient repeat information to verify comprehension.

Communication Theory

Communication conveys values and beliefs among people and between people and organizations. Communication clarity and congruence promote positive behavior. Lack of communication clarity leads to dysfunction or poor coping. Communication is both verbal and nonverbal.

▶ Process

  ▷ Establish rapport.

  ▷ Present a caring manner.

  ▷ Ask open-ended questions: "What brought you to the clinic today?"

  ▷ Quickly assess patient's abilities: hearing, sight, language, cognitive ability.

  ▷ Identify supportive or inhibiting communication in the presence of family members.

  ▷ Assure confidentiality and privacy (HIPAA).

▶ Active Listening

  ▷ Maximize understanding: "Are you saying that…?"

  ▷ Clarify: "How many times a day do you take that medication?"

  ▷ Maintain eye contact; take brief notes but don't focus more on the chart than on the patient.

  ▷ Follow a train of thought through to completion: "…and if you get dizzy, what do you do next?"

▶ Summarize

  ▷ "So I'm thinking if we work on treating your pain and get you walking a bit more, you might do better at home."

Difficult Communication

▶ Poor prognosis and end-of-life choices

  ▷ Assess patient and family understanding, advance directives, living will, healthcare proxy

  ▷ Appropriate use of scarce resources (aggressive care, palliative care, hospice)

  ▷ Involve interdisciplinary team; avoid medical jargon

▶ Loss of independence

  ▷ Patient safety versus ability to live alone; appropriate use of professional and family caregivers

▶ Safety concerns

  ▷ Unstable patients; cognitive or physical impairment

▶ Driving

  ▷ Frequent accidents or near-accidents, sensory or cognitive impairment; psychotropics or narcotics

- ▶ Medication issues
  - ▷ Cognitive impairment; medication adherence; complicated medication regimens; drug toxicity; multiple prescribers; financial issues.
  - ▷ Know your state laws for reporting unsafe drivers.
- ▶ Other safety concerns
  - ▷ Unstable patients; frequent monitoring or observation needs; cognitive or physical impairment needs more supportive care

Communication Challenges

- ▶ Cognitively impaired
  - ▷ Continually adjust approach; get patient's attention; assess hearing; communicate nonverbally; keep it simple; repeat; give time to respond; monitor reaction
- ▶ Older patient
  - ▷ Nurse-patient age gap; consider patient biases and prejudices; avoid paternalism; address by surname (Mr., Mrs., Ms., Miss)
- ▶ Bias
  - ▷ Avoid stereotyping, gendered terminology, and using labels.
  - ▷ Respectful communication regardless of religion, age, race, gender, physical appearance, or sexual preference.
- ▶ Cultural sensitivity
  - ▷ Be aware of cultural differences in verbal and nonverbal communication.
  - ▷ Be aware of your own cultural assumptions.
  - ▷ Check for understanding.
  - ▷ Avoid talking down or too slowly.
  - ▷ Be aware of patients' traditions and beliefs.
- ▶ Adolescents
  - ▷ * Because adolescents' major morbidity is due to increased risky behaviors, an interview tool called the HEADSS should be used to assess their psychosocial risk. This psychosocial risk assessment instrument is an interview tool to evaluate the adolescent's home, employment/education, activities, drugs, sexuality, and suicidality and depression (HEADSS; Cohen, Mackenzie, and Yates 2017).
- ▶ Risk factor identification
  - ▷ General principles; healthy lifestyle choices (e.g., cardiac, obesity, suicide)
- ▶ Third-party interview
  - ▷ Often critical for obtaining information from patients with dementia; need 15–20 percent more time; maintain patient's autonomy in presence of third party; allow private time with patient (exam); negotiate family involvement when possible

► Urgent situations

▷ Suspected abuse or mistreatment

▶ Unexplained bruises in various stages of healing without explanation; suspicion of diversion of financial resources, denial of physical care, or verbal abuse or intimidation.

▶ Unexplained withdrawal from normal activities, a sudden change in alertness, and unusual depression may be indicators of emotional abuse.

▶ Bruises around the breasts or genital area can occur from sexual abuse.

▶ Bedsores, unattended medical needs, poor hygiene, and unusual weight loss are indicators of possible neglect.

▶ Strained or tense relationships, frequent arguments between the caregiver and elderly person are also signs (Administration for Community Living 2015).

▷ Expressing suicidal ideation

▶ Ask direct questions: Do you ever want to hurt yourself? Do you have a plan?

▷ Concerns of self-neglect

▶ "Failure to perform essential self-care tasks and that such failure threatens his/her own health or safety" (Administration for Community Living 2015)

▶ May be difficult or challenging as patients have a right to autonomy and self-actualization and may be choosing behaviors that cause self-neglect

▶ May be a sign of abuse

▶ Must question whether patient is abusing substances

▷ Questionable drug use

Good Communication Techniques

▶ Basis for therapeutic relationship.

▶ Take time to communicate with patients and families.

▶ Remember HIPAA, privacy, confidentiality.

▶ Share information appropriately with interdisciplinary team by effectively charting.

▶ Be a good listener, nonjudgmental, open-minded.

▶ Listen to patients. They are trying to relay what is wrong.

▶ Techniques for older adults

▷ Quiet setting

▷ Anticipate hearing and vision loss

▷ Attempt to correct problems (pocket amplifiers, clean glasses, etc.)

▷ Adequate light

▷ Same level as patient and look at patient when speaking

▷ Slow, clear speech

▷ Avoid shouting

▶ ◄ Aphasic patients

    ▷   Ask yes-or-no questions; note writing.

    ▷   Have patient's attention.

    ▷   Eliminate background stimuli.

    ▷   Keep voice at regular level.

    ▷   Give patient time to speak and do not finish sentences.

    ▷   Use alternative methods of communicating such as writing, drawings, and gestures.

    ▷   Confirm accurate communication with "yes" or "no" questions (National Aphasia Association, n.d.).

REFERENCES

Accreditation Commission for Health Care. N.d. "About Accreditation." http://www.achc.org/getting-started/what-is-accreditation.

Administration for Community Living, Administration on Aging. 2015. "What is Elder Abuse?" https://www.acl.gov/programs/elder-justice/what-elder-abuse .

Agency for Healthcare Research and Quality. 2015. *2014 National Healthcare Quality and Disparities Report.* AHRQ Publication No. 15-0007. Rockville, MD: Department of Health and Human Resources. https://www.ahrq.gov/sites/default/files/wysiwyg/research/findings/nhqrdr/nhqdr14/2014nhqdr.pdf.

American Association of Colleges of Nursing. 2010. *Adult-Gerontology Primary Care Nurse Practitioner Competencies.* Washington, DC: American Association of Colleges of Nursing. http://www.aacn.nche.edu/geriatric-nursing/adultgeroprimcareNPcomp.pdf.

American Association of Nurse Practitioners. 2013. "Standards of Practice for Nurse Practitioners." https://www.aanp.org/images/documents/publications/standardsofpractice.pdf.

———. 2015. "Scope of Practice for Nurse Practitioners." https://www.aanp.org/images/documents/publications/scopeofpractice.pdf.

American Health Lawyers Association. N.d. "Health Care Quality Improvement Act of 1986." https://www.healthlawyers.org/hlresources/Health Law Wiki/HCQIA.aspx.

American Nurses Association. 2010. *Nursing's Social Policy Statement: The Essence of the Profession.* 3rd ed. Silver Spring, MD: American Nurses Association.

———. 2015a. *Code of Ethics for Nurses with Interpretive Statements.* Silver Spring, MD: American Nurses Association.

———. 2015b. *Nursing: Scope and Standards of Practice.* 3rd ed. Silver Spring, MD: American Nurses Association.

———. 2016. "Know Your Disaster." http://www.nursingworld.org/MainMenuCategories/WorkplaceSafety/Healthy-Work-Environment/DPR/KnowYourDisaster.

American Nurses Credentialing Center. 2017. "Credentialing Definitions." http://www.nursecredentialing.org/FunctionalCategory/ANCC-Awards/Grants/Credentialing-Definitions.html.

APRN Consensus Work Group and NCSBN APRN Advisory Committee. 2008. *Consensus Mode for APRN Regulation: Licensure, Accreditation, Certification, and Education*. http://www. aacn.nche.edu/education-resources/APRNReport.pdf.

Bandura, A. 1986. *Social Foundations of Thought and Action: A Social Cognitive Theory*. Englewood Cliffs, NJ: Prentice Hall.

Graduate Student Instructor Teaching and Resource Center. 2017. "Overview of Learning Theories." Berkeley Graduate Division. http://gsi.berkeley.edu/gsi-guide-contents/ learning-theory-research/learning-overview/.

Buppert, C., and T. A. Klein. 2017. "Dilemmas in Mandatory Reporting for Nurses." Medscape. http://www.medscape.org/viewarticle/585562_2.

Frieden, T. 2011. Foreword in *CDC Health Disparities and Inequalities Report—United States, 2011,* supplement, *Morbidity and Mortality Weekly Report* 60. https://www.cdc.gov/mmwr/ pdf/other/su6001.pdf.

Centers for Disease Control and Prevention. 2016. "Progress Reviews for Healthy People 2020." https://www.cdc.gov/nchs/healthy_people/hp2020/hp2020_progress_reviews.htm.

Centers for Medicare and Medicaid Services. N.d. "The Center for Consumer Information and Insurance Oversight: Patient's Bill of Rights." https://www.cms.gov/CCIIO/Programs-and-Initiatives/Health-Insurance-Market-Reforms/Patients-Bill-of-Rights.html.

———. 2016. *Long-Term Care Minimum Data Set (MDS)*. https://www.healthdata.gov/dataset/ long-term-care-minimum-data-set-mds.

CMF Group. 2001. "Don't Make These Mistakes When Buying Your Malpractice Insurance." http:// www.npcentral.net/malpractice/buying.mistakes.shtml.

Cohen, E., R. G. MacKenzie, and G. L. Yates. 1991. "HEADSS, A Psychosocial Risk Assessment Instrument: Implications for Designing Effective Intervention Programs for Runaway Youth." *Journal of Adolescent Health* 12 (7): 539–44.

Dunphy, L., J. Winland-Brown, B. Porter, and D. Thomas, eds. 2015. *Primary Care: The Art and Science of Advanced Practice Nursing*. 4th ed. Philadelphia: F. A. Davis.

Hashmi, K. N.d. "Introduction and Implementation of Total Quality Management (TQM)." iSixSigma.com. https://www.isixsigma.com/methodology/total-quality-management-tqm/ introduction-and-implementation-total-quality-management-tqm/.

Health Insurance Portability and Accountability Act of 1996, Pub. L. 104–191, 110 Stat. 1936, 104 Cong. https://www.gpo.gov/fdsys/pkg/PLAW-104publ191/pdf/PLAW-104publ191.pdf.

Health Resources and Services Administration. 2011. *Quality Improvement*. Rockville, MD: Department of Health and Human Services. http://www.hrsa.gov/quality/toolbox/ methodology/qualityimprovement.

Janz, N., and M. Becker, M. 1984. "The Health Belief Model: A Decade Later." *Health Education and Behavior* 11 (1): 1–47. doi:10.1177/109019818401100101.

Kerr, M. E. 2000. "One Family's Story: A Primer on Bowen Theory." Bowen Center for the Study of the Family. http://thebowencenter.org/theory/.

Kohn, L., Corrigan, J., and Donaldson, M. 2000. *To Err Is Human: Building a Safer Health System*. Washington, DC: National Academies Press.

Maslow, A. 1954. *Motivation and Personality*. New York: Harper and Row.

Morrison, A. 1985. "The World Health Organization and 'Health for All.'" *Health Affairs* 4 (1): 102–13. doi:10.1377/hlthaff.4.1.102.

National Aphasia Association. N.d. "Communication Tips." http://www.aphasia.org/aphasia-resources/communication-tips/.

National Committee on Quality Assurance. N.d.a. "About NCQA." http://www.ncqa.org/AboutNCQA.aspx.

———. N.d.b. "HEDIS® and Quality Compass®." http://www.ncqa.org/HEDISQualityMeasurement/WhatisHEDIS.aspx.

National Council of State Boards of Nursing. 2011. "What You Need to Know about Nursing Licensure and Boards of Nursing." https://www.ncsbn.org/Nursing_Licensure.pdf.

———. 2012. "2012 APRN model and Rules." https://www.ncsbn.org/2012_APRN_Model_and_Rules.pdf.

———. 2017. "Licensure: About Nursing Licensure." https://www.ncsbn.org/licensure.htm.

National Council on Aging. 2016. "Older Americans Act." https://www.ncoa.org/public-policy-action/older-americans-act/.

National Organization of Nurse Practitioner Faculties. 2012. "Nurse Practitioner Core Competencies." http://c.ymcdn.com/sites/www.nonpf.org/resource/resmgr/competencies/npcorecompetenciesfinal2012.pdf?hhSearchTerms=%22%22Nurse+practitioner+core+competencies%22%22.

———. 2015. "The Doctorate of Nursing Practice NP Preparation: NONPF Perspective." http://c.ymcdn.com/sites/www.nonpf.org/resource/resmgr/DNP/NONPFDNPStatementSept2015.pdf.

National Practitioner Data Bank. 2015. *The NPDB Guidebook.* Rockville, MD: Department of Health and Human Services. http://www.npdb.hrsa.gov/resources/aboutGuidebooks.jsp.

National Task Force on Quality Nurse Practitioner Education. 2016. *Criteria for Evaluation of Nurse Practitioner Programs.* 5th ed. Washington, DC: American Association of Colleges of Nursing.

National Wellness Institute. 2017. "The Six Dimensions of Wellness." http://www.nationalwellness.org/?page=Six_Dimensions.

Nielsen-Bolhman, L., A. Panzer, and D. Kindig, eds. 2004. *Health Literacy: A Prescription to End Confusion.* Washington, DC: National Academies Press.

Office for Civil Rights. 2003. "OCR Privacy Brief: Summary of the HIPAA Privacy Rule." Department of Health and Human Services. http://www.hhs.gov/sites/default/files/privacysummary.pdf.

———. 2013. *HIPAA Administrative Simplification: Regulation Text.* Department of Health and Human Services. https://www.hhs.gov/sites/default/files/hipaa-simplification-201303.pdf.

Office of Disease Prevention and Health Promotion. 2008. *Quick Guide to Health Literacy.* Rockville, MD: Department of Health and Human Services. http://health.gov/communication/literacy/quickguide/Quickguide.pdf.

Office of Minority Health. 2008. *A Strategic Framework for Improving Racial/Ethnic Minority Health and Eliminating Racial/Ethnic Health Disparities.* Rockville, MD: Department of Health and Human Services. https://minorityhealth.hhs.gov/Assets/PDF/Checked/OMH%20Framework%20Final_508Compliant.pdf.

Patient Self Determination Act of 1990, H.R. 4449, 101 Cong. (1990). https://www.congress.gov/bill/101st-congress/house-bill/4449.

Prochaska, J., and W. Velicer. 1997. "The Transtheoretical Model of Health Behavior Change." *American Journal of Health Promotion* 12 (1): 38–48. doi:10.4278/0890-1171-12.1.38.

Scudder, L. 2006. "Prescribing Patterns of Nurse Practitioners." *Journal for Nurse Practitioners* 2 (2): 98–106. doi:10.1016/j.nurpra.2005.12.019.

Siu, A. L. 2015. "Abnormal Blood Glucose and Type 2 Diabetes Mellitus: Screening." *Annals of Internal Medicine* 163 (Clinical Guideline): 861–68. https://www.uspreventiveservicestaskforce.org/Page/Document/UpdateSummaryFinal/screening-for-abnormal-blood-glucose-and-type-2-diabetes.

Smith, M. K. 2002. "Malcolm Knowles, Informal Adult Education, Self-Direction and Andragogy." Infed.org. http://www.infed.org/thinkers/et-knowl.htm.

Walonick, D. S. 1993. "General Systems Theory." StatPac Research Library. http://www.statpac.org/walonick/systems-theory.htm.

CHAPTER 3

HEALTHCARE ISSUES

EPIDEMIOLOGY

Defines Causes of Disease

▶ ● "Prevalence rate refers to the number of cases of a particular disease at a particular point in time divided by the percentage of the population at a point in time. The prevalence rate does not distinguish between new and old cases" (Dunphy et al. 2015, 39).

▶ ● Incidence is "the number of new cases of a disease diagnosed at a point in time (e.g., 1 year)" (39).

▶ ● An epidemic is "the presence of an event (illness or disease) at a much higher rate than expected on the basis of past history" (40).

▶ ● Endemic: "When the presence of an event is constant at or about the same frequency as expected based on past history" (40).

▶ ● A pandemic is "the presence of an event in epidemic proportions affecting many communities and countries in a short period of time" (40).

Stages of Natural Course of Disease

▶ Susceptibility

▶ Presymptomatic disease

▶ Clinical disease

▶ Disability

Goal

▶ Prevent disease and disability.

▶ Interventions are directed against the reservoir.

▷ Isolation or quarantine

▷ Water purification, pasteurization, inspection, immunization

Prevention through Primary, Secondary, and Tertiary Prevention Strategies

▶ Primary

 ▷ "The prevention of disease" (Dunphy et al. 2015, 25)

 ▷ Intervention started at the susceptibility stage of disease to prevent disease from occurring

 ▷ Strategies: Education, healthy lifestyle and diet, environmental control, water purification, regulation of food handling procedures, immunization

▶ Secondary

 ▷ "Early screening and detection of disease" (Dunphy et al. 2015, 25)

 ▷ Intervention started at the subclinical stage of disease to detect early stages of disease to abate disease complications and severity

 ▷ Strategies: Screening for diseases such as heart disease, lipids, diabetes, vision and hearing problems, cancers; genetic testing for inherited diseases; interventions for smoking cessation, substance abuse

▶ Tertiary

 ▷ "The restoration of health after illness or disease has occurred" (Dunphy et al. 2015, 25)

 ▷ Intervention started at the clinical stage of disease to reduce complications resulting from disease, and slow disease progression through treatment and provide rehabilitative initiatives

CULTURAL INFLUENCES ON HEALTH

▶ To ensure racial and ethnic minorities obtain needed health care, providers need to address language barriers and cultural beliefs, practices, and values, and empower patients in healthcare planning. Improved communication can bridge the gap between the culture of medicine and beliefs and practices of patients' value systems. Individual value systems can be based on ethnicity, age, religion, sexual orientation, disability, or socioeconomic status. Every healthcare encounter can have a positive effect on patient health potential by helping providers learn more about individual cultures. Family teaches beliefs, religion, culture, and societal mores. Ethnicity provides identity within a group, race, tribe, or nation and influences beliefs and behaviors. Culture provides beliefs, symbolic behaviors, and social characteristics common among its members.

Improving Communication

▶ Inquire how patient wants to be identified.

▶ Determine what components of culture are important.

▶ Use individualized assessment.

▶ Use open-ended questions.

▶ Involve patients and families in planning care, if desired.

▶ Be knowledgeable of culture-specific resources.

Cultural Sensitivity

▶ Sensitivity to patients' traditions and beliefs enhances care

▶ Awareness of how cultural groups understand life processes and define health and illness

▶ What cultural groups do to maintain wellness and believe about causes of illness

▶ How healers cure and care for members of cultural groups

▶ Ethnocentrism: How one's own culture influences care

▶ Multiculturalism: Patient-centered nursing to understand cultural needs

▶ Cultural relativism: Recognize other ways of doing things as equally valid

▶ Spirituality: People search for life's meaning via participation in various activities (e.g., religion, belief in a god or gods, family). Relation between spiritual beliefs and health can influence perceptions of health and illness.

▶ High-risk groups reflect individual, social, and environmental factors associated with race, ethnicity, socioeconomic status, age, geographic location, language, gender, disability status, citizenship status, gender identity, and sexual orientation. High-risk groups are more likely to be uninsured or underinsured, have limited access to care, receive poorer quality of care, and experience worse health outcomes.

TABLE 3–1.
CULTURAL GROUPS AND HEALTH RISKS

CULTURAL GROUP	HIGHER RISK DISEASES
Asian American	Stroke, heart disease, tuberculosis, hepatitis B, certain types of cancer (Russell 2010)
Asian women	Osteoporosis, cervical cancer, suicide (older Asian women have the highest rate of all women over 65 in the United States; National Osteoporosis Foundation [NOF] 2017; Russell 2010)
White women	Osteoporosis (NOF 2017)
White men	Suicide (Centers for Disease Control and Prevention [CDC] 2017)
African American	Obesity, diabetes, hypertension, heart disease, stroke, asthma, undiagnosed cancer (Russell 2010)
Hispanic/Latinx	Obesity, diabetes, heart disease, end-stage renal disease, cervical cancer (Russell 2010)
Native American or Alaska Native	Obesity, diabetes, stroke, heart disease, cancer, suicide, smoking (Russell 2010)
Native Hawaiian or Pacific Islander	Obesity, diabetes, stroke, heart disease, cancer, smoking, alcohol consumption (Russell 2010)

ILLNESS PRESENTATION AND AGING CHANGES

▶ Consider normal and abnormal age-related changes when caring for older adults. Typical signs and symptoms of illness often are not present among older adults. Symptoms are often vague or functional status declines and may present as

▷ Confusion, delirium, mental changes, or worsening dementia

▷ Falls

▷ Incontinence

▷ Nonspecific, vague pain

▷ Slow to finish activities of daily living (ADLs)

▷ Dizziness

▷ Loss of appetite, weight loss, failure to thrive

▶ Common presentations

▷ Mental changes

▷ Confusion

▷ Worsening dementia

▷ Delirium

▶ **Multimorbidity** presents as conditions with common risk factors (chronic obstructive pulmonary disease [COPD] and cardiovascular disease [CVD]), or one condition complicating another (diabetes and CVD).

▷ Multimorbidity increases with age, compounds complexity of care, and is associated with poorer outcomes, decreased quality of life, depression, extended hospitalizations, more complications, and higher mortality.

▷ Analyzing the effects of multimorbid conditions on physical, psychological, and social functioning, and assessing risks, benefits, and applicability of treatment is basic to mutual patient–healthcare provider treatment priorities.

▷ Management of multiple concurrent disease states includes identifying risks common among multiple disease states, developing goals acceptable to patients, engaging patients, implementing plans of care, reviewing care effectiveness and medication adherence, and referring patients for specialized care as needed.

Aging Changes and Transitions

▶ Cognitive: No amount of decrease in cognition is normal with age. Immediate and remote memory are rarely impaired. Recent short-term memory decreases. Distant long-term memories remain intact and more retrievable than more recent memories. Decreased mental functioning with illness is often a result of vascular changes. Cognitive decline is a measure of speed performance, problem-solving ability, or organizational skills.

▶ Functional: Reaction time to sensory stimuli slows with age and is an area of most disparity in older populations. Some older adults function similar to middle-aged adults, while others may not function at all. Functional status is one tool used to guide how to care for patients in this cohort. Robust older persons may be offered

TABLE 3–2.
NORMAL AGING CHANGES

Universal	Changes occur in all. If a disease occurs primarily in older adults, do not assume that the disease is secondary to aging; it varies greatly from person to person.
Intrinsic	Changes are processes that occur within the body and do not result from external factors.
Progressive	Changes are processes, not events. Chronologic age as a marker of functional capacity becomes less accurate with aging.
Deleterious	Changes are processes that are negative and decrease person's ability to survive.

different options for care than the frail older person. Performance capacity declines; hurrying older adults causes frustration and decreased performance.

▶ Personality: No personality change is seen with age. Mood, orientation, and memory should be assessed for a baseline. Pathology often has an effect, making accurate assessment difficult.

▶ Learning: Verbal and abstract abilities remain constant. Basic intelligence is not changed. Spatial awareness and intuitive, creative thought declines. Use simple association rather than analysis.

▶ Psychosocial: Sexuality and sexual patterns persist throughout life. Sexual function is necessary for wellness, a sense of normalcy, and well-being. Normal age variations, disability, medications, and treatments affect sexual activity. Close relationships have a positive effect and result in less stress, better mental health, and life satisfaction. Social network of friends shrinks with age. Loss can result in social change that requires older adults to learn new roles and how to manage tasks of daily living. Spiritual search for meaning is common and may cause crisis of faith and questioning meaning of life.

▶ See the article by Constance Smith and Valerie Cotter (2012) for an excellent review of normal age-related changes.

Transitions

▶ Physical, social, familial, spiritual transitions: Life events viewed as losses

▶ Status and role issues: Perceptions of exclusion and devaluation

▶ Relocation: Major psychosocial adjustment

▶ Territoriality and personal space: Need to gain, maintain, and defend space to preserve integrity

Assessment Considerations

▶ Functional status determines quality of life

▶ Need for systematic assessment

▶ Use appropriate standardized assessment instruments

▶ Cognitive, mood, and functional assessments complement physical assessment

▶ Spirituality and religion

▶ Bowel and bladder continence

▶ Drug use including prescription, over-the-counter (OTC), recreational drugs, supplements, herbals

▶ Substance abuse: alcohol, drugs, tobacco use

▶ Sexuality, sexual orientation, gender identity

▶ Support systems and social network

▶ Living arrangements and ADLs

▶ Culture and education

Transitions in Relationships

Relationships provide the opportunity to express passion, affection, admiration, and loyalty. Relationship may be:

▶ Short- or long-term

▷ Personal: companionship; spousal; life partners; family members; friends.

▷ Isolation: Common as older adults outlive others in their cohort. Isolation is a risk factor for depression, malnutrition, self-neglect, and abuse by others.

▷ Intergenerational: Intergenerational involvement improves quality of life regardless of functional status, and includes community programs promoting child–older adult interaction.

▷ Intimate: Sexual dysfunction and disruption of satisfactory sexual activity (e.g., women experience dry vaginal tissue, dyspareunia because of decreased estrogen; men experience erectile dysfunction, longer time between erections because of decreased testosterone).

▷ Therapeutic relationships with healthcare providers.

▷ Socioeconomic: Ask about expenses that may affect compliance with medications or other treatments; sometimes patients run up credit card debt to cover needed medical expenses.

Employment

▶ Many working longer or reentering workforce to meet expenses

Housing

▶ Independent living

▶ Assisted living

▶ Group homes

▶ Retirement communities

▶ Adult foster care

Support Systems

► Nursing assessment should include type and source of support (siblings, children, organized religious support, significant other).

Disease Processes

► Osteoporosis, arthritis, dementia

Geriatric Syndromes

► Patterns of symptoms in older adults that do not fit into particular disease categories, have more than one cause, can contribute to each other, and complicate treatment and management. Pressure ulcers, incontinence, falls, functional decline, and delirium increase in older age, cognitive and functional impairment, and impaired mobility.

► Other common factors of geriatric syndromes are frailty, dizziness, syncope, gait disorders, hearing and vision impairment, sleep disorders, dysphagia, and malnutrition.

► Being cognizant of risk factors can expedite diagnosis, appropriate interventions, and prevention strategies, but a gap remains in guidelines for effective treatment.

► When multiple conditions are present, treatment evaluation and care modification according to outcomes and response to treatment are crucial.

HOSPICE, PALLIATIVE, AND RESPITE CARE

► Medical care, pain management, emotional and spiritual support for life-limiting illness or injury.

► Belief in the right to die pain-free, with dignity, with support for patients and family.

► • **Hospice**: Must be terminally ill or within 6 months of death. Medicare does not recognize certification by a nurse practitioner that a hospice patient is terminally ill and has a life expectancy of 6 months or less. Certification can only be authorized by hospice or attending physicians.

► • **Palliative care**: No time restrictions, available any time and at any stage of illness whether terminal or not. Services are available concurrently or independent of curative or life-prolonging care.

► • **Respite**: Short-term accommodation for a dependent family member in a facility outside the home to provide caregiving relief to family caregivers.

LEADERSHIP AND ADVOCACY

Leadership Skills

► Develop, communicate, and guide change.

► Establish, nurture, and maintain interpersonal relationships.

► Influence, motivate, inspire, and instill confidence.

▶ Use critical thinking skills in problem-solving and making decisions.

▶ Demonstrate flexible adaptation in behaviors and resources to match situation.

Advocacy Skills

▶ Prerequisite knowledge of political climate and processes, clinical expertise, communication and negotiation skills.

▶ Process: Communicate with families and professionals; provide information to patient, assist and support patient decisions; change health systems, develop public policy, and overcome barriers to advocacy.

▶ Goals: Improve patients' situations and assist patients to receive needed information and services.

▶ NPs can advocate for health through prevention and health promotion strategies such as health screenings, counseling, and immunizations, and provide early diagnosis, education, and treatment in a variety settings (community centers, worksites, schools, and residential facilities) so that those at highest risk (frail, older, disabled, minorities) may be reached.

NP Full Practice Authority

The Institute of Medicine (IOM) report asserts that APRNs should practice to the fullest extent of their education and training (IOM 2010). NPs can improve health outcomes of diverse populations. Independent NP practice will lead to better care, better health, and lower healthcare costs.

Informatics

Health care has been transformed by the Internet and information technology. Electronic data have improved process and outcomes evaluation. Computerized clinical decision support systems improve clinical decision-making in prevention, diagnostics, prescribing, dosing, and disease management. Information transfer is advanced via electronic health records (EHRs). Telehealth allows expedited transfer of health information. Electronic communication of medical information is a high priority for HIPAA regulation.

▶ Technological clinical tools such as smartphones, tablet computers, Dopplers, and oximeters are used for diagnosis and treatment, medications, and measurement.

Government Incentives to Use Electronic Health Records (EHRs) and Meaningful Use

▶ Not using electronic health records results in penalties of Medicare reimbursement reduction by 1 percent in 2015, 2 percent in 2016, 3 percent in 2017, and 4 percent in 2018.

▶ "Meaningful use is using certified electronic health record (EHR) technology to:

▷ Improve quality, safety, and efficiency and reduce health disparities

▷ Engage patients and family

▷ Improve care coordination, and population and public health

▷ Maintain privacy and security of patient health information"
(HealthIT.gov 2015)

Minimum Data Set (MDS)

▶ "The Long-Term Care Minimum Data Set (MDS) is a standardized, primary screening and assessment tool of health status that forms the foundation of the comprehensive assessment for all residents in a Medicare and/or Medicaid-certified long-term care facility. The MDS contains items that measure physical, psychological and psychosocial functioning. The items in the MDS give a multidimensional view of the patient's functional capacities and helps staff to identify health problems" (Centers for Medicare and Medicaid Services [CMS] 2016).

▶ Standardized, comprehensive instrument that includes demographics, fractures, falls, behavior and depression, cognitive status, medications, incontinence, infections, nutrition, dehydration, and activities of nursing home residents.

▶ Monitors quality of care in nursing homes and evaluates residents' functional capability and clinical status with the goal of focusing treatment plans.

▶ Items reflect residents' acuity levels, including diagnoses, treatments, and functional status.

▶ Assessment data used for Medicare reimbursement system and many state Medicaid reimbursement systems.

EVIDENCE-BASED PRACTICE (EBP)

Evidence-based practice is the integration of clinical judgment and best scientific evidence with patient preferences and values to improve patient outcomes. It is a shift from practice grounded in habit or intuition to practice grounded in clinical evidence. EBP uses a variety of sources, including research, expert opinion, and patient preferences.

Research

▶ "A systematic inquiry that uses disciplined methods to answer questions or solve problems" (Polit and Beck 2012).

▶ "The purpose of conducting research is to generate new knowledge or to validate existing knowledge based on a theory" (Connor 2014).

▶ **Quantitative**: Think numbers.

▷ An exploration of relationships between variables related to the phenomenon (Connor 2014)

▶ **Qualitative**: Think words.

▷ An exploration of life experiences to give them meaning (Connor 2014)

Levels of Evidence

A hierarchy helps determine the strength of evidence when analyzing and evaluating EBP. Determining the strength of the evidence helps guide patient care. There are multiple hierarchies of evidence, which are similar to some degree (Connor 2014).

▶ The highest (strongest) level of evidence typically comes from a systematic review, a meta-analysis, or an established evidence-based clinical practice guideline based on a systematic review (Connor 2014).

▶ Other levels of evidence come from randomized controlled trials (RCTs), other types of quantitative studies, qualitative studies, and expert opinion and analyses (Connor 2014).

Evidence-Based Skills: Using PICOT

PICOT is a process technique used in evidence-based practice to formulate an answerable clinical question related to a patient or problem.

P – Population: Describe as accurately as possible patient or group of patients (older, diabetic)

I – Intervention: Dimension of interest (increased exercise)

C – Comparison: Statins to lower cholesterol

O – Outcomes: Desired clinical outcomes (prevention of cardiovascular disease)

T – Timeframe: In 6 months' time

DOCUMENTATION

Documentation provides a record of a patient's medical history, care, hospitalizations, surgeries, medications, procedures, results of diagnostic tests, and referrals. It is a means of making information explicit to other healthcare professionals, and is a legal document that can be used to ascertain whether standards of care have been met. Documentation methods includes handwritten records, dictation systems, electronic records, electronic prescriptions, email, the Internet, and a variety of electronic devices such as smart phones, tablets, laptops, and computers. Some basic tenets of documentation are below:

▶ If it is not documented, it was not done.

▶ Documentation must be clear and concise.

▶ State pertinent facts.

▶ Be objective, not emotional.

▶ Documentation must meet regulatory and payer requirements.

REFERENCES

Centers for Disease Control and Prevention. N.d.. "Can Lifestyle Modifications Using Therapeutic Lifestyle Changes (TLC) Reduce Weight and the Risk for Chronic Disease?" https://www.cdc.gov/nutrition/downloads/R2P_life_change.pdf.

———. 2015. "Assessing Your Weight." Healthy Weight. http://www.cdc.gov/healthyweight/assessing/.

———. 2016. "Progress Reviews for Healthy People 2020." https://www.cdc.gov/nchs/healthy_people/hp2020/hp2020_progress_reviews.htm.

———. 2017. "Fatal Injury Reports, National, Regional, and State, 1981–2015." Web-Based Injury Statistics Query and Reporting System. https://webappa.cdc.gov/sasweb/ncipc/mortrate.html.

Centers for Medicare and Medicaid Services. 2016. *Long-Term Care Minimum Data Set (MDS)*. Rockville, MD: Department of Health and Human Services. https://www.healthdata.gov/dataset/long-term-care-minimum-data-set-mds.

Connor, B. T. 2014. "Differentiating Research, Evidence-Based Practice, and Quality Improvement." *American Nurse Today* 9 (6). https://www.americannursetoday.com/differentiating-research-evidence-based-practice-and-quality-improvement/.

Dunphy, L., J. Winland-Brown, B. Porter, and D. Thomas, eds. 2015. *Primary Care: The Art and Science of Advanced Practice Nursing*. 4th ed. Philadelphia: F. A. Davis.

HealthIT.gov. 2015. "EHR Incentives and Certification: Meaningful Use Definition." https://www.healthit.gov/providers-professionals/meaningful-use-definition-objectives.

Institute of Medicine. 2010. *The Future of Nursing: Leading Change, Advancing Health*. Washington, DC: National Academies Press. http://books.nap.edu/openbook.php?record_id=12956&page=R1.

National Human Genome Research Institute. 2015. "Frequently Asked Questions about Genetic Testing." http://www.genome.gov/19516567.

National Osteoporosis Foundation. 2017. "What Women Need to Know." https://www.nof.org/preventing-fractures/general-facts/what-women-need-to-know/.

Polit, D., and C. Beck. 2012. *Nursing Research: Generating and Assessing Evidence for Nursing Practice*. 9th ed. Philadelphia: Wolters Kluwer Health/Lippincott Williams and Wilkins.

Russell, L. 2010. "Fact Sheet: Health Disparities by Race and Ethnicity." Center for American Progress, December 16. https://www.americanprogress.org/issues/healthcare/news/2010/12/16/8762/fact-sheet-health-disparities-by-race-and-ethnicity/.

Smith, C., and V. Cotter. 2012. "Nursing Standard of Practice Protocol: Age-Related Changes in Health." Hartford Institute for Geriatric Nursing, Age Related Changes. https://consultgeri.org/geriatric-topics/age-related-changes.

CHAPTER 4

HEALTH PROMOTION AND DISEASE PREVENTION

LEARNING OBJECTIVES

- ▶ Discuss health promotion strategies to enhance individual health
- ▶ Identify demographics of health status by age and ethnicity
  - ▷ Incidence
  - ▷ Risk factors
- ▶ Prevention and screening
  - ▷ Immunization

HEALTHY PEOPLE 2010–2020

- ▶ Increase quality and years of healthy life.
- ▶ Eliminate health disparities.
- ▶ Older adult areas of importance.
  - ▷ Access to quality health care, food safety, medical product safety, injury, violence prevention
- ▶ Health indicators reflect high-priority health issues and actions to address them.
- ▶ Priority areas: Nutrition, fitness, screening, immunizations, self-care skills, and complementary health models; greater need for geriatric specialist healthcare providers, focus switch to chronic disease and rising healthcare costs.
  - ▷ Renew focus on identifying, measuring, tracking, and reducing health disparities through determinants of approach.
- ▶ Assess health of nation over decade, facilitate collaboration across sectors, and motivate action to improve health of US population at national, state, and community levels.
- ▶ Objectives are available on the web at https://www.healthypeople.gov/2020/topics-objectives.

HEALTH MAINTENANCE AND GOALS

▶ Maximize functional status

▶ Minimize morbidity, limit disease progression

▶ Maintain independence

▶ Increase satisfaction and quality of life

▶ Gerontology: Mobility, bowel and bladder continence, mental status, self-care, safety, social support

SCREENING GUIDELINES

▶ Established by US Preventive Services Task Force (USPSTF; http://www. uspreventiveservicestaskforce.org).

▶ • USPSTF is an independent panel of experts in primary care and prevention that systematically reviews evidence of effectiveness and develops recommendations for clinical preventive services, and focuses on the critical need to define the efficacy of specific preventive measures.

AVERAGE LIFE EXPECTANCY

▶ Women: 81.2 years of age

▶ Men: 76.3 years of age (Xu et al. 2016, 1)

  ▷ Why the difference?

    ▶ Women pay more attention to their own health.

    ▶ Women more apt to see a provider early on when they have a symptom.

HEALTH BEHAVIORS AMENABLE TO INTERVENTION

▶ Exercise, nutrition, weight loss, serum cholesterol

▶ Calcium, aspirin

▶ Smoking cessation, alcohol, drugs

▶ Safety, injury, abuse prevention

▶ Vaccinations: Influenza, pneumonia, tetanus, zoster

DIET, EXERCISE, AND HEALTH

▶ General nutritional guidelines (Department of Health and Human Services [HHS] and Department of Agriculture [USDA] 2015):

▶ A variety of vegetables from all of the subgroups—dark green, red and orange, legumes (beans and peas), starchy, and other.

▶ Fruits, especially whole fruits.

▶ Grains, at least half of which are whole grains.

- ► Fat-free or low-fat dairy, including milk, yogurt, cheese, and fortified soy beverages.
- ► A variety of protein foods, including seafood, lean meats and poultry, eggs, legumes (beans and peas), and nuts, seeds, and soy products.
- ► Oils.
- ► Consume less than 2,300 milligrams (mg) per day of sodium.
- ► Limit alcohol consumption
    - ▷ 1 drink per day for women
    - ▷ 2 drinks per day for men
- ► Limit trans fatty acids.
    - ▷ Found in partially hydrogenated vegetable oils and foods (e.g., commercially prepared fried foods, some margarines, prepackaged cookies and crackers, baked goods)
- ► Consume less than 10 percent of calories per day from added sugars.
- ► Consume less than 10 percent of calories per day from saturated fats.

Nutritional Considerations for Older Adults

- ► Assess for protein energy malnutrition (PEM).
- ► Decreased lean body mass because of decreased protein consumption.
- ► Decreased lean body mass can
    - ▷ Delay healing,
    - ▷ Shorten life span,
    - ▷ Diminish functional capacity, and
    - ▷ Lower quality of life.

Protein Energy Malnutrition (PEM)

- ► Marasmus: Develops gradually over months or years; skeletal muscle metabolized (rather than plasma or visceral proteins); insufficient protein intake leads to weight loss
- ► Kwashiorkor (hypoalbuminemic): Develops over days to weeks because of acute illness; often superimposed on marasmus; causes serum protein depletion leading to edema; usually no weight loss

Malnutrition Risk Factors

- ► Poor dentition; dysphagia
- ► Neurological or musculoskeletal issues (food preparation or eating difficulties)
- ► Inability to obtain food, low income
- ► Gastrointestinal problems (constipation, anorexia, malabsorption)
- ► Taste alterations (chemotherapy, aging changes, medications)
- ► Cultural dietary influences

▶ Cognitive impairment; mood disorders; isolation

▶ Inadequate knowledge

▶ Effects of medication

▶ Alcohol or substance abuse

Nutrition Assessment

▶ History

▷ Dietary intake; medical history; drug history; social history

▶ Assess risk:

▷ "The Mini-Nutritional Assessment Short Form (MNA®-SF) is a screening tool used to identify older adults (>65 years) who are malnourished or at risk of malnutrition" (DiMaria-Ghalili and Amella 2012).

▷ • Anthropometric measurements:

▶ • BMI (body-mass index): under 22 or over 27 problematic

▶ • Weight changes: unintentional weight loss over 5 percent in last 30 days or over 10 percent in last 180 days

▶ • Midarm circumference

▶ • Triceps skinfold

▷ Additional nutrition assessment measures:

▶ • Waist circumference: Abdominal obesity

▶ • Prealbumin: Early marker and changes rapidly but unrelated to albumin

▶ • Anemia: Early manifestation; total lymphocyte count

▶ • Serum albumin: In absence of liver disease, proteinuria, protein-losing enteropathies; low indicates malnutrition; normal may be misleading

Nutritional Interventions

▶ Monitor weight and albumin.

▶ Monitor for pressure ulcers.

▶ Teach about My Plate (https://www.choosemyplate.gov).

▶ Obesity is difficult to treat.

▷ Questionable need to treat otherwise healthy older adults unless they have risk factors for hypertension (HTN), diabetes mellitus (DM), or malignancy

▶ Calorie intake needed to maintain weight:

▷ • Women:

▶ Not physically active needs about 1,600 calories

▶ Somewhat active needs about 1,800 calories

▶ Active lifestyle needs about 2,000–2,200 calories

▷ ● Men (Greenberg 2012):

    ▶ Not physically active needs about 2,000 calories

    ▶ Somewhat active needs about 2,200–2,400 calories

    ▶ Active lifestyle needs about 2,400–2,800 calories

▷ Add fiber slowly.

▷ May need vitamins.

    ▶ ● Thiamine in alcoholics

    ▶ ● B12 in many older adults (may require injections)

    ▶ ● Vitamin C to enhance iron absorption

▷ For bones:

    ▶ ● At least 1,200 mg calcium plus 400–800 IU vitamin D per day

    ▶ Limit caffeine (National Osteoporosis Foundation [NOF] 2014)

    ▶ Referrals as needed

▷ Dentist; healthcare provider; dietician, nutritionist; psychological support.

▷ Social services (Meals on Wheels, Senior Centers).

Exercise and Fitness

Lack of exercise increases risk of

▶ Obesity; diabetes;

▶ HTN; coronary disease; lung disease;

▶ Osteoporosis;

▶ Cancer; and

▶ Ineffective immune system.

Benefits of Exercise

▶ Improved appetite

▶ Improved cardiac function

▶ Improved muscle strength

▶ Increased bone density

▶ Improved balance

▶ Lowered cholesterol

▶ Improved glucose tolerance

▶ Better emotional health

▶ Fewer medical problems

▶ Psychological and physical benefits: improved self-esteem, reduced stress, decreased low-density lipoproteins (LDLs), increased basal metabolic rate (BMR), anti-aging effects, cardiopulmonary conditioning

▶ Principles to guide initiation of an exercise program:

  ▷ Adults should exercise 150 minutes per week.

  ▷ For maximum cardiopulmonary conditioning, a patient's heart rate (HR) should remain in the target zone (based on a person's age) for 30 minutes during exercise (American Heart Association [AHA] 2015).

Exercise and Health

▶ Older adults with health risk factors (such as cardiovascular disease) should have a complete history, physical exam, and exercise stress test before implementing an exercise program.

▶ Cardiovascular risk factors (high blood pressure, abnormal cholesterol levels, family history of heart disease, smoking habit, obesity, and abnormal glucose tolerance) may indicate danger in beginning an exercise program and warrant physical examination and screenings.

▶ Caution with exercise with family history of heart disease, diabetes, valve or large vessel disease, hypertension, or severe anemia, taking beta blockers or digitalis, or smoking cigarettes.

▶ Exercise programs contraindicated with complete atrioventricular (AV) block, embolic conditions, decompensated congestive heart failure (CHF), unstable angina, hemodynamically significant aortic stenosis, and uncontrolled DM.

ACHIEVE A HEALTHY BODY WEIGHT

▶ Balance caloric intake and physical activity.

  ▷ 30 minutes of continuous moderate to vigorous activity, at least 10 minutes at a time, most days of week

▶ Reduce weight.

  ▷ Energy expenditure should exceed caloric intake to lose weight.

▶ Limit high-calorie and low nutritional quality foods.

  ▷ Avoid refined sugars, trans fatty acids.

▶ Limit high saturated fat.

  ▷ Choose grains and unsaturated fat, vegetables, fish, legumes, and nuts.

  ▷ Consume less than 10 percent of calories per day from added sugars.

▶ Consume less than 10 percent of calories per day from saturated fats. (HHS and USDA 2015).

Ideal Body Weight (IBW) Estimation of Caloric Needs

The My Plate eating guide is exactly that—a guide. Each patient is a different individual. The NP can estimate ideal body weight and estimate patient caloric needs. (See table 4–1.)

TABLE 4–1.
DETERMINATION OF IDEAL BODY WEIGHT

BUILD	WOMEN	MEN
Medium	100 lb for first 5 ft plus 5 lb for each additional inch	106 lb for first 5 ft plus 6 lb for each additional inch
Small	Subtract 10 percent	Subtract 10 percent
Large	Add 10 percent	Add 10 percent

Example: Estimate ideal body weight (IBW)

John is 6 feet, 0 inches tall and has a large frame.

> 106 lb for first 5 ft = 106
>
> 6 lb × 12 additional in. = 72 lb
>
> 106 + 72 = 178 lb

Add 10 percent for large body frame: 178 × 0.10 = 18

> 178 + 18 = 196 lb IBW

Estimate Caloric Needs

▶ Daily caloric needs equal the sum of basal caloric needs plus activity caloric needs. To determine basal need, multiply IBW by 10.

Body Mass Index (BMI)

▶ Calculation requires only height and weight

▶ Used to identify possible adult weight problems

BMI formula: (Weight ÷ (Height^2)) × 703

▶ Example: A man weighs 220 lb and is 6 ft, 3 in. tall.

▷ Height = 72 + 3 = 75 in.

▷ (220 ÷ (75^2)) × 703 = 27.5 BMI

TABLE 4–2.
BMI LEVELS ₰

BMI	WEIGHT STATUS
Below 18.5	Underweight
18.5–24.9	Normal
25.0–29.9	Overweight
30.0 and above	Obese

ADULT HEALTH SCREENINGS

Health Screening

TABLE 4–3.
GENERAL SCREENING TESTS [a]

EXAM	FREQUENCY	SOURCE
Blood pressure (BP)	BP screening should be done in adults age 18 years and older every 2 years if BP < 120/80 mm Hg and every year if BP 120–139/80–89 mm Hg.	USPSTF
Cholesterol	20 years or older: Every 5 years.	NCEP
Colorectal Screening	Can use any of these three regimens for ages 50–75 (people at average risk): 1. Annual high-sensitivity fecal occult blood testing (FOBT) 2. Sigmoidoscopy every 3 years combined with high-sensitivity FOBT every 3 years 3. Screening colonoscopy at intervals of every 10 years	USPTF
Visual acuity	Current evidence is insufficient to assess the balance of benefits and harms of screening for impaired visual acuity in older adults.	USPSTF
Hearing	Adults age > 50 years: Current evidence is insufficient to assess the balance of benefits and harms of screening for hearing loss in asymptomatic adults aged 50 years or older.	USPSTF
Oral cancer	Asymptomatic adults over 18 years: Current evidence is insufficient to assess the balance of benefits and harms of screening for oral cancer in asymptomatic adults.	USPSTF
Glucose	Testing should be considered in overweight or obese (BMI ≥ 25 kg/m^2 or ≥ 23 kg/m^2 in Asian Americans) adults who have one or more of the following risk factors: • A1C ≥ 5.7 percent (39 mmol/mol), IGT, or IFG on previous testing • First-degree relative with diabetes • High-risk race/ethnicity (African American, Latinx, Native American, Asian American, Pacific Islander) • Women diagnosed with GDM • History of CVD • Hypertension (≥140/90 mmHg) or on therapy for hypertension • HDL cholesterol level <35 mg/dL (0.90 mmol/L) and/or a triglyceride level >250 mg/dL (2.82 mmol/L) • Women with polycystic ovary syndrome • Physical inactivity • Other clinical conditions associated with insulin resistance (e.g., severe obesity, acanthosis nigricans).	ADA

EXAM	FREQUENCY	SOURCE
Glucose (cont'd)	For all patients, testing should begin at age 45.	
	If results are normal, testing should be repeated at a minimum of 3-year intervals, with consideration of more frequent testing depending on initial results (e.g., those with prediabetes should be tested yearly) and risk status.	
Thyroid function	Current evidence is insufficient to assess the balance of benefits and harms of screening for thyroid dysfunction in nonpregnant, asymptomatic adults.	USPSTF ATA/AACE
	Screening for hypothyroidism should be considered in patients over the age of 60 years (recommendation B).	
Electrocardiogram (ECG)	USPSTF recommends against screening asymptomatic adults at low risk for coronary heart disease (CHD) with resting or exercise ECG for the prediction of CHD events (recommendation D).	USPSTF
Glaucoma	Current evidence is insufficient to assess the balance of benefits and harms of screening for primary open-angle glaucoma (POAG) in adults.	USPSTF
Mental status	Current evidence is insufficient to assess the balance of benefits and harms of screening for cognitive impairment.	USPSTF
Skin cancer	Routine self-examination.	ACS, USPSTF
	Regularly scheduled dermatologist screening.	
	Current evidence is insufficient to assess the balance of benefits and harms of using a whole-body skin examination by a primary care clinician or patient skin self-examination for the early detection of cutaneous melanoma, basal cell cancer, or squamous cell skin cancer in the adult general population.	
Bone mineral density	Women: Recommend screening for osteoporosis in women aged 65 years and older and in younger women whose fracture risk is equal to or greater than that of a 65-year-old white woman who has no additional risk factors (recommendation B).	USPSTF, NOF
	Men: Current evidence is insufficient to assess the balance of benefits and harms of screening for osteoporosis in men (recommendation I).	
	NOF recommends bone mineral density testing on women age 65 and older and men age 70 and older, in postmenopausal women and men age 50–69 based on risk factor profile, and in men and women age 50 years and older who have had an adult-age fracture.	

(continued)

EXAM	FREQUENCY	SOURCE
Prostate-specific antigen (PSA)	At age 50, men should make an informed decision about testing. Insufficient evidence to recommend screening. AUA recommends against PSA screening in men under age 40 years. Not recommended to routinely screen in men between ages 40 and 54 years at average risk. For men ages 55–69 years, shared decision-making should be used for PSA screening, proceeding based on the man's values and preferences. To reduce the harms of screening, a routine screening interval of 2 years or more may be preferred over annual screening in those men who have participated in shared decision-making and decided on screening. Not recommended to routinely check PSA in men age 70+ years or any man with less than a 10- to 15-year life expectancy.	ACS, USPSTF, AUA
Testicular cancer	Recommends against screening for testicular cancer in adolescent or adult men (recommendation D).	USPSTF
Abdominal aortic aneurysm (AAA)	Men age 65–75 years: One-time screening by ultrasonography for men who ever smoked (recommendation B). Recommends that clinicians selectively offer screening for AAA in men ages 65–75 years who have never smoked rather than routinely screening all men in this group (recommendation C). The current evidence is insufficient to assess the balance of benefits and harms of screening for AAA in women ages 65 to 75 years who have ever smoked (recommendation I). Recommends against routine screening for AAA in women who have never smoked (recommendation D).	USPSTF
Mammography (Applies to women of average risk)	Women aged 50–74 years: Biennial screening (recommendation B). Women aged 40–49 years: The decision to start screening mammography in women prior to age 50 years should be an individual one. Women who place a higher value on the potential benefit than the potential harms may choose to begin biennial screening between the ages of 40 and 49 years. Women age 75 years and older: Current evidence is insufficient to recommend for or against mammography screening in women aged 75 years or older (recommendation I).	USPSTF
BRCA 1, 2 genetic mutations testing	Only when an person has personal or family cancer history that suggests a hereditary susceptibility.	USPSTF

EXAM	FREQUENCY	SOURCE
Cervical cancer screening	Women 21 to 65: The USPSTF recommends screening for cervical cancer in women age 21 to 65 years with cytology (Pap smear) every 3 years or, for women age 30 to 65 years who want to lengthen the screening interval, screening with a combination of cytology and human papillomavirus (HPV) testing every 5 years. (recommendation A).	USPSTF
	Women younger than 21: The USPSTF recommends against screening for cervical cancer in women younger than age 21 years (recommendation D).	
	Women younger than 30 years: The USPSTF recommends against screening for cervical cancer with HPV testing, alone or in combination with cytology, in women younger than age 30 years (recommendation D).	
	Women Older than 65: The USPSTF recommends against screening for cervical cancer in women older than age 65 years who have had adequate prior screening and are not otherwise at high risk for cervical cancer (recommendation D).	
	Women who have had a hysterectomy: The USPSTF recommends against screening for cervical cancer in women who have had a hysterectomy with removal of the cervix and who do not have a history of a high-grade precancerous lesion (cervical intraepithelial neoplasia [CIN] grade 2 or 3) or cervical cancer (recommendation D).	
Atherosclerotic cardiovascular disease (ASCVD)	It is reasonable to assess traditional ASCVD risk factors every 4 to 6 years in adults 20–79 years of age who are free from ASCVD and to estimate 10-year ASCVD risk every 4 to 6 years in adults 40 to 79 years of age who are free from ASCVD. NHLBI grade: B (Moderate).	ACC/AHA, USPSTF
	Assessment of 30-year or lifetime ASCVD risk on the basis of traditional risk factors may be considered in adults 20–59 years of age who are free from ASCVD and are not at high short-term risk. NHLBI grade: C.	

Note: ACC/AHA = American College of Cardiology/American Heart Association; ACS = American Cancer Society; ADA = American Diabetes Association; AHA = American Heart Association; AHCPR = Agency for Health Care Policy and Research; ATA/AACE = American Thyroid Association/American Association of Clinical Endocrinologists; AUA = American Urological Association; JNC-8 = Eighth Report of the Joint National Committee on Prevention, Detection, Evaluation, and Treatment of High Blood Pressure; NCEP = National Cholesterol Education Program; NOF = National Osteoporosis Foundation; USPSTF = US Preventive Services Task Force

TABLE 4–4.
SCREENING EFFECTIVENESS

MOST EFFECTIVE WHEN	LEAST EFFECTIVE WHEN
• Directed to high-risk groups	• Past screening results consistently negative
o Recent hospitalization	
o Recent bereavement	• Person is frail, has dementia, or is not a candidate for treatment
o Socially isolated	• Person has limited remaining quality and quantity of life
o Financially stressed	
o Genetic predisposition	• Person unable or unwilling to cooperate with the intervention
• Diagnosed with comorbid conditions	
• Diagnosis and treatment improve quality of life	

▶ Genes are one of several factors related to development of disease. Genetic testing can help determine risks of developing diseases, help healthcare providers assess treatment options, provide information to lower disease risks, facilitate individual treatment decisions, and discuss possible responses to treatment. Most genetic tests are used to diagnose rare genetic disorders.

▶ Newer tests can identify multiple genes that affect risks for developing particular diseases and possibly prevent them.

▶ • Cervical Cancer Screening:

   ▷ Begin screening 3 years after sexual activity begins or after age 21 years.

   ▷ Screen sexually active women with cervixes who are 21–65 years old.

   ▷ Can extend screening interval if 3 consecutive negative Pap smears or negative HPV testing.

   ▷ Stop screening at 65 years if history of normal Pap smears.

   ▷ No screening if total abdominal hysterectomy (TAH) for benign disease; screen if secondary to malignancy.

Wound Risk Assessment

▶ Diabetic foot wound, assess for:

   ▷ Neuropathy

   ▷ Deformity

   ▷ Repetitive stress

   ▷ Nonhealing factors

      ▶ Wound depth

      ▶ Infection

      ▶ Ischemia

- Pressure ulcers
  - ▷ Assess bony prominences
  - ▷ Prediction tool: Braden scale
  - ▷ Identification and staging guidelines: National Pressure Ulcer Advisory Panel criteria (Haesler 2014)
  - ▷ Assess for pressure, friction, shear
  - ▷ Documentation and reassessment

Assessing Safety and Environment

- Fire safety; home safety; automobile safety; helmet safety; personal safety; aging adult safety; biological, chemical, physical, sociological, psychological safety

Falls

Annually, more than a third of adults 65 years or older fall, with five percent of falls resulting in fracture or hospitalization. Adults over age 85 are at highest risk and falls are the leading cause of injury-related death in this age group.

Risk Factors for Falls

- Previous falls or injuries
- Impaired cognition and judgment or altered level of consciousness
- Sensory disturbances
- Dehydration, infection, electrolyte imbalances
- Incontinence
- Medication toxicity
- Depression
- Assistive devices
- Inappropriate footwear
- Restraint
- Use of nonsturdy furniture or equipment
- Poor lighting
- Uneven or slippery surfaces
  (Boltz 2016; Moyer 2012; Hartford Institute for Geriatric Nursing, n.d.)

Falls Assessment

Falls are not normal. "The American Geriatric Society (AGS) recommends a multifactorial risk assessment for patients with a history of falls each year. The assessment should include a focused medical history, physical examination, functional assessment, and environmental assessment to evaluate patients' balance, gait, mobility, vision, medications, and home environment" (Hartford Institute for Geriatric Nursing, n.d.).

- Ask about history of falls
- Balance examination
- Gait evaluation

Fall History

▶ Description of fall (all recent events)

▷ Location, time of day, activity, symptoms, assistive device use

▶ Onset and course of balance problem

▶ Medication history

▶ Fear of falling: "postfall syndrome"

▶ Home environment

▶ Social support

▶ Positional vital signs; BP in both arms (rule out subclavian steal); hearing and vision (acuity and fields); vestibular function; cardiac and peripheral vasculature; musculo-skeletal assessment

▶ Neurological assessment: Cognition (orientation, memory, language), sensation (vibratory), deep tendon reflexes, tone (passive range of motion [ROM] all limbs), coordination (finger to nose, rapid alternating movements)

▶ Gait evaluation; history of falls, fear of falling

▶ Balance: Static balance; Romberg; semitandem (heel to arch) or tandem walk for robust patients; functional reach; reach for objects in different directions and across midline; dynamic balance–robust; pelvic tug or push

Interdisciplinary Management

▶ Reduce dose or number of medications (if more than four meds); exercise program; interventions for medical problems; training on assistive devices to promote safety

Interventions to Prevent Falls

▶ Exercise

▷ For balance and strength

▶ Medication adjustments

▶ Vestibular rehabilitation

▶ Vision

▷ Annual eye exams

▷ Corrected prescription

▷ Avoid bifocals

▶ Footwear modification

▶ Household modifications

▷ Provide adequate lighting

▷ Remove tripping hazards

▷ Eliminate walkway clutter

▷ Install railings as needed

▶ Postural hypotension

▷ Medication adjustment

▷ Compression stockings

▷ Salt loading

▷ ● Florinef (fludrocortisone)

▶ Evaluate for

▷ Bedroom and hallway clutter,

▷ Improper walking devices and wheelchairs (inappropriate size or use),

▷ Faulty footwear (slippery soles, improper fit),

▷ Poorly maintained walking aids (canes and walkers), and

▷ Lack of safety equipment, such as grab bars and other durable medical equipment.

Fall Risk Assessment Tools

▶ ● Timed get up and go

▷ From chair, stand up and walk 10 feet (3 m) and return to seated position.

▷ Under 10 seconds = normal mobility

▷ Over 29 seconds = mobility problems

▶ ● Berg functional balance

▷ Measures balance among older people with impairment in balance function by assessing performance of functional tasks

▶ ● Falls efficacy scale

▷ An instrument to measure fear of falling

▶ Home assessment checklist

▷ Checklist to identify potential hazards in the home that may increase the risk of falls

▶ Personal risk factors checklist

▷ Assess fall history and risk for falls

▶ The Hendrich II Fall Risk Model

▷ To be used in the acute care setting

▷ Brief and includes "risky" medication categories and interventions for specific areas of risk rather than a single, summed general risk score (Hendrich 2013)

▶ Additional fall screening and assessment tools: http://fallpreventiontaskforce.org/resourcetools/screening-assessment-tools/

Domestic Violence Screening

Domestic violence (DV) is a crime that can present as a pattern of assaultive and coercive behavior that includes physical, sexual, and psychological attacks. It is also known as partner abuse, spouse abuse, battering, or intimate partner violence. Healthcare providers have a duty to victims to be aware of legal obligations in diagnosing and reporting domestic abuse. Reporting laws vary state to state.

Interview Alone at Each Visit

Three validated questions can be used to screen for DV and can identify up to 75 percent of women who are at risk for DV (Feldhaus et al. 1997; Dunphy et al. 2015):

1. Have you been hit, kicked, punched, forced to have sex, or otherwise hurt by someone within the past year? If so, by whom?

2. Do you feel safe in your current relationship?

3. Do you feel threatened or controlled by a partner or ex-partner or anyone else in your life?

Elder Abuse

This term refers to any knowing, intentional, or negligent act by a caregiver or any other person that causes harm or a serious risk of harm to a vulnerable older adult (Administration on Aging [AoA] 2016).

Elder Abuse and Neglect Screening

▷ Do you feel safe where you live?

▷ Who helps you with your meals and medication?

▷ Who takes care of your bills?

▷ Does anyone at home frighten, threaten, or hurt you?

▷ Does anyone touch you without your consent?

▷ Does anyone make you do things you don't want to do?

▷ Does anyone take your things without asking?

▷ Have you had to sign documents that you did not understand?

▷ Are you alone a lot?

► Many cases are overlooked: signs are mistaken for changes of aging or declining health; injury or illness can mask or mimic signs; bone loss, weight loss, overmedication, and nonadherence to medication regimens can result in disorientation, somnolence, fractures, and exacerbation of chronic illnesses.

► Many cannot provide accurate information because of cognitive impairments from dementia or depression; depression, confusion, fearfulness, changes in behavior, loss of sleep are common.

► ∘ Suspect abuse when there are significant delays between time of injury and time treatment is requested; patient's and caregiver's explanations are contradictory or vague; there have been repeated visits the emergency department (ED); or if the patient uses a variety of facilities or changes healthcare professionals frequently.

Elder Abuse Screening Tools

► BASE: Brief Abuse Screen for the Elderly: http://www.nicenet.ca/tools-base-brief-abuse-screen-for-the-elderly

► CASE: Caregiver Abuse Screen: http://www.nicenet.ca/tools-case-caregiver-abuse-screen

► EASI: Elder Abuse Suspicion Index: http://www.nicenet.ca/tools-easi-elder-abuse-suspicion-index

▶ Elder Assessment Instrument: http://www.cgakit.com/eai

▶ Health Attitudes toward Aging, Living Arrangements, Finances: https://gme.medicine.uiowa.edu/familymedicine/familymedicine/sites/medicine.uiowa.edu.familymedicine/files/wysiwyg_uploads/HALF.pdf

Driving Assessment

▶ There are more than 40 million licensed drivers ages 65 and older in the United States (Office of Highway Policy Information 2016).

▶ "Older drivers made up 16 percent of all licensed drivers in 2011, compared with 15 percent in 2002" (National Highway Traffic Safety Administration [NHTSA] 2014, 3).

▶ "Among drivers involved in fatal crashes in 2012, older drivers had the lowest involvement rate per population as compared to other driver age groups" (NHTSA 2014, 4).

▶ In 2012 fatal crashes, "the involvement rate for male drivers (65+) was 21.73 [per 100,000] and the involvement rate for female drivers (65+) was 6.80" (NHTSA 2014, 4).

Predictors of Adverse Driving Events

▶ History of falls past 1–2 years.

▶ Visual and cognitive deficits.

▶ History of motor vehicle crashes.

▶ Current medication use (e.g., tricyclic antidepressants, benzodiazepines).

▶ No single battery of tests is available.

▶ ● Inability to draw a pentagon is an independent predictor of adverse driving events.

▶ Snellen assessment and confrontation reveal vision issues.

▶ Gait, balance, mobility, neck range of motion identify neuromuscular issues.

REFERENCES

Carr, D., J. Schwartzberg, L. Manning, and J. Sempek. 2010. *Physician's Guide to Assessing and Counseling Older Drivers*. 2nd ed. Washington, DC: National Highway Traffic Safety Administration. https://www.nhtsa.gov/staticfiles/nti/older_drivers/pdf/811298.pdf.

Administration on Aging. 2016. *Administration for Community Living*. https://www.acl.gov/programs/elder-justice/what-elder-abuse.

American Cancer Society. 2016a. "The American Cancer Society Guidelines for the Prevention and Early Detection of Cervical Cancer." http://www.cancer.org/cancer/cervicalcancer/moreinformation/cervicalcancerpreventionandearlydetection/cervical-cancer-prevention-and-early-detection-cervical-cancer-screening-guidelines.

———. 2016b. "American Cancer Society Recommendations for Prostate Cancer Early Detection." http://www.cancer.org/cancer/prostatecancer/moreinformation/prostatecancerearlydetection/prostate-cancer-early-detection-acs-recommendations.

———. 2016c . "Breast Cancer Signs and Symptoms." http://www.cancer.org/cancer/breastcancer/detailedguide/breast-cancer-signs-symptoms.

———. 2017a . "ACS Guidelines for Nutrition and Physical Activity." http://www.cancer.org/healthy/eathealthygetactive/acsguidelinesonnutritionphysicalactivityforcancerprevention/acs-guidelines-on-nutrition-and-physical-activity-for-cancer-prevention-guidelines.

———. 2017b. "American Cancer Society Recommendations for the Early Detection of Breast Cancer." https://www.cancer.org/cancer/breast-cancer/screening-tests-and-early-detection/american-cancer-society-recommendations-for-the-early-detection-of-breast-cancer.html.

———. 2017c. "Colorectal Cancer Screening Tests." http://www.cancer.org/cancer/colonandrectumcancer/moreinformation/colonandrectumcancerearlydetection/colorectal-cancer-early-detection-screening-tests-used.

———. 2017d. "Hodgkin Lymphoma Stages." http://www.cancer.org/cancer/hodgkindisease/detailedguide/hodgkin-disease-staging.

American College of Cardiology/American Heart Association Task Force on Practice Guidelines. 2014. "2013 ACC/AHA Guideline on the Treatment of Blood Cholesterol to Reduce Atherosclerotic Cardiovascular Risk in Adults." *Journal of the American College of Cardiology* 63 (25): 2889–934. http://dx.doi.org/10.1016/j.jacc.2013.11.002.

American Diabetes Association. 2017. "Standards of Medical Care in Diabetes—2017," supplement, *Diabetes Care* 40 (S1). http://care.diabetesjournals.org/content/40/Supplement_1.

American Heart Association. 2016. "Target Heart Rates." http://www.heart.org/HEARTORG/HealthyLiving/PhysicalActivity/FitnessBasics/Target-Heart-Rates_UCM_434341_Article.jsp#.WOQMdl61vu0.

American Urological Association. 2010. *American Urological Association Guideline: Benign Prostatic Hyperplasia (BPH)*. N.p.: American Urological Association. https://www.auanet.org/education/guidelines/benign-prostatic-hyperplasia.cfm.

Association of Reproductive Health Professionals. 2012. "Making Sense of Cervical Cancer." Health Matters. http://www.arhp.org/uploadDocs/makingsenseofcervicalcancer.pdf.

Boltz, M. 2016. *Evidence-Based Geriatric Nursing Protocols for Best Practice*. 5th ed. New York: Springer Publishing Company.

Centers for Disease Control and Prevention. 2016. "HPV-Associated Cancers and Precancers." In "2015 Sexually Transmitted Diseases Treatment Guidelines," *Morbidity and Mortality Weekly Report* 64 (3). http://www.cdc.gov/std/tg2015/hpv-cancer.htm.

Department of Health and Human Services and Department of Agriculture. 2015. *Dietary Guidelines for Americans 2015–2020*. 8th ed. http://health.gov/dietaryguidelines/2015/guidelines/.

DiMaria-Ghalili, R. A., and E. Amella. 2012. "Assessing Nutrition in Older Adults." *Try This: Best Practices in Nursing Care to Older Adults*, no. 9, edited by S. Greenberg. https://consultgeri.org/try-this/general-assessment/issue-9.pdf.

Dunphy, L., J. Winland-Brown, B. Porter, and D. Thomas, eds. 2015. *Primary Care: The Art and Science of Advanced Practice Nursing*. 4th ed. Philadelphia: F. A. Davis.

Feldhaus, K., J. Koziol-McClain, H. Amsbury, I. Norton, S. Lowenstein, and J. Abbott. 1997. "Accuracy of 3 Brief Screening Questions for Detecting Partner Violence in the Emergency Department." *Journal of the American Medical Association* 277 (17): 1357–61. http://dx.doi.org/10.1001/jama.1997.03540410035027.

Forbes, G., and J. Reina. 1970. "Adult Lean Body Mass Declines with Age: Some Longitudinal Observations." *Metabolism* 19:653–63.

Garber. J., R. Cobin, H. Gharib, J. Hennessey, I. Klein, J. Mechanick, R. Pessah-Pollack, P. Singer, and K. Woeber. 2012. "Clinical Practice Guidelines for Hypothyroidism in Adults: Cosponsored by the American Association of Clinical Endocrinologists and the American Thyroid Association." *Endocrine Practice* 18 (6). https://www.aace.com/files/hypothyroidism_guidelines.pdf.

Haesler, E., ed. 2014. *Prevention and Treatment of Pressure Ulcers: Clinical Practice Guideline*. Osborne Park, Aus.: Cambridge Media. http://www.npuap.org/resources/educational-and-clinical-resources/prevention-and-treatment-of-pressure-ulcers-clinical-practice-guideline/.

Hartford Institute for Geriatric Nursing. N.d. "Falling." https://consultgeri.org/patient-symptoms/falling.

Hendrich, A. 2013. "Fall Risk Assessment for Older Adults: The Hendrich II Fall Risk Model™." *Try This: Best Practices in Nursing Care to Older Adults*, no. 8. https://consultgeri.org/try-this/general-assessment/issue-8.pdf.

Melanoma Research Foundation. 2017. "The ABCDEs of Melanoma." http://www.melanoma.org/understand-melanoma/diagnosing-melanoma/detection-screening/abcdes-melanoma.

Morley, J. E. 1986. "Nutritional Status of the Elderly." *American Journal of Medicine* 81: 679–95

Moyer, V. 2012. "Prevention of Falls in Community-Dwelling Older Adults: U.S. Preventive Services Task Force Recommendation Statement." *Annals of Internal Medicine* 157 (3): 197–204. doi:10.7326/0003-4819-157-3-201208070-00462.

National Cancer Institute. 2017. "Colon Cancer Treatment (PDQ®)–Patient Version: Stages of Colon Cancer." http://www.cancer.gov/types/colorectal/patient/colon-treatment-pdq#section/_112.

National Cholesterol Education Panel. 2002. "Third Report of the Expert Panel on Detection, Evaluation, and Treatment of High Blood Cholesterol in Adults (Adult Treatment Panel III)." Washington, DC: National Heart, Lung and Blood Institute.

National Highway Traffic Safety Administration. 2014. "Traffic Safety Facts: 2012 Data; Older Population." DOT HS 812 005. https://crashstats.nhtsa.dot.gov/Api/Public/ViewPublication/812005.

National Human Genome Research Institute. 2017. "Frequently Asked Questions about Genetic Testing." http://www.genome.gov/19516567.

National Osteoporosis Foundation. 2014. "What Happens Next?" In *Healthy Bones for Life: Patient's Guide*, 26–29. https://www.nof.org/wp-content/uploads/2016/11/NOF-Health-Bones-For-Life-Patients-Guide.pdf.

Office of Highway Policy Information. 2016. "Table DL-20." From *Highway Statistics 2015*. Federal Highway Administration. https://www.fhwa.dot.gov/policyinformation/statistics/2015/dl20.cfm

Tabloski, P., ed. 2006. *Gerontological Nursing*. Upper Saddle River, NJ: Prentice Hall.

US Preventive Services Task Force. 2012. "Cervical Cancer: Screening." https://www.uspreventiveservicestaskforce.org/Page/Document/UpdateSummaryFinal/cervical-cancer-screening.

———. 2013. "BRCA-Related Cancer: Risk Assessment, Genetic Counseling, and Genetic Testing." https://www.uspreventiveservicestaskforce.org/Page/Document/UpdateSummaryFinal/brca-related-cancer-risk-assessment-genetic-counseling-and-genetic-testing?ds=1&s=breast.

————. 2014a. "Abdominal Aortic Aneurysm: Screening." https://www.uspreventiveservicestaskforce.org/Page/Document/UpdateSummaryFinal/abdominal-aortic-aneurysm-screening?ds=1&s=Abdominal%20aortic%20aneurysm:%20Screening.

————. 2014b. *Guide to Clinical Preventive Services 2014: Recommendations of the U.S. Preventive Services Task Force*. https://www.ahrq.gov/sites/default/files/publications/files/cpsguide.pdf.

————. 2015a. "Abnormal Blood Glucose and Type 2 Diabetes Mellitus: Screening." https://www.uspreventiveservicestaskforce.org/Page/Document/UpdateSummaryFinal/screening-for-abnormal-blood-glucose-and-type-2-diabetes?ds=1&s=Abnormal%20blood%20glucose%20and%20type%202%20diabetes%20mellitus:%20Screening.

————. 2015b. "Osteoporosis: Screening." https://www.uspreventiveservicestaskforce.org/Page/Document/UpdateSummaryFinal/osteoporosis-screening?ds=1&s=osteoporosis%20screening.

————. 2015c. "Thyroid Dysfunction: Screening." https://www.uspreventiveservicestaskforce.org/Page/Document/UpdateSummaryFinal/thyroid-dysfunction-screening?ds=1&s=thyroid%20disease.

Wilson, J. A. P. 2010. "Colon Cancer Screening in the Elderly: When Do We Stop?" *Transactions of the American Clinical and Climatological Association* 121: 94–103.

Xu, J., S. Murphy, K. Kochanek, and E. Arias. 2016. "Mortality in the United States, 2015." NCHS Data Brief No. 267. https://www.cdc.gov/nchs/products/databriefs/db267.htm.

CHAPTER 5

INFECTIOUS DISEASES

LEARNING OBJECTIVES

- ▶ Recognize common infectious diseases
  - ▷ Risk factors
  - ▷ Signs and symptoms
  - ▷ Diagnostic tests
  - ▷ Differential diagnoses
- ▶ Describe treatment and management of common infectious diseases
  - ▷ Management
  - ▷ Prevention

TYPES OF INFECTIONS

- ▶ Acute
  - ▷ Short term
  - ▷ Relatively severe course
- ▶ Chronic
  - ▷ Long term
  - ▷ May last a lifetime (e.g., hepatitis B [HBV] or C [HCV], human immunodeficiency virus [HIV])
  - ▷ May also require treatment for acute infections
- ▶ Localized
  - ▷ Confined to identified site
  - ▷ Exhibit heat, erythema, swelling, and pain

▶ Systemic

▷ Involve entire body

▷ Symptoms include fever, fatigue, general malaise

INFECTION TRIGGERS

▶ Inflammatory response

▶ Second line of defense that works to destroy invaders

▷ Humoral immune response: Immunoglobulin antibodies signal immune cells to destroy harmful substances.

▷ Cell-mediated response: White blood cells (including B cells and T cells) destroy foreign invaders.

CHAIN OF INFECTION

▶ Infectious agents

▶ Reservoirs

▶ Portals of exit

▶ Mode of transmission

▶ Portal of entry

▶ Hosts

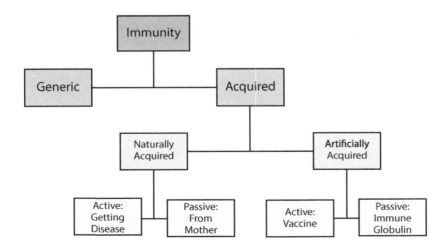

FIGURE 5–1.
TYPES OF IMMUNITY

INFECTIOUS AGENTS

▶ Bacteria

▶ Fungi

▶ Viruses

▶ Protozoa

Pathogenicity and Virulence

▶ Pathogenicity

▷ Ability of a microorganism to enter, survive in a host, and produce disease

▶ Virulence

▷ Severity of infectious agent

▷ How harmful infectious agent will be

▷ Must colonize host: Invade, live, and grow

Reservoirs, Carriers, and Portals of Exit

▶ Reservoirs

▷ Any place where the infectious agent can survive, grow, or multiply (e.g., plants, animals, soil, water, medical equipment, devices). The human body is the most common reservoir.

▶ Carrier

▷ Persons who carry the infectious agent and can spread disease but may not have disease themselves

▶ Portals of exit

▷ Pathway by which infectious agents leave the reservoir (e.g., body fluids, mouth and nose, respiratory tract)

Transmission and Susceptibility

▶ Primary transmission modes

▷ Contact

▶ Direct: person to person

▶ Indirect: object, surface, or droplet to person

▷ Airborne

▷ Ingestion

▷ Vector

▶ Living creature (e.g., insects)

▶ Infectious agent pathway to enter host

    ▷   Any opening in body can be a portal of entry

    ▷   Infectious agent enters host via a break in skin, ears, eyes, respiratory tract, gastrointestinal (GI) tract, genitourinary (GU) tract, and so forth

▶   Barriers to infection generally compromised

    ▷   Immunosuppression

    ▷   Level of susceptibility depends on various factors

▶   Age (infants and older adults are at greatest risk), nutritional status, stress, environment, preexisting conditions

▶   Immune status

    ▷   Humoral immunity is immunity conferred upon the body (e.g., vaccination; see table 5–1); includes passive and active immunity.

    ▷   Cell-mediated immunity is immunity that body has inherently; generally three types of cell-mediated immunities: helper, suppressor, and cell-mediated immunity.

TABLE 5–1.
IMMUNIZATIONS FOR ADULTS

IMMUNIZATION	TIMING
Influenza	Annually
Tetanus, diphtheria (Td), and pertussis (Tdap)	One dose Tdap, then booster Td every 10 years; women should get a Tdap vaccine during every pregnancy to protect the baby
Human papillomavirus (HPV; for adults and adolescents)	Two doses of HPV vaccine are recommended for most persons starting the series before their fifteenth birthday. • The second dose of HPV vaccine should be given 6–12 months after the first dose. • Adolescents who receive two doses less than 5 months apart will require a third dose of HPV vaccine. Three doses of HPV vaccine are recommended for teens and young adults who start the series at ages 15–26 years, and for immunocompromised persons. • The recommended three-dose schedule is 0, 1–2, and 6 months. • Three doses are recommended for immunocompromised persons (including those with HIV infection) aged 9–26 years. (Centers for Disease Control and Prevention [CDC] 2016g)
Measles, mumps, rubella (MMR)	One or two doses at ages 19–26. Adults born before 1957 are considered immune to measles and mumps. MMR is contraindicated in pregnancy, immunocompromising conditions, and persons with HIV and CD4 count < 200.

IMMUNIZATION	TIMING
Pneumococcal	One dose of PCV13 is recommended for adults • 65 years or older who have not previously received PCV13, and • 19 years or older with certain medical conditions and who have not previously received PCV13. One dose of PPSV23 is recommended for adults 65 years or older, regardless of previous history of vaccination with pneumococcal vaccines. No additional doses of PPSV23 should be administered to adults immunized with PPSV23 at age 65 or older. A second dose may be indicated for adults 19–64 years with certain medical conditions. Timing between PCV 13 and PPSV23 for adults age 65 years and older should be at least 8 weeks for adults who are immunocompromised or have cochlear implants or cerebrospinal fluid leaks. See https://www.cdc.gov/vaccines/vpd/pneumo/downloads/pneumo-vaccine-timing.pdf for recommendations for pneumococcal vaccine timing.
Herpes zoster	Adults should get zoster vaccine at 60 years old even if they previously had zoster (shingles). Zoster vaccines are contraindicated in pregnancy, immunocompromising conditions, and persons with HIV and CD4 count < 200.
Varicella	Two doses, 4–8 weeks apart, if no evidence of immunity. (Evidence of varicella immunity: US-born before 1980 except healthcare personnel and pregnant women; documentation of two doses of varicella vaccine at least 4 weeks apart; verification of varicella or herpes zoster diagnosed by healthcare provider; lab evidence of immunity or lab confirmation of disease.) Varicella vaccine is contraindicated in pregnancy, immunocompromising conditions, and persons with HIV and CD4 count < 200.
Meningococcal	One or more doses at ages 19–65+ years; schedule varies according to type of vaccine and indication.
Hepatitis A	Two doses at ages 19–65+ years.
Hepatitis B	Three doses for intermediate or high-risk patients, one series per lifetime. See http://www.cdc.gov/vaccines/schedules/downloads/adult/adult-schedule-easy-read.pdf for an easy-to-read adult immunization schedule.

Source: CDC 2016h

Effects of Aging on Immunity

▶ Immune system function declines with age.

▶ Macrophages have decreased ability to clear antigens and attack tumor cells.

▶ T-cell function and specific antibody responses decline.

▶ Thymus becomes small (fewer B and T cells).

▶ B cells produce antibodies that do not bind antigens well, causing suboptimal antibody response to vaccines and delayed hypersensitivity response.

▶ Decreased complement levels.

▶ Increase in autoantibodies.

Aging Changes in Immune Response

▶ Decreased resistance to infection

▶ Increased chance of latent infections reactivating (e.g., tuberculosis [TB], shingles)

▶ Absent or diminished classic signs and symptoms of infection

▶ Pneumonia without fever

▶ Urinary tract infection (UTI) presenting with nausea and vomiting or altered mental status and sepsis

▶ Inability or muted cutaneous hypersensitivity reactions

▶ Decreased vaccine response

Infections in Older Adults

▶ Older adults with chronic disease are at increased risk for infectious processes.

▶ Institutionalized older adults are at increased risk for infectious processes.

▶ Older adults experience increased incidence of autoimmune disorders.

▶ Usual symptoms of infections may be absent or diminished.

▶ Higher mortality from infection.

▶ Infections account for 40 percent of deaths in geriatric patients.

Common Pathogens

▶ Methicillin-resistant *Staphylococcus aureus* (MRSA)

▶ Vancomycin-resistant *Enterococcus* (VRE)

▶ Pseudomembranous colitis from *Clostridium difficile* toxin

Common Life-Threatening Infections in Older Adults

▶ Bacterial pneumonia and influenza

▶ Urinary tract infection (most common)

▶ Skin infections (cellulitis)

▶ MRSA

▶ VRE

▶ Sepsis

▶ Herpes zoster

▶ Infective endocarditis, increasingly seen because of degenerative valvular disorders and prosthetic valves

▶ Prosthetic device infections

▶ HIV

Etiology

▶ Gram-negative bacilli more common in older people

▶ VRE in urinary tract and on skin

▶ MRSA resistant to quinolones

Risk Factors for Infections

▶ Decreased physiologic reserve, including immune system

▶ Immobility

▶ Decreased fluid intake

▶ Malnourishment

▶ Invasive procedures

▶ Immunosuppressive agents (e.g., steroids, chemotherapy)

▶ Nosocomial infections and increased exposure to antibiotics

Comorbid Conditions that Predispose Older Adults to Infection

▶ Diabetes mellitus

▶ Chronic obstructive pulmonary disease (COPD)

▶ Malignancy

▶ Bladder outlet obstruction (BOO)

History

▶ Nonspecific presentation of illness is most common scenario.

▶ Delirium or decrease in activities of daily living (ADLs).

▶ Sudden onset of functional decline, falls, incontinence, fatigue, or anorexia.

▶ Usual symptoms of particular infection may be blunted or absent.

INFLUENZA (FLU)

▶ Infectious disease caused by influenza viruses (orthomyxoviruses) and transmitted via respiratory route.

▶ Human flu virus types A, B, and C; mutations produce new strains each flu season.

▶ Flu infections often lead to pneumonia in older adults (fifth leading cause of death).

▶ Occurs in epidemics; incubation 1–4 days; usually occurs in fall and winter.

Risk Factors

▶ Living in long-term care facilities

▶ Living with children

Signs and Symptoms

▶ Fever or chills

▶ Malaise, myalgia

▶ Headache

▶ Nausea and vomiting

▶ Anorexia

▶ Coryza

▶ Nonproductive cough

Diagnostic Tests

▶ Rapid flu test

▶ White blood count (WBC)

Differential Diagnoses

▶ Upper respiratory infection (URI)

▶ Pneumonia

Management

▶ Supportive

▶ Analgesics, hydration

▶ Rimantadine 100 mg b.i.d. × 7 days

After Exposure to Influenza A

• ▶ Amantadine (Symmetrel) 200 mg daily × 2 days

After Exposure to Influenza A or B

• ▶ Peramivir (Rapivab) one 600 mg dose, via intravenous (IV) infusion for 15–30 minutes

▶ Zanamivir (Relenza) 10 mg (2–5 mg inhalations) b.i.d. × 5 days

▶ Oseltamivir (Tamiflu) 75 mg b.i.d. × 5 days

Prevention

▶ Influenza vaccine: 85 percent develop immunity.

▶ Protection begins about 2 weeks after injection and lasts a few months.

▶ Trivalent influenza vaccine 0.5 cc intramuscularly (IM).

INFECTIOUS MONONUCLEOSIS (MONO)

▶ Acute infectious disease caused by the Epstein-Barr virus (EBV); usually affects persons 10–35 years of age.

▶ Mono is transmitted via saliva.

▶ Incubation period is 5 to 15 days.

Risk Factors

▶ Lowered immune resistance because of other illness, stress, or fatigue

▶ Living in close quarters with a large number of people, such as in a college dormitory

▶ Sharing drinking glasses, eating utensils, dishes, or a toothbrush with an infected person

▶ Intimate contact with someone who has mononucleosis

Signs and Symptoms

▶ Fever

▶ Sore throat

▶ Malaise, anorexia, myalgia

▶ Cervical lymphadenopathy

▶ White exudate on tonsils

▶ Splenomegaly

▶ Maculopapular or petechial rash

Diagnostic Tests

▶ Lymphocytic leukocytosis

▶ Positive heterophil monospot

▶ Early rise in IgM

▶ Permanent rise in IgG

Differential Diagnoses

▶ Human herpesvirus

▶ Acute HIV disease

▶ Toxoplasmosis

▶ Acute cytomegalovirus

▶ Viral pharyngitis

Management

▶ Supportive

▶ Nonsteroidal anti-inflammatory drugs (NSAIDs)

▶ Warm saline gargles

▶ Corticosteroids

▷ When enlarged lymph tissue threatens airway obstruction

▶ Penciclovir has some anti-EBV properties, but not routinely used

Prevention

▶ Avoid kissing or sharing drinks, food, or personal items, such as toothbrushes, with people who have infectious mononucleosis.

LYME DISEASE

▶ Lyme disease is the most common vector-borne disease in the United States and is caused by the *Borrelia burgdorferi* spirochete.

▶ Northeast, upper Midwest, and Pacific Coast most affected.

▶ Mice and deer tick are major animal reservoirs. Birds may also be a source.

Risk Factors

▶ Living in Northeast and Midwest regions

▶ Walking through bushes or other vegetation

Signs and Symptoms

▶ Rash up to 30 cm at tick bite site after 3–30 days

▷ Average 7 days

▷ ● "Bull's-eye" appearance

▶ Fatigue, chills, fever, headache, muscle and joint aches, lymphadenopathy

Diagnostic Tests

▶ Diagnosis is made when the patient has been exposed to a tick habitat within last 30 days and has erythema migrans or one late manifestation and lab confirmation.

▶ Three phases:

1. Early localized: Skin inflammation

2. Early disseminated: Heart and nervous system involvement

3. Late: Motor and sensory nerve damage, brain inflammation, and arthritis

▶ •Indirect fluorescent antibody (IFA) or enzyme-linked immunosorbent assay (ELISA); screening.

▶ • Confirmed with Western blot assay.

▷ Detects antibody to *B. burgdorferi*

▶ *B. burgdorferi* may be cultured from skin aspirate.

▶ Polymerase chain reaction (PCR) for *B. burgdorferi* DNA.

▶ Elevated erythrocyte sedimentation rate (ESR).

▶ Mild liver function test (LFT) abnormalities.

Differential Diagnoses

▶ Rocky Mountain spotted fever

▶ Rheumatic fever

▶ Viral disease

▶ Fibromyalgia

▶ Human granulocytic anaplasmosis

▶ Babesiosis

Management

▶ • Doxycycline 100 mg b.i.d. × 14 days

▶ Amoxicillin 500 mg t.i.d. × 14 days

▶ Cefuroxime axetil 500 mg b.i.d. × 14 days

Prevention

▶ Avoid walking in brush and foliage.

▶ Wear protective clothing.

▶ Use tick repellant.

▶ Inspect skin for ticks after walking in wooded or brushy areas.

VIRAL HEPATITIS

▶ Liver inflammation caused by a viral infection resulting in liver dysfunction

▶ Symptoms mild and self-limiting (lasting <6 months), chronic (lasting >6 months), or profound and life-threatening

Hepatitis A

▶ Can cause mild to severe illness.

▶ ● The hepatitis A virus (HAV) is transmitted through ingestion of contaminated food and water or through direct contact with an infectious person.

▶ Almost everyone recovers fully from hepatitis A and develops lifelong immunity. However, a very small proportion of people infected with hepatitis A could die from fulminant hepatitis.

▶ The risk of hepatitis A infection is associated with a lack of safe water, and poor sanitation and hygiene (such as dirty hands; World Health Organization [WHO] 2016a).

Hepatitis B

▶ More than 686,000 people die every year because of complications of hepatitis B, including cirrhosis and liver cancer (GBD 2013 Mortality and Causes of Death Collaborators 2015).

▶ Insidious onset.

▶ Risk of fulminant hepatitis is <1 percent, but 60 percent mortality if it occurs.

▶ ● Transmitted via blood, saliva, semen, vaginal secretions.

Hepatitis C

▶ Leading cause of chronic liver disease in the United States.

▶ ● Most common modes of infection are unsafe injection practices, inadequate sterilization of medical equipment, and the transfusion of unscreened blood and blood products (WHO 2017b).

▶ Transmission rarely sexual or perinatal.

▶ Acute infection asymptomatic 75 percent of time.

Hepatitis D

▶ ● Requires hepatitis B virus (HBV) for its replication

▶ ● Primarily transmitted among IV drug users

▶ Transmitted sexually in endemic areas (Mediterranean, Middle East, South America, and Africa)

▶ Often results in fulminant hepatitis and high mortality (WHO 2016b)

Hepatitis E

▶ Usually self-limiting but some cases may develop into fulminant hepatitis

▶ Transmitted via the fecal-oral route, principally via contaminated water

▶ Found worldwide, but the prevalence is highest in East and South Asia (WHO 2017c)

Hepatitis G

▶ The role of hepatitis G in causing human disease is unclear.

▶ Present in 50 percent of IV drug users, 30 percent of hemodialysis patients, 20 percent of people with hemophilia. (Reshetnyak, Karlovich, and Ilchenko 2008).

Risk Factors

▶ Poor sanitation, contaminated water

▶ Unprotected sex

▶ Intravenous or intranasal drug use

▶ Living in a household with an infected person

▶ Healthcare workers and others who may be exposed to blood and blood products through their work

Signs and Symptoms

▶ **Preicteric**

▷ Fatigue, malaise, anorexia, nausea and vomiting, headache, aversion to smoking and alcohol

▶ **Icteric**

▷ Weight loss, jaundice, pruritus, right upper quadrant (RUQ) pain, clay-colored stool, dark urine

▷ Physical appearance depends on virulence and type; mildly ill to very toxic

▷ Low-grade fever

▶ Hepatosplenomegaly

▶ Cough, pharyngitis

▶ Elevated WBC, aspartate aminotransferase (AST) and alanine aminotransferase (ALT), actate dehydrogenase (LDH), bilirubin, alkaline phosphatase, prothrombin time (PT)

Diagnostic Tests

▶ Viral titers

▶ WBC, AST, and ALT

▶ LDH, bilirubin, alkaline phosphatase, PT

▶ Computed tomography (CT) scan

▶ Sonogram

▶ Liver biopsy

Differential Diagnoses

▶ Cirrhosis

▶ Cholecystitis

▶ Coxsackievirus

▶ Toxoplasmosis

Management

▶ Generally supportive.

▶ Bed rest.

▶ 3,000–4,000 cc fluids daily.

▶ Avoid alcohol and drugs.

▶ Refer all patients with hepatitis B, C, or D.

▶ Liver transplant for hepatitis B–, C–, or D–caused liver failure.

▶ Most with hepatitis A and E get well on their own after a few weeks.

▶ Considerations for older adults:

▷ Inform of all risks and benefits of evaluation

▷ Many diagnostics very invasive and require much preparation

▷ *No* evaluation may be most appropriate, especially if significant risk or if physical or functional status unstable or not ideal

▶ Rest during active phase.

▶ Pharmacologic treatment.

▷ Acute, uncomplicated: No treatment

▷ Hepatitis B: lamivudine (Epivir), adefovir (Hepsera), telbivudine (Tyzeka), and entecavir (Baraclude)

▷ Hepatitis C: Rebetron (interferon and ribavirin), simeprevir (Olysio), sofosbuvir (Sovaldi), ombitasvir/paritaprevir/ritonavir, and dasabuvir (Viekira Pak) for the treatment of genotype 1 chronic hepatitis C infection in adults

▷ Vitamin K IM for PT more than 1.5 times normal

▷ Avoid sedatives—possible hepatic encephalopathy

▷ Chronic hepatitis B and C: Recombinant human interferon alpha with or without nucleoside analogs

Prevention

▶ Hepatitis A prevention: Proper food handling and avoiding contaminated water.

▶ Hepatitis A immunization.

▷ Two doses, 6 months apart

▶ Hepatitis B immunization.

▷ Three doses: at start, 1 month, 6 months

▶ Nonconverters: Up to three additional doses at 1–2 month intervals with serologic testing after each dose.

▶ Postvaccination testing for immunity is advised only for persons whose subsequent clinical management depends on knowledge of their immune status: infants born to HBsAg-positive mothers, health care and public safety workers, chronic hemodialysis patients, HIV-infected persons, other immunocompromised persons, and sex partners of persons with chronic hepatitis B infection (CDC 2016c).

▶ Counseling.

Psychosocial Factors in Hepatitis

▶ Multiple psychosocial factors influence adherence and treatment effectiveness.

▶ Patients with chronic hepatitis B and C are more stigmatized.

▶ Educate about importance of effective treatment as method to engage patients in their care.

▶ Screening and prevention strategies can improve patient outcomes.

▶ Education, pretreatment preparation, and support can increase adherence to medication regimens and improve outcomes and quality of life.

HIV AND AIDS

▶ Human immunodeficiency virus (HIV) is a sexually transmitted viral infection that causes acquired immune deficiency syndrome (AIDS). Incubation period is months to 10 years from HIV infection to AIDS.

▶ About 1.2 million people in the United States were living with HIV at the end of 2012 (CDC 2016b).

▶ In 2014, an estimated 44,073 people were diagnosed with HIV. The annual number of new diagnoses declined by 19 percent from 2005 to 2014 (CDC 2016d).

▶ In 2013, people aged 50 and over accounted for 18 percent (8,575) of an estimated 47,352 HIV diagnoses in the United States. Of these, the largest number (44 percent, 3,747) were among those aged 50–54 (CDC 2016d).

▶ Highest risk sexual behavior is anal sex, second is vaginal sex (CDC 2016a).

TABLE 5–2.
VIRAL HEPATITIS TYPES

TYPE	CAUSATIVE VIRUS	TRANSMISSION	INCUBATION	SYMPTOM ONSET	INFECTIVITY	COMMENTS
Hep A (HAV) (WHO 2016a)	Enteral virus RNA	Fecal-oral route Contaminated water or food	2–6 weeks 15–45 days	2–6 weeks after infection	Blood or stool 2–6 weeks	Rare complications No chronic state
Hep B (HBV) (WHO 2017a)	DNA with an inner core protein and outer surface coat component	Blood or blood products, sexual activity, and mother-fetus Blood, blood products, and body fluids	6 weeks–6 months 30–180 days	1–4 months	Any time after infected	Chronic infection common
Hep C (HCV) (WHO 2017b)	RNA, six genotypes	Bloodborne virus Usually IV drug use or blood transfusion Blood, blood products, and body fluids	15–180 days (average 50)	2 weeks–6 months 15–160 days	Any time after infected	Acute infection is usually mild, most cases become chronic
Hep D (HDV) (WHO 2016b)	Defective RNA	Bloodborne, sexual, percutaneous Occurs only in persons with hepatitis B	30–90 days	1–4 months 30–180 days	Only occurs if infected with Hep B	HBV must be present for HDV infection to occur
Hep E (HEV) (WHO 2017c)	RNA virus	Fecal-oral Waterborne contamination Contaminated food and water	10–60 days (average 40 days)	30–90 days postexposure 14–60 days	One week prior to onset up to 30 days Always acute but self-limiting	Course follows Hep A Rare in United States
Hep G (HGV) flavivirus (Dunphy et al. 2015)	Recently identified	Percutaneous transmission Blood, blood products, body fluids	15–150 days	Asymptomatic Unknown	Antibody to HBeAg (anti-HBe) becomes detectable when HBeAg is lost and is associated with low infectivity of serum	Often coinfection of Hep B or Hep C

TABLE 5–3.
HEPATITIS SEROLOGY

HEPATITIS TYPE	LAB TEST	NAME	INDICATES	COMMENTS
A	Anti-HAV IgM	IgM antibody to hepatitis A	Acute disease; resolves in 3–6 months	Diagnostic for HAV
A	Anti-HAV IgG	IgG antibody to hepatitis A	Early infection; peaks in 1 month	Indicates previous exposure; lifetime immunity
B	HBsAg	Hepatitis B surface antigen	Appears first, persists through illness; remains positive in chronic illness and in carriers	Establishes infection
B	Anti-HBs	Antibody to hepatitis B surface antigen (IgM and IgG)	Appears as surface antigen is disappearing; present after HBV vaccine	Indicates recovery; lifetime immunity
B	Anti-HBc	Antibody to hepatitis B core antigen (IgM and IgG)	IgM appears as patient is ill (when surface antigen is present); IgG antibodies appear during acute illness and persist for life despite recovery	Indicates acute infection; may be window of time when only IgM antibodies to core detectable (after surface antigen clears and before surface antibodies present)
B	HBeAg	Hepatitis B antigen	Appears almost simultaneously with antibodies to the core	Indicates viral replication and infectivity
B	Anti-HBe	Antibody to hepatitis B antigen	Appears as person begins to clear the virus	Indicates decreased viral replication and no infectivity
B	HBV DNA	Hepatitis B viral load	Will be present when Be antigen is present	Most accurate measure of HB virus
C	Anti-HCV	Antibody to hepatitis C	Screening test; looks for antibodies	Indicates infection (acute or chronic), not immunity
C	HCV RIBA	Recombinant immunoblot assay	Positive in HCV, confirm with HCV RNA	Indicates infection
C	HCV RNA	Hepatitis C virus by RNA	Ongoing viremia; measures viral load	Most sensitive to detect infection
D	Anti-HDV	Antibodies to hepatitis D	Detects infection	Most have concomitant HBsAg
E or G	Serologic markers not widely available			

Source: Dunphy et al. 2015

TABLE 5–4.
ABNORMAL LIVER FUNCTION TESTS

TEST	ELEVATION CAUSE	CONDITIONS
Gamma-glutamyl Transferase (GGT)	Hepatic excretion	Sensitive for acute alcohol ingestion Differentiates origin of an elevated alkaline phosphatase (bone or liver)
ALT	Acute hepatocellular injury from necrosis or inflammation; ALT is specific for hepatocyte	**Mild**: Biliary obstruction, mild viral or alcoholic hepatitis, cirrhosis, liver metastases **High**: Acute viral hepatitis, drug-induced liver injury
AST	Acute hepatocellular injury from necrosis or inflammation	**Mild:** Biliary obstruction, mild viral or alcoholic hepatitis, cirrhosis, liver metastases **High**: Acute viral hepatitis, drug-induced liver injury
Direct bilirubin	Impaired excretion of bilirubin from liver	Hepatocellular disease; biliary tract obstruction; drugs
Indirect bilirubin (unconjugated; not processed by liver)	Hepatic bilirubin uptake decreased	Hemolysis; drugs; heart failure
Alkaline phosphatase	Impaired biliary tract function; cholestasis	**Mild:** Hepatitis, cirrhosis, early cancer **High**: Biliary tract obstruction, cholestasis
Prothrombin time	Impaired hepatic synthesis of coagulation factors	Significant liver disease
Albumin	Impaired hepatic protein synthesis Excess protein loss	Chronic liver disease; malnutrition

Source: Limdi 2003

Stages of Infection

▶ **Stage 1: Acute HIV infection**

▷ Within 2–4 weeks of infection; flu-like illness or may not feel sick.

▶ **Stage 2: Clinical latency (HIV inactivity or dormancy)**

▷ Asymptomatic or may be sick at end of this stage; viral load increases and CD4 count decreases.

▶ **Stage 3: Acquired immune deficiency syndrome (AIDS)**

▷ Opportunistic illnesses occur; without treatment patient may survive 3 years. CD4 count < 200.

Opportunistic Infections and Related Complications

▶ **Bacterial and mycobacterial**

▷ Mycobacterium avium complex, salmonellosis, syphilis and neurosyphilis, tuberculosis

▶ **Fungal**

▷ Aspergillosis, candidiasis, coccidioidomycosis, cryptococcal meningitis, histoplasmosis

▶ **Malignancies**

▷ Kaposi's sarcoma, non-Hodgkin lymphoma, primary central nervous system, lymphoma

▶ **Protozoal**

▷ Cryptosporidiosis, isosporiasis, microsporidiosis, pneumocystis carinii pneumonia, toxoplasmosis

▶ **Viral**

▷ Cytomegalovirus, hepatitis, herpes simplex, herpes zoster, human papillomavirus, molluscum contagiosum

▶ **Oral**

▷ Hairy leukoplakia, progressive multifocal leukoencephalopathy

▶ **Neurological**

▷ AIDS dementia complex, peripheral neuropathy

▶ **Other conditions**

▷ Aphthous ulcers, malabsorption, depression, diarrhea, thrombocytopenia, wasting syndrome, idiopathic thrombocytopenic purpura (ITP)

▶ Refer cases to an infectious disease specialist for evaluation and management. The average disease progression without treatment from seroconversion to death in younger persons is 10–12 years. Older adults experience a more rapid downhill course, perhaps because of impaired T-cell replacement.

AIDS (CDC Definitions)

▶ HIV-positive person with opportunistic infection (OI) such as esophageal candidiasis, tuberculosis, *Cryptococcus* meningitis, *Pneumocystis jirovecii* (formerly *carinii*) pneumonia, or HIV-positive person with CD4 cell count < 200/mL or CD4 < 14 percent

Initiating Antiretroviral Medications

▶ History of AIDS-defining illness *or*

▶ CD4 T-cell count < 350 *or*

▶ CD4 T-cell count < 200, *and*

▶ Pregnant women

▶ Patients with HIV-associated neuropathy

▶ Coinfection with HPV when treatment for HBV indicated

▶ May consider for patients with CD4 T-cell counts > 350 but rapidly declining

▶ Viral load

▶ Viral resistance testing

▶ Discuss patient adherence and barriers to adherence

▶ Use drug cocktails (combination therapy)

Antiretroviral Medications Classes

▶ Thirty-one antiretroviral drugs (ARVs) are approved by the Food and Drug Administration (FDA).

▷ Nucleoside reverse transcriptase inhibitors

▷ Nonnucleoside reverse transcriptase inhibitors

▷ Protease inhibitors

▷ Transcriptase inhibitors

▷ Protease inhibitors

▷ Entry infusion inhibitors

▷ Integrase inhibitors

▷ Fixed-dose combination

Recommendations for Initial Antiretroviral Therapy

▶ Current US HIV treatment guidelines recommend antiretroviral treatment (ART) for all persons with HIV, regardless of CD4 cell count, to improve their health, prolong their lives, and reduce their risk of transmitting HIV to others (CDC 2014)

▶ AIDS Info (treatment information): National Institutes of Health (NIH) Clinical Guidelines Portal (Panel on Antiretroviral Guidelines for Adults and Adolescents 2016a, 2016b)

▶ Integrase strand transfer inhibitor–based regimen

▷ Dolutegravir/abacavir/lamivudine: *only* for patients who are HLA-B*5701-negative

▷ Dolutegravir plus tenofovir disoproxil fumarate (tenofovir)/emtricitabine

▷ Elvitegravir/tenofovir/emtricitabine: *only* for patients with pre-antiretroviral therapy CrCl > 70 mL/min

▷ Raltegravir plus tenofovir/emtricitabine

▶ Protease inhibitor–based regimen

▷ Darunavir/ritonavir plus tenofovir/emtricitabine

▶ Medication management principles

▷ Must receive each dose of antiretroviral prescription.

▷ Dose should be taken at the same time each day.

▷ Cannot substitute one medication for another.

▷ Attempt to initiate once-daily or b.i.d. dosing.

▷ Observe patient for signs and symptoms of drug therapy.

▷ Monitor lab values; treat abnormal lab values or a change in patient condition.

▷ Refer as needed.

▶ Preexposure prophylaxis (PrEP; CDC 2017)

▷ To help prevent HIV infection in people at very high risk

▷ ●A combination of two HIV medicines (tenofovir and emtricitabine)

▷ If taken daily, can significantly reduce risk of HIV infection from

▶ Sex by more than 90 percent and

▶ Injection drug use by more than 70 percent.

▶ Postexposure prophylaxis (PEP)

▷ Should be used only in emergency situations and must be started within 72 hours after possible exposure to HIV

▷ Occupational transmission of HIV to healthcare workers

▶ Extremely rare, and exposure can be minimized by proper use of safety devices and barriers (CDC 2017).

▶ If exposed to potentially infectious body fluids, determine the patient's HIV status if possible.

▶ Start PEP medication regimen as soon as possible after occupational exposure to HIV and continue for 4 weeks.

▷ ●Regimen should contain three (or more) antiretroviral drugs

▶ Expert consultation is recommended.

▶ Provide close follow-up that includes counseling, baseline and follow-up HIV testing, and monitoring for drug toxicity. Follow-up appointments should begin within 72 hours after HIV exposure.

▶ Continue follow-up testing for 4 months after exposure if a newer fourth-generation combination HIV p24 antigen–HIV antibody test is used, or for 6 months if antigen-antibody testing is not available (Kuhar et al. 2013).

Laboratory Testing

▶ HIV tests

▷ Antibody tests

▶ Enzyme-linked immunosorbent assays (ELISAs) that detect antibody to HIV are used as an initial test to screen for HIV infection.

▷ Laboratory-based

▷ Rapid tests

  ▷ Combination tests (antibody/antigen tests)

  ▶ Fourth-generation HIV tests; detect both HIV antibody and antigens

  ▷ Nucleic acid tests (NATs)

  ▶ Detect HIV the fastest by looking for HIV in the blood. It can take 7 to 28 days for NATs to detect HIV. Very expensive.

  ▷ Confirmatory tests

  ▶ HIV-1/HIV-2 differentiation immunoassay

  ▶ Western blot (CDC 2016e; Bartlett and Sax 2016)

▶ See CDC's Quick Reference Guide: https://stacks.cdc.gov/view/cdc/23446

HIV Resources

▶ HIV.gov: http://www.hiv.gov/federal-response/

▶ FDA (antiretroviral drugs used in the treatment of HIV): http://www.fda.gov/ForPatients/Illness/HIVAIDS/Treatment/ucm118915.htm

▶ CDC: https://www.cdc.gov/hiv/

▶ University of California, San Francisco (HIV InSite): http://hivinsite.ucsf.edu/

▶ International AIDs Society: http://www.iasociety.org/

▶ The Body: http://www.thebody.com/

▶ Panel on Antiretroviral Guidelines for Adults and Adolescents (2016b)

ROCKY MOUNTAIN SPOTTED FEVER

▶ Systemic febrile illness caused by *Rickettsia rickettsii* bacterium that is transmitted by the bite of the American dog tick, Rocky Mountain dog tick, and brown dog tick. The tick must attach for 4–6 hours to transmit infection. Incubation is 2–14 days. It is not transmitted person to person. The disease confers immunity.

▶ Predominantly in southeastern and central states; more than 50 percent of cases are in South Atlantic region. It is also in Rocky Mountain states, Canada, Mexico, and South and Central America. Peak season is in late spring. Two-thirds of the cases are among children and adolescents less than 15 years old.

Risk Factors

▶ Tick bite

▶ Outdoor activities

▶ Clothing that exposes skin

▶ Not using repellant

Signs and Symptoms

- ► Triad: History of tick bite, fever, rash—may not all be present together at initial assessment

- ► Sudden onset of fever higher than 104°F

- ► Conjunctival injection

- ► Rash

    - ▷ 90 percent have some type of rash during the course of illness, but some do not develop the rash until late in the disease process.

    - ▷ Classically, appears 2–5 days after the onset of fever as small, flat, pink, nonitchy spots (macules) on the wrists, forearms, and ankles, and spreads to include the trunk and sometimes the palms and soles.

    - ▷ The red-to-purple spotted (petechial) rash is usually not seen until the sixth day or later after onset of symptoms and occurs in 35–60 percent of patients with the infection. This is a sign of progression to severe disease, and every attempt should be made to begin treatment before petechiae develop.

- ► Lymphadenopathy, severe headache, myalgia (especially calf and thigh), splenomegaly (50 percent of cases)

- ► Nausea, vomiting, abdominal pain

- ► Cough, confusion

- ► Titers: acute and convalescent sera

    - ▷ Fourfold antibody increase; may not appear for 10–14 days

- ► Complete blood count (CBC) may show thrombocytopenia, variable WBC, mild anemia

- ► Prolonged PT, partial thromboplastin time (PTT)

- ► Elevated blood urea nitrogen (BUN)/creatinine ratio in renal insufficiency

- ► Hyponatremia

- ► Elevated LFTs in hepatitis

Diagnostic Tests

- ► Titers: Acute and convalescent sera (fourfold antibody increase) may not appear for 10–14 days.

- ► Complete blood count (CBC), PT, PTT, BUN/creatinine, electrolytes, LFTs.

Differential Diagnoses

- ► Viral infection, mononucleosis

- ► Bacterial sepsis

- ► Meningitis, meningococcemia

- ► Lyme disease

▶ Rubella, scarlet fever, rheumatic fever

▶ Erythema multiforme

▶ Ehrlichiosis

Management

▶ Rest and fluids

▶ Antibiotic therapy at least 3 days after the fever subsides and until there is evidence of clinical improvement. Standard duration of treatment is 7–14 days.

▷ Treatment should begin within first 5 days of illness

▷ • Doxycycline 200 mg, then 100 mg q12h

▷ If allergic to tetracyclines:

▶ • Amoxycillin 100 mg t.i.d., *or*

▶ Cefuroxime 500 mg b.i.d.

▶ Late stage: Ceftriaxone 2 g intravenously (IV) daily

▶ Pregnant women

▷ • Chloramphenicol 500 mg q6h

Prevention

▶ Patient education (CDC 2016i):

▷ Know where ticks live.

▷ Use DEET repellent on skin.

▷ Treat clothing and gear with permethrin.

▷ Treat pets for ticks.

▷ Check clothing for ticks.

▷ Check dogs for ticks after returning from tick habitats.

▷ Shower soon after being outdoors.

▷ Check body for ticks after being outdoors.

▷ Remove any attached ticks from people or pets immediately.

WEST NILE VIRUS

▶ Viral infection caused by the arbovirus of family *Flaviviridae*. Transmitted by infected mosquitos to birds, and from infected birds to mosquitos that bite humans, who are then infected. Infected mosquitos may infect domestic animals and horses, but there is no documented case of spread from animal to animal or animal to human.

▶ West Nile virus (WNV) was first reported in Asia, Africa, Europe, and the United States in 1999. Incubation period is 5–15 days. Mild illness occurs in 3–6 days in

20 percent of infected persons. Though rare, the virus can be spread via blood transfusion, organ transplant, and prenatal transmission. Every 1 in 150 develops neurological disease (encephalitis more than meningitis). Adults older than 50 years are at higher risk and mortality is highest in persons older than 65 years.

Risk Factors

▶ Outdoor activities during high mosquito activity

▶ Outdoor occupations

▶ Blood transfusion and organ transplants

▶ Advanced age

Signs and Symptoms

▶ Most symptomatic persons experience an acute systemic febrile illness that often includes headache, weakness, myalgia, or arthralgia; gastrointestinal symptoms and a transient maculopapular rash also are commonly reported.

▶ Less than 1 percent of infected persons develop neuroinvasive disease, which typically manifests as meningitis, encephalitis, or acute flaccid paralysis.

Diagnostic Tests

▶ Spinal tap: Cerebrospinal fluid (CSF) for IgM antibody for WNV and lymphocytes.

▶ Serum WNV presumptive of recent exposure in persons with central nervous system (CNS) infection. Antibody titer increasing four times original titer 2–4 weeks later confirms WNV infection.

Differential Diagnoses

▶ Encephalitis

▶ Colorado tick fever

▶ Dengue fever

Management

▶ Supportive care.

▶ Monitor for complications.

▶ Treat symptoms and complications.

▶ Refer to infectious disease specialist.

▶ Report WNV encephalitis cases to the state health department.

▶ Immediate hospitalization for deteriorating mental status (CDC 2015).

Prevention

▶ Use insect repellents when going outdoors.

▶ Wear long sleeves, long pants, and socks when outdoors.

▶ Install or repair screens on windows and doors to keep mosquitos outside.

▶ Reduce the number of mosquitos around the home by emptying standing water.

REFERENCES

Bartlett, J. G., and P. E. Sax. 2016. "Screening and Diagnostic Testing for HIV Infection." UpToDate. https://www.uptodate.com/contents/screening-and-diagnostic-testing-for-hiv-infection?source=machineLearning.

Centers for Disease Control and Prevention. 2011. "Lyme Disease (*Borrelia burgdorferi*): 2011 Case Definition." National Notifiable Diseases Surveillance System (NNDSS). http://wwwn.cdc.gov/nndss/conditions/lyme-disease/case-definition/2011/.

———. 2014. *Recommendations for HIV Prevention with Adults and Adolescents with HIV in the United States, 2014: Summary for Clinical Providers*. https://stacks.cdc.gov/view/cdc/26063.

———. 2015. "Clinical Evaluation and Disease." West Nile Virus. https://www.cdc.gov/westnile/healthcareproviders/healthcareproviders-clinlabeval.html.

———. 2016a. "About HIV/AIDS." http://www.cdc.gov/hiv/basics/whatishiv.html.

———. 2016b. "Basic Statistics." HIV/AIDS. http://www.cdc.gov/hiv/basics/statistics.html.

———. 2016c. "Hepatitis B FAQs for Health Professionals." http://www.cdc.gov/hepatitis/hbv/hbvfaq.htm#vaccFAQ.

———. 2016d. "HIV among People Aged 50 and Over." HIV/AIDS. http://www.cdc.gov/hiv/group/age/olderamericans/index.html.

———. 2016e. "HIV Testing." HIV/AIDS. http://www.cdc.gov/hiv/testing/index.html.

———. 2016f. "HPV-Associated Cancers and Precancers." http://www.cdc.gov/std/tg2015/hpv-cancer.htm.

———. 2016g. "HPV Vaccine Recommendations." https://www.cdc.gov/vaccines/vpd/hpv/hcp/recommendations.html.

———. 2016h. "Recommended Adult Immunization Schedule—United States—2016." http://www.cdc.gov/vaccines/schedules/downloads/adult/adult-schedule.pdf.

———. 2016i. "RMSF Is Deadly, yet Preventable." http://www.cdc.gov/features/rmsf/.

———. 2016j. "VaxView." https://www.cdc.gov/vaccines/vaxview/index.html.

———. 2017. "PrEP." https://www.cdc.gov/hiv/basics/prep.html.

Dunphy, L., J. Winland-Brown, B. Porter, and D. Thomas, eds. 2015. *Primary Care: The Art and Science of Advanced Practice Nursing*. 4th ed. Philadelphia: F. A. Davis.

GBD 2013 Mortality and Causes of Death Collaborators. 2015. "Global, Regional, and National Age–Sex Specific All-Cause and Cause-Specific Mortality for 240 Causes of Death, 1990–2013: A Systematic Analysis for the Global Burden of Disease Study 2013." *Lancet* 385:117–71. http://www.thelancet.com/pdfs/journals/lancet/PIIS0140-6736(14)61682-2.pdf.

Kuhar, D., D. Henderson, K. Struble, W. Heneine, V. Thomas, L. Cheever, A. Gomaa, and A. Panlilio. 2013. *Updated U.S. Public Health Service Guidelines for the Management of Occupational Exposures to HIV and Recommendations for Postexposure Prophylaxis.* https://stacks.cdc.gov/view/cdc/20711.

Limdi, J. 2003. "Evaluation of Abnormal Liver Function Tests." *Postgraduate Medical Journal* 79 (932): 307–12. http://dx.doi.org/10.1136/pmj.79.932.307.

National Center on Elder Abuse. 2010. "Frequently Asked Questions: Why Should I Care about Elder Abuse?" https://ncea.acl.gov/faq/#faq14.

Panel on Antiretroviral Guidelines for Adults and Adolescents. 2016a. "Initiation of Antiretroviral Therapy." In *Guidelines for the Use of Antiretroviral Agents in HIV-1-Infected Adults and Adolescents*, pp. C-2–C-4. N.p.: Department of Health and Human Services. https://aidsinfo.nih.gov/guidelines/html/1/adult-and-adolescent-arvguidelines/10/initiation-of-antiretroviral-therapy.

———. 2016b. "What to Start: Initial Combination Regimens for the Antiretroviral-Naïve Patient." In *Guidelines for the Use of Antiretroviral Agents in HIV-1-Infected Adults and Adolescents*, p. F-1. N.p.: Department of Health and Human Services. https://aidsinfo.nih.gov/guidelines/html/1/adult-and-adolescent-arv-guidelines/11/what-to-start. Reshetnyak, V. I., T. I. Karlovich, and L. U. Ilchenko, 2008. "Hepatitis G virus." *World Journal of Gastroenterology,* 14 (30): 4725–34. https://dx.doi.org/10.3748%2Fwjg.14.4725

World Health Organization. 2015. *Guideline on When to Start Antiretroviral Therapy and on Pre-exposure Prophylaxis for HIV.* Geneva: World Health Organization. http://apps.who.int/iris/bitstream/10665/186275/1/9789241509565_eng.pdf.

World Health Organization. 2016a. "Hepatitis A." http://www.who.int/mediacentre/factsheets/fs328/en/.

———. 2016b. "Hepatitis D." http://www.who.int/mediacentre/factsheets/hepatitis-d/en/.

———. 2017a. "Hepatitis B." http://www.who.int/mediacentre/factsheets/fs204/en/.

———. 2017b. "Hepatitis C." http://www.who.int/mediacentre/factsheets/fs164/en/.

———. 2017c. "Hepatitis E." http://www.who.int/mediacentre/factsheets/fs280/en/.

CHAPTER 6

DERMATOLOGICAL DISORDERS

LEARNING OBJECTIVES

▶ Recognize common dermatological disorders and then analyze processes useful to providing differential diagnosis among them.

▷ Risk factors

▷ Signs and symptoms

▷ Diagnostic tests

▷ Differential diagnoses

▶ Describe treatment and management of dermatological disorders.

▷ Management

▷ Prevention

ABOUT DERMATOLOGICAL DISORDERS AND CONDITIONS

Dermatological disorders can be indicative of dermatological conditions or symptomatic of systemic problems. A thorough history is key to establishing exposure, time of onset, recent trips, new products used, or if anyone else has it. Patient presentation (comfortable, agitation, pain, toxic) and vital signs assist in distinguishing minor from serious skin signs in sick patients (4S). Determine whether it is an infection or inflammatory process.

▶ For the most efficient and thorough examination, a designated area should include

▷ Well-lit room,

▷ Penlight to illuminate,

▷ Wood's lamp to fluoresce certain lesions,

▷ Magnifying glass,

▷ Glass slides to identify blanching (diascopy) and skin scrapings,

▷ 10–20 percent potassium hydroxide (KOH) to illuminate hyphae,

▷   5 percent acetic acid to illuminate human papilloma virus lesions,

▷   Mineral oil to collect scabies or lice,

▷   Giemsa or Wright's stains to identify herpes simplex and varicella zoster, and

▷   Microscope.

Making a Dermatologic Diagnosis

▶   Dermatologic diagnosis is a visual task that requires practice and good references.

▶   Two distinct clinical situations:

▷   Incidental findings or important skin lesions that cannot be overlooked on routine exam

▷   A chief complaint of skin changes

General Signs to Evaluate and Document

▶   **Morphology:** Types of lesions (abscess, bulla, comedone, cyst, ecchymosis, macule, papule, patch, plaque, pustule, purpura, vesicle, wheal, nodule, telangiectasis, etc.)

▷   Primary lesions include macule, patch, papule, plaque, nodule, tumor, vesicle, bulla, pustule.

▷   Secondary lesions are atrophy, lichenification, scale, excoriation, crust, fissure, erosion, ulcer.

▶   **Distribution**: Extent, pattern, characteristic patterns, asymmetric, central, generalized, intertriginous areas, localized, peripheral, predilection to certain body areas (e.g., extensor or flexor surfaces), symmetric, sun-exposed, pressure, bony prominences

▶   **Arrangement:** Arcuate, clustered, confluent, discrete, disseminated, linear, patchy, polycyclic, reticular, scarlatiniform, zosteriform

▶   **Configuration**: Annular, gyrate, iris, nummular, oval, pedunculated, umbilicated, serpiginous, verrucous

▶   **Margination**: Demarcated (can be traced with the tip of a pencil) or ill-defined

▶   **Color**: Depigmented, erythematous, flesh-colored, hypomelanotic, hypermelanotic, uniform, variegated, violaceous (white, pink, blue, red, yellow, etc.)

▶   **Measurements**: Diameter, depth (depression), elevation, length, width

▶   **Descriptors**: Atrophied, crusted, excoriated, friable, hyperkeratotic, hypertrophic, keloidal, lichenified, pigmented, sclerosed, weeping

▶   **Palpation:** Consistency (soft, firm, hard, fluctuant, smooth, rough), depth (dermal or squamous), induration, mobile or fixed, temperature (cool, warm, hot), tenderness

▶   **Associated symptoms:** Hair, nails, mucus membranes, lymphadenopathy, hepatosplenomegaly, ophthalmic or neurologic involvement

Normal Aging Changes of the Skin

▶ **Epidermis**: Thinner; dermis connection less adhesive and more easily traumatized; susceptible to blisters, tears, protective barrier diminished; keratinocytes proliferate more slowly leading to slower healing; fewer melanocytes for ultraviolet (UV) light protection; fewer Langerhan cells weaken immune system; fewer Merkel cells and Meissner corpuscles diminish pressure sensation; fewer Pacini cells decrease pain sensation

▶ **Dermis**: Skin transparency, skin feels thin (20 percent thinner), decreased capillaries cause skin atrophy, fewer fibroblasts lead to decreased collagen production

▶ **Subcutaneous layer**: Thinned; less protection from trauma and cold

▶ **Nails**: Thinner and brittle or thick and dystrophic, rate of growth slows

▶ **Hair**: Graying, thinning, balding

▶ **Sebaceous glands**: Reduced function causes dry skin, may hypertrophy

▶ **Wound healing**: Delayed, and protective scarring is weaker; multiple medical issues add to compromised healing process

Dermatological Psychosocial Issues

▶ Dermatologic conditions may result in

▷ Self-esteem and body image issues

▷ Anxiety, fear, social phobias

▷ Major depression, suicidal thoughts

Management

▶ Psychotropic medication

▶ Stress management

▶ Psychiatric referral

COMMON BACTERIAL SKIN INFECTIONS

Impetigo

▶ Highly contagious local bacterial infection caused by *Staphylococcus aureus* or Group A strep (GAS), found mainly in children, but may occur in teens and adults

Risk Factors

▶ Contact with infected people

▶ Sharing towels and linens with infected people

Signs and Symptoms

▶ Small vesicles or bullae

▶ Honey-colored, crusted pustules

Diagnostic Tests

▶ Visual exam of lesions

▶ Culture of lesions

Differential Diagnoses

▶ Contact dermatitis

▶ Atopic dermatitis

▶ Herpes simplex

▶ Bullous pemphigus

Management

▶ Cool compresses

▶ Topical antibiotics

   ▷ Mupirocin (Bactroban) ointment to affected areas t.i.d. × 3–5 days

▶ Systemic antibiotics for severe cases

   ▷ Amoxicillin/clavulanate (Augmentin) 250–500 mg b.i.d. × 10 days (adults); cephalosporins and macrolides

Prevention

▶ Avoid contact with infected people.

▶ Good handwashing.

▶ Keep fingernails short to avoid self-inoculation.

▶ Refrain from contact sports.

▶ Do not share towels, razors, or linens.

Cellulitis

▶ Spreading infection of epidermis, subcutaneous tissue, and superficial lymphatic system caused by *S. aureus* and GAS

Risk Factors

▶ Preexisting skin infections

▶ Break in the skin

▶ Diabetes mellitus

▶ Human immunodeficiency virus (HIV)

▶ Chronic steroid use

- ▶ Peripheral vascular disease
- ▶ Drug or alcohol use
- ▶ Lymphatic blockage
- ▶ Saphenous vein grafting

Signs and Symptoms

- ▶ Bright red plateau, with sharply demarcated surrounding areas
- ▶ Red streak to lymph nodes

Diagnostic Tests

- ▶ CBC, blood culture.
- ▶ X-ray.
- ▶ Check for foreign object in skin or possible bone infection.

Differential Diagnoses

- ▶ Deep vein thrombosis (DVT)
- ▶ Necrotizing fasciitis
- ▶ Herpes zoster
- ▶ Contact dermatitis
- ▶ Drug reaction
- ▶ Osteomyelitis

Management

- ▶ May need incision and drainage (I&D).
- ▶ Antibiotic therapy
  - ▷ Dicloxacillin 250–500 mg oral q.i.d. × 7–10 days
  - ▷ Cephalexin 250–500 mg oral q.i.d. × 7–10 days
  - ▷ Erythromycin 250–500 mg oral q.i.d. × 7–10 days if allergic to penicillin
  - ▷ MRSA: Clindamycin 300–400 mg oral q 6–8h
  - ▷ Trimethoprim/sulfamethoxazole, 2 double-strength tablets q12h
  - ▷ Doxycycline or minocycline 100 mg oral daily
- ▶ Nonsteroidal anti-inflammatory drugs (NSAIDs) for fever, analgesia, and inflammation (risk for gastrointestinal [GI] bleed, gastritis).
- ▶ Treat for 7–10 days depending on extent of involvement.
- ▶ Reevaluate in 48 hours.

Prevention

- ▶ Keep skin moisturized.
- ▶ Excellent hand hygiene.

▶ Prompt treatment of superficial skin infections.

▶ Monitor superficial skin infections or breaks in the skin for signs of infection.

Superficial Fungal (Dermatophyte) Infections (Tinea)

▶ Tinea capitis: Hair and scalp (trichomycosis)

▶ Tinea barbae: Beard (trichomycosis)

▶ Tinea corporis: Body, glabrous skin

▶ Tinea manus: Hand

▶ Tinea unguium: Nails (onychomycosis)

▶ Tinea cruris: Genitalia, pubic, perineal, and perianal (jock itch)

▶ Tinea pedis: Feet (athlete's foot)

▶ Tinea versicolor: Identified by multicolored appearance; usually on torso and neck

Risk Factors

▶ Heat and humidity

▶ Obesity (skin folds)

▶ Close contact with infected animals and humans

▶ Mechanical pressure in shoes can cause onychomycosis

Signs and Symptoms

▶ Depends on body area

▶ Ringworm: Red, ringed rash

▷ Scalp ringworm: Itchy, red patches; can leave bald spots

▶ Athlete's foot: Itching, burning, cracked skin between toes

▶ Jock itch: Itchy, burning groin rash

▶ Tinea corporis: Glabrous skin (palms, soles, and groin)

Diagnostic Tests

▶ KOH mount 10–20 percent preparation test

▷ Slide-mounted skin scrapings warmed for 30–60 minutes show mycelia and hyphae

▷ Capitis: Spores invading hair follicles

▷ Cruris: Mycelia and septate hyphae and buds

▷ Versicolor: Long hyphae and buds (spaghetti and meatball appearance)

▶ Wood's lamp fluoresces:

▷ Capitis: Green-yellow

▷ Versicolor: Copper or orange

TABLE 6-1
TINEA DIFFERENTIAL DIAGNOSES

BARBAE	CAPITIS	CORPORIS	CRURIS	MANUS	PEDIS	TRICHOMYCOSIS
Folliculitis	Seborrheic dermatitis	Atopic dermatitis	Erythrasma	Atopic dermatitis	Candidiasis	Paronychia
Acne vulgaris	Psoriasis	Contact dermatitis	Inverse pattern psoriasis	Contact dermatitis	Contact dermatitis	Herpetic whitlow
Acne rosacea	Atopic dermatitis	Annular erythema	Candidiasis	Psoriasis	Dyshidrotic eczema	Eczematous dermatitis
Furunculosis	Alopecia areata	Psoriasis		Lichen simplex chronicus	Erythrasma	Allergic contact dermatitis
	Lichen simplex chronicus	Seborrheic dermatitis		In situ squamous cell carcinoma	Impetigo	Lichen planus
	Chronic systemic lupus erythematosus (SLE)	Erythema migrans		Pityriasis rubra pilaris	Psoriasis	Pseudomonal nail infection (black-green color)
	Impetigo	Pityriasis				Reiter syndrome
	Ecthyma					Traumatic nail injury
	Crusted scales					

- ▶ Less common tests
  - ▷ Fungal cultures identify specific fungi.
    - ▶ Fungi slow-growing; results take weeks
    - ▶ Indicated only when infection is resistant to treatment
  - ▷ Susceptibility testing from a culture to determine which antifungal is appropriate.
    - ▶ Antigens and antibodies testing

Management

- ▶ Treat predisposing conditions.
  - ▷ Obesity
  - ▷ Diabetes
  - ▷ Immunosuppression
- ▶ Avoid tight, occlusive clothing.
- ▶ Dry completely after bathing.
- ▶ ◉ Topical or systemic antifungals:
  - ▷ Topical
    - ▶ Clotrimazole 1 percent cream, lotion, solution
    - ▶ Econazole 1 percent cream
    - ▶ Ketoconazole 2 percent cream, shampoo
    - ▶ Miconazole 2 percent cream
    - ▶ Oxiconazole1 percent solution
    - ▶ Sulconazole 1 percent cream, solution
    - ▶ Naftifine 1 percent gel, cream
    - ▶ Tolnaftate 1 percent cream, gel, powder, aerosol, solution
    - ▶ Terbinafine 1 percent cream, gel
- ▶ Onychomycosis:
  - ▷ Terbinafine 250 mg daily × 12 weeks for toenails, 6 weeks for fingernails
  - ▷ Topical treatments usually ineffective alone, but may help in combination with oral preparations
  - ▷ Ciclopirox 8 percent nail lacquer
- ▶ Tinea capitis and barbae:
  - ▷ Griseofulvin 500 mg oral in single or 2 divided doses daily
- ▶ Tinea versicolor:
  - ▷ Selenium sulfide lotion applied from neck to waist, leave on for 10 minutes, daily for 2 weeks.
  - ▷ Ketoconazole shampoo for weekly maintenance.

▷ Oral antifungal agents (e.g., ketoconazole, griseofulvin) should be reserved for severe cases.

▷ Follow up every 4 weeks for reevaluation and liver function tests (LFTs).

▷ LFTS before treatment and every 4–6 weeks.

▷ Systemic antifungals may cause hepatotoxicity, lower serum testosterone.

Candidiasis

► Pathologic cutaneous yeast (*Candida albicans* most common) that are normal flora in mucus membranes and intestinal tract but can cause infections in the mouth, throat, intertriginous, vagina, male genitalia, and nails.

Risk Factors

► Immunosuppression

► Diabetes

► Chemotherapy

► Broad-spectrum antibiotics

► Corticosteroids

► Moisture

► Obesity (skin folds)

► Chronic debility and inability to perform personal hygiene

► Occlusive clothing

► Hyperhidrosis

Signs and Symptoms

► Pruritic or burning rash in areas that are moist and warm.

▷ Such as skinfolds, under breasts, axillae, anogenital area

► Lesions are bright red, smooth macules, with scaling, elevated border.

► Macerated skin in intertriginous infection.

► Satellite pustules may be present outside of main lesion.

► Painful "stuck-on" white, friable lesions in oral mucosa (thrush) that are removable.

► Painful "stuck-on" white, friable lesions in vagina with white curd-like vaginal discharge, pruritis, dysuria, and dyspareunia.

► Painful fissures in penile foreskin with dysuria and dyspareunia.

► Painful, inflamed nail folds, nail discoloration, creamy nail discharge.

► Painful, congested, edematous, macerated ear canal with moist, white, scaly exudate.

Diagnostic Tests

- ▶ Culture
- ▶ KOH test
- ▶ Saline wet mount
- ▶ pH paper

Differential Diagnoses

- ▶ Contact dermatitis
- ▶ Bacterial intertrigo
- ▶ Trichomoniasis
- ▶ Bacterial vaginosis
- ▶ Genital warts

Management

- ▶ Burrow's solution compresses to affected areas.
- ▶ Oral candidiasis:
  - ▷ Treatment for 10–14 days
  - ▷ Nystatin suspension 200,000–400,000 units, swish in mouth and swallow, five times daily
  - ▷ Clotrimazole 10 mg troches orally, five times daily
  - ▷ Fluconazole 200 mg orally once, then 100 mg daily
- ▶ Cutaneous candidiasis:
  - ▷ Treatment for 1 to several weeks depending on infection extent and immune status
- ▶ Paronychial candidiasis:
  - ▷ Treat for 2–4 weeks
  - ▷ Clotrimazole 1 percent, miconazole 2 percent, or econazole 1 percent cream applied twice daily or
  - ▷ Ketoconazole 2 percent cream applied once daily
  - ▷ Ciclopirox applied twice daily
  - ▷ Nystatin cream or powder applied twice daily
- ▶ Vulvovaginal candidiasis:
  - ▷ Diflucan 150 mg p.o., one dose.
  - ▷ May use topical antifungal.
  - ▷ Oral antifungal therapy may be required in recurrent or extensive infections or when the patient's immunity is compromised.
- ▶ Follow up in 2–4 weeks to evaluate progress.

▶ Bacterial superinfections of excoriated areas may occur.

▶ Esophagitis and odynophagia may result in weight loss.

Prevention

▶ Treat underlying factors.

▶ Expose affected areas to air.

▶ Carefully and thoroughly dry skin and skinfolds.

▶ Wear cotton undergarments.

▶ Change incontinence briefs frequently.

VIRAL SKIN INFECTIONS

Herpes Simplex

▶ Herpes simplex viruses (HSV) cause a wide variety of diseases. There are two types, HSV I and HSV II. Both types belong to the family *Herpesviridae*. Though they are closely related, they differ in epidemiology. HSV infection occurs via inoculation into mucous membranes (e.g., oropharynx, cervix, conjunctiva) or through small cracks in the skin. HSV I is associated with orofacial disease. HSV II is associated with genital disease. However, lesion location is not necessarily indicative of viral type.

▶ Most oral and genital herpes infections are asymptomatic.

▶ HSV is transmitted via close personal contact. Reactivation and replication of latent HSV is always in the ganglia of origin. Reactivation can be induced by fever, trauma, stress, sunlight, or menses. Reactivation is more common and severe in immunocompromised persons. Prompt diagnosis and early treatment are important in management (World Health Organization [WHO] 2017).

Herpes Simplex I: Fever Blister

▶ Cold sore; oral herpes simplex; herpes labialis; herpes simplex.

▶ The trigeminal ganglia are usually involved in orofacial HSV infections. HSV I reactivates more frequently in the oral region and is mainly transmitted by contact with infected saliva.

Herpes Simplex II: Genital Herpes

▶ The sacral nerve root ganglia (S2–S5) are usually involved in genital HSV infections. HSV II reactivates more frequently in the genital region and is transmitted sexually or from a mother's genital tract infection to her newborn.

Risk Factors

▶ Contact with infected person

▶ Immunocompromised state

▶ Multiple sexual partners

▶ Not using condoms

Signs and Symptoms

▶ Single or multiple clusters of small, painful vesicles on red base that sequence as follows:

▷ Prodrome: tingling, burning, itching, pain at the site

▷ Erythematous papules

▷ Tiny vesicles become pustular and ulcerate

▷ Dry to yellow crust within 5–7 days

Diagnostic Tests

▶ Viral culture

▶ Viral DNA test

▶ Tzanck test to check for HSV

Differential Diagnoses

▶ Candidiasis

▶ Chancroid

▶ Hand, foot, and mouth disease

▶ Herpes zoster

▶ Syphilis

Management

▶ Ice or warm cloth to affected areas.

▶ Saltwater rinse to affected areas.

▶ Wash area gently with germ-fighting (antiseptic) soap and water.

▷ Prevents spreading virus to other body areas

▶ Avoid hot, citrus, spicy, and salty foods and drinks.

▶ Gargle with cool water or eat popsicles.

▶ UV light exposure.

▶ Antiviral skin creams are expensive and only shorten outbreak by few hours to a day.

▶ Oral medications:

▷ Acyclovir 200–400 mg five times a day for 5 days

▷ Acyclovir 400 mg t.i.d. *or* 200 mg oral five times a day for 7–10 days

▷ Famciclovir 125–500 mg for 5 days

▷ Famciclovir 250 mg t.i.d. for 7–10 days

▷ Valacyclovir 2000 mg b.i.d. for 1 day

▷ Valacyclovir 1 g b.i.d. for 7–10 days

▷ Acetaminophen 650 q4h p.r.n. for pain

- ▶ Immunocompromised:
  - ▷ Consult with physician
  - ▷ High-dose intravenous acyclovir
- ▶ Topical creams:
  - ▷ Penciclovir cream applied in first hour of symptoms, and q2h for 4 days
  - ▷ Acyclovir cream applied at first sign of pain or tingling, and q2h for 4 days
  - ▷ Docosanol cream (nonprescription) ointment applied at first sign of pain or tingling, then five times a day
- ▶ Topical anesthetics provide modest relief.
  - ▷ Anbesol gel, Blistex lip ointment, Camphophenique, Herpecin-L, Viractin, Zilactin, lidocaine 5 percent gel or ointment

Prevention

- ▶ Zinc oxide sunblock or lip balm containing zinc oxide to lips.
- ▶ Lip moisturizing balm to prevent the lips from becoming too dry.
- ▶ Avoid direct contact with herpes sores.
- ▶ Wash towels and linens in boiling hot water after each use.
- ▶ Do not share utensils, straws, glasses, or other items with someone with oral herpes.

Herpes Zoster (Shingles)

Acute unilateral cutaneous infection in dorsal root ganglia of a unilateral dermatome caused by reactivation of HSV II varicella zoster virus (VZV) that usually infects as chicken pox in childhood, then remains dormant in a nerve ganglion until it is reactivated and erupts along a nerve. Reactivation is age-related and due to decline in immune function. HSV II varicella zoster infection is most prevalent in persons older than 50 years of age. About half of all cases occur in men and women 60 years old or older (Centers for Disease Control and Prevention [CDC] 2016).

Risk Factors

- ▶ Immunosuppressed or immunocompromised
- ▶ Advanced age
- ▶ Stress

Signs and Symptoms

- ▶ Pain: Piercing, stabbing, boring.
- ▶ Paresthesia along single root: Tingling, burning, itching.
- ▶ Allodynia: Heightened sensitivity to mild tactile stimuli.
- ▶ Vesicular eruptions appear 48 hours after pain.
- ▶ Grouped along a unilateral dermatome followed by bullae within 2 days.
- ▶ Bullae become pustules by day 4.

▶ Crusting appears in 7–10 days.

▶ Lesions are erythematous on edematous base.

▶ Malaise, headache, fever.

Diagnostic Tests

▶ Tzanck test, VZV antibodies, viral culture

▶ Electrocardiogram (ECG) to rule out cardiac etiology

▶ X-ray to rule out pleural or abdominal etiology

▶ Ultrasound to rule out cholelithiasis and nephrolithiasis

Differential Diagnoses

▶ Migraine

▶ Cardiac or pleuritic pain

▶ Acute abdomen

▶ Disc disease

▶ Vesicular-crusting stage

▷ Herpes simplex

▷ Contact dermatitis

▷ Erysipelas

▷ Bullous impetigo

▷ Necrotizing fasciitis

Management

▶ Moist, warm saline, water, or Burrow's solution dressings

▶ Analgesics

▷ Gabapentin 100 mg daily

▷ Capsaicin cream 0.025–0.075 percent applied to affected area three to four times daily

▶ Antiretroviral therapy for 7–10 days

▷ Acyclovir 800 mg oral five times daily

▷ Valacyclovir 1000 mg oral t.i.d.

▷ Famciclovir 500 mg q8h

▶ Ophthalmology consult if cranial nerve V is involved

▶ Immunocompromised: Consult physician

▶ Resolves in 2–3 weeks but postherpetic neuralgia can persist for months to years

Prevention

▶ Shingles vaccination

DERMATITIS

Contact Dermatitis

▶ Acute or chronic inflammatory reaction from substances that come in contact with the skin and cause irritant contact dermatitis (ICD) or allergic contact dermatitis (ACD). ICD accounts for 70 percent of cases of contact dermatitis, while ACD is more common among persons younger than 70 years of age.

▶ ICD results from direct contact–triggered toxic effect that damages a component of the water-protein-lipid matrix of the epidermal layer of skin.

▶ ACD results from a delayed hypersensitivity reaction to a contact allergen that causes a cell-mediated hypersensitivity response. There are two phases:

1. Initial exposure phase sensitizes the skin and causes proliferation of T lymphocytes.

2. Elicitation phase causes antigen-specific T lymphocytes to combine with the allergen, thus producing an inflammatory response.

  ▶ Common allergens are rhus plants (poison ivy, oak, sumac), nickel (jewelry), chemicals (rubber, chemicals in personal products such as cosmetics, shampoos, drugs).

Risk Factors

▶ ICD

  ▷ History of atopic dermatitis

  ▷ White skin

  ▷ Low-temperature, low-humidity climates

  ▷ Occupational exposure to abrasives, cleaning agents, oxidizing or reducing agents, plants

▶ ACD

  ▷ Exposure to metal salts, antibiotics, dyes, plants.

  ▷ Frequent exposure to topical medications may trigger reactions in older adults.

Signs and Symptoms

▶ History of exposure to irritant or allergen

▶ ICD

  ▷ Erythematous rash is limited to the exposed area and may progress to vesicles, erosions, or crusting. Initial rash develops within a few hours of contact.

▶ ACD

  ▷ Initial rash is limited to the exposed area, but may spread to areas not exposed. Eruption may become generalized. Papules, vesicles, erosions, and crusts may develop.

  ▷ Metal allergy (nickel most common)

    ▶ Locations: neck, wrists, waist, strap line

    ▶ Generally mild, chronic with scaling, pigment changes, and pruritis

▷ Plant allergy (poison ivy, oak sumac most common)

▶ Often linear pattern

▶ May be weeping, scaling, edema, crusting, excoriations

Diagnostic Tests

▶ Skin examination, paying close attention to lesions

▶ History of current and past health issues, recent exposures

▶ Patch test if allergy suspected or in severe recurrent episodes

Differential Diagnoses

▶ Psoriasis

▶ Candidiasis

▶ Phytophotodermatitis

▶ Drug reaction

▶ Insect bite

Management

▶ Remove and avoid causative irritant or allergen.

▶ Wash objects that were in contact with irritant or allergen.

▶ Bathe in tepid water with mild soap.

▶ Moisturize with colloidal suspension (such as Aveeno).

▶ Topical or systemic steroids 2–3 times daily.

▶ Antibiotics if infected.

▶ Antihistamines for itching.

Prevention

▶ Avoid causative irritant.

▶ Wash skin immediately after contact with irritant.

▶ Wear protective clothing.

▶ Use skin moisturizer.

Nummular Eczema/Dermatitis

▶ Nummular (meaning round or "coin shaped") dermatitis or eczema (NE) is an inflammatory skin condition characterized by the presence of well-demarcated round-to-oval erythematous plaques.

▶ The cause is likely to be a combination of epidermal lipid barrier dysfunction and an immunologic response.

▶ Prevalence of nummular eczema is 2 cases per 1,000 people.

▶ More common in males than in females.

- Two peaks of age distribution (Miller 2017):
  - The most common is in the sixth to seventh decade of life.
  - A smaller peak occurs in the second to third decade of life.

Risk Factors

- Atopic history
- Male
- Xerosis

Signs and Symptoms

- Intense pruritis is a hallmark sign.
- Well-demarcated 4–5 cm coin-shaped plaques of grouped papules or vesicles on erythematous base.
- Lower legs (older males), trunk, hands and fingers (young females).
- Exudate, crusting, scales, and excoriations may be seen.
  - Later: scaling, lichenification, and pigmentation

Diagnostic Tests

- Skin biopsy

Differential Diagnoses

- Contact dermatitis
- Fungal infection
- Psoriasis

Management

- Skin emollients
- Topical steroids twice daily until lesions resolve
- Systemic antibiotics if staph present

Prevention

- Avoid any triggers.
- Keep skin moist and use gentle cleansers.
- Avoid skin irritants.

Seborrheic Dermatitis

- Chronic, recurrent, pruritic inflammation of skin where sebaceous glands are most active (face, scalp, body folds). Its cause is unknown, but *Malassezia furfur* yeast species may be linked.

Risk Factors

▶ Family history

▶ Human immunodeficiency virus (HIV) infection

▶ Zinc or niacin deficiency

▶ Parkinson's disease

Signs and Symptoms

▶ Scaly rash on lateral sides of nose, nasolabial folds, brows, glabella, and scalp

▷ May also see dandruff, an inflammatory base, sticky crusting (mostly in ears), and fissures (where ear attaches to scalp)

▶ Lesions greasy, yellow or red, erythematous, sharply marginated, 5–20 mm scaling macules and papules

Diagnostic Tests

▶ Clinical diagnosis

Differential diagnoses

▶ Psoriasis

▶ Rosacea

▶ Impetigo

▶ Pemphigus

▶ Dermatophyte infection

▶ Lupus erythematosus

Management

▶ Over-the-counter (OTC) selenium sulfide shampoos (Selsun Blue, Tegrin)

▶ Tar-based soap or shampoo preparations

▶ 2 percent ketoconazole shampoo

▶ Low-potency steroid topical solution or gel following shampoo

▶ Follow-up every 2 months during maintenance to monitor for signs of atrophy, candida and bacterial infections

Prevention

▶ The severity of seborrheic dermatitis can be lessened by controlling the risk factors and by paying careful attention to skin care (MedlinePlus 2017).

OTHER DERMATOLOGIC CONDITIONS

Acne Vulgaris

▶ Endogenous skin disorder characterized by open and closed comedones because of increased sebum release by sebaceous gland. More common in adolescents and young adults but may persist into middle age.

Risk Factors

► Hormonal changes

► Skin friction

► Using skin products that are not noncomedogenic or are irritating to skin

► Touching skin frequently

► Certain medications

Signs and Symptoms

► Three stages

► **Stage I:** Comedones

▷ Open: Whiteheads

▷ Closed: Blackheads

▷ Plugged follicles, no inflammation

► **Stage II:** Inflammatory lesions, follicles rupture, creating a pustule

► **Stage III:** Scarring

Diagnostic Tests

► Hormone evaluation: Elevated total testosterone, dehydroepiandosterone sulphate (DHEA-S), luteinizing hormone (LH), follicle-stimulating hormone (FSH); bacterial culture

► Skin examination

► Skin culture

Differential Diagnoses

► Rosacea

► Folliculitis

► Dermatitis

Management

► Skin cleansing

► Benzoyl peroxide

► Topical antibiotics

► Systemic antibiotics

► Retinoic acid

► Education

Prevention

► Use noncomedogenic products.

► Do not wash skin excessively.

► Avoid touching skin.

Psoriasis

▶ Psoriasis is chronic, hyperproliferative disorder that involves vasculature and epidermis of the skin. It develops from increased production of epidermal cells, an autoimmune response that results in psoriatic lesions. Psoriasis presents as erythematous papules and plaques with silver scales in a characteristic distribution on lower back, trunk, knees, elbows, and scalp. Psoriasis is a disease of exacerbations and remissions, and has a genetic predisposition.

Risk Factors

▶ Genetics

▶ Physical trauma

▶ Strep infection

▶ Stress

▶ Medications

▷ Systemic glucocorticoids, lithium, antimalarials, interferon, and beta blockers known to cause flare-ups in existing psoriasis

Signs and Symptoms

▶ Epidermal thickening

▶ Erythematous plaques (<1–10 cm) with demarcated margins and silver scales

▶ Erythema under scales

▶ Removal of scale results in tiny blood droplets

▶ Pitting fingernails

▶ Possible pruritis

▶ Variations

▷ Guttate psoriasis: Scaly plaques begin on trunk and spread to extremities; lesions 3–10 cm; occurs after strep infection

▷ Pustular psoriasis: Severe form; acute onset of widespread disease; more common in persons older than 50 years; may be precipitated by infection and recent systemic corticosteroid use

▷ Psoriatic arthritis: Presents similarly to inflammatory arthritis

▷ Distal interphalangeal joints common site for arthralgia

▶ Variable symptoms may precede skin lesions

Diagnostic Tests

▶ Skin examination

▶ Lesion biopsy when unsure of origin (resembles eczema)

▶ Auspitz's sign: Positive if droplets of blood form when scales removed from psoriatic lesions

Differential Diagnoses

- ▶ Seborrheic dermatitis
- ▶ Nummular eczema
- ▶ Atopic dermatitis
- ▶ Lichen planus
- ▶ Pityriasis rubra pilaris

Management

- ▶ Tar-based shampoo and steroid lotions.
- ▶ Steroid creams for face and trunk.
- ▶ Phototherapy using ultraviolet B light.
- ▶ Photochemotherapy with PUVA: Light therapy causing interaction of long wavelength ultraviolet light (UVA, 320–400 nm) with psoralens plant molecule.
- ▶ Systemic steroids.
- ▶ Refer to dermatologist if 10 percent body affected.

Prevention

- ▶ Minimize triggers such as stress, medications, or infection.

Pityriasis Rosea

- ▶ Mild, acute, self-limiting, inflammatory disorder of unknown origin that may cause pruritis
- ▶ Currently thought to be viral in origin; more common in spring and fall; frequently follows recent upper respiratory infection (URI)
- ▶ Affects females more than males; more common in persons 10–35 years of age
- ▶ Usually lasts 3–8 weeks

Risk Factors

- ▶ Possibly recent URI.
- ▶ Close physical contact with infected person.
- ▶ Immunocompromise.
- ▶ Ampicillin increases eruption distribution, resembling its effect on the rash of infectious mononucleosis.

Signs and Symptoms

- ▶ Herald patch = initial lesion
- ▶ Usually macular, oval, fawn-colored lesions, crinkled appearance, and collarette scale
- ▶ Lesions follow Christmas tree pattern
- ▶ Proximal extremities frequently involved

Diagnostic Tests

▶ Rapid plasma reagin (RPR) or Venereal Disease Research Laboratory (VDRL)

▶ WBC and differential, erythrocyte sedimentation rate (ESR)

▶ Total serum protein level, globulin level, albumin level

▶ Rheumatoid factor (RF), cold agglutinins, and cryoglobulins

▶ KOH test

▶ When only the herald patch is present, may be difficult to diagnose

Differential Diagnoses

▶ Ringworm

▶ Eczema

▶ Syphilis

▶ HIV

▶ Viral exanthems

▶ Cutaneous T-cell lymphoma

▶ Drug eruptions

▶ Guttate psoriasis

▶ Kaposi sarcoma

▶ Lichen planus

▶ Dermatitis

▶ Dermaphyte infection

Management

▶ None usually required

▶ Daily UVB light

▶ Medium-strength topical steroids for pruritus

Prevention

▶ No known cause or prevention

SKIN CANCER

▶ Abnormal growth of skin cells that most often develops on skin exposed to UV light but can also occur on skin not ordinarily exposed to sunlight.

▶ Three major types of skin cancer are basal cell carcinoma, squamous cell carcinoma, and melanoma. Skin cancer is the most common cancer, with more than one million new cases in the United States annually.

▶ Melanoma is the most serious form of skin cancer. Nonmelanomas (usually basal or squamous cell) are the most common forms of skin cancer and are highly curable.

Skin Cancer Screening (for all types)

- ▶ Routine self-examinations of the skin
- ▶ Regularly scheduled skin screening exams by a dermatologist
- ▶ Photo history to aid early in detection of changing pigmented lesions

Risk Factors (for all types)

- ▶ Excessive sun exposure
- ▶ Family history
- ▶ Fair skin
- ▶ Sunburn
- ▶ Sunny high-altitude climates
- ▶ Moles
- ▶ Radiation exposure
- ▶ History of skin cancer
- ▶ Immunocompromise
- ▶ Exposure to toxins
- ▶ Precancerous lesions

Prevention (for all types)

- ▶ Sunscreen
- ▶ Avoid the sun during midday hours
- ▶ Wear protective clothing
- ▶ Avoid tanning beds
- ▶ Report any mole changes

Basal Cell Carcinoma

- ▶ Most common type of cutaneus cancer
- ▶ Slow-growing and rarely metastasizes, but can become invasive and cause local destruction and disfigurement if neglected

Signs and Symptoms

- ▶ Pearly or waxy bump
- ▶ Flat, flesh-colored or brown scar-like lesion

Diagnostic Tests

- ▶ Clinical diagnosis
- ▶ Biopsy suspicious lesions

Differential Diagnoses

▶ Molluscum contagiosum

▶ Solar lentigo

▶ Actinic keratosis

▶ Squamous cell cancer

▶ Malignant melanoma

▶ *Verruca vulgaris*

Management

▶ Excision, cryosurgery, or electrosurgery.

▶ ◉ Mohs surgery.

▶ Microscopic surgery for lesions in danger zones of nasolabial folds, around eyes, ear canal, posterior auricle sulcus.

▷ Radiation therapy

▶ Alternative treatment in areas of cosmetic disfigurement:

▷ Some topical treatments are available but have low cure rates.

▷ 5 percent 5-flourouracil (for superficial lesions), imiquimod cream when surgery is inappropriate.

▶ Tumors on nose and in "T zone" have higher recurrence rates.

Squamous Cell Carcinoma

▶ Second most common cutaneous cancer

▶ Capable of local infiltrative growth, spread to regional lymph nodes, and distant metastasis

Signs and Symptoms

▶ Firm, red nodule

▶ Flat lesion with a scaly, crusted surface

Diagnostic Tests

▶ Skin biopsy

Differential Diagnoses

▶ Nummular eczema

▶ Psoriasis

▶ Paget's disease

▶ Pyroderma gangreosum

▶ Actinic keratosis

▶ Basal cell cancer

Management

▶ Surgery or radiation depending on the size, shape, and tumor location

▶ Surgical excision via cryotherapy, electrodessication and curettage, excision, or Mohs microscopic surgery

▶ Some topical treatments are available but have low cure rates.

▶ 5 percent 5-flourouracil (superficial lesions), imiquimod cream when surgery is inappropriate.

▶ Patients who develop squamous cell carcinoma have 40 percent risk of developing additional lesions within the next 2 years.

Malignant Melanoma

Signs and Symptoms

▶ Usually small brown-black or larger multicolored patches, plaques, or nodules with irregular outline

▶ Surface may crust or bleed

▶ May arise in preexisting moles

▶ Sudden or progressive change in pigmented lesion

▶ Increase in size of pigmented lesion

▶ Sudden appearance of new mole-like growth

▶ Asymmetry

▷ One half does not match other

▶ Irregular borders or edges

▷ Ragged, notched, or blurred

▶ Uneven pigmentation

▷ Varied shades: tan, brown, black

▶ Diameter > 6 millimeters

▷ Larger than a pencil eraser (Melanoma Research Foundation 2017)

Diagnostic tests

▶ Skin exam

▶ Biopsy

Differential diagnoses

▶ Benign nevi

▶ Solar lentiginous

▶ Seborrheic keratosis (Dunphy et al. 2015)

Management

▶ Removal of the melanoma by surgical excision

▶ Chemotherapy

▶ Biological therapies such as high-dose interferon and interleukin-2

Other, Less Common Types of Skin Cancer

Kaposi Sarcoma

▶ Rare form

▶ Develops in blood vessels of skin and causes red or purple patches on skin or mucous membranes

▶ Mainly occurs with immune systems weakened by AIDS, chemotherapy, immunosuppressants

▶ Increased risk in African, Mediterranean, Middle Eastern, and Eastern European males

Merkel Cell Carcinoma

▶ Causes firm, shiny nodules that occur on or just beneath the skin and in hair follicles

▶ Most often found on the head, neck, and trunk

Sebaceous Gland Carcinoma

▶ Aggressive cancer of sebaceous glands

▶ Mostly appears on eyelid as hard, painless nodules

Precancerous Conditions

▶ Actinic (solar) keratosis

▷ Rough, scaly, slightly raised lesions

▷ Color ranges from brown to red

▷ Up to 1 inch in diameter

▷ Appear mostly in older adults

▶ Actinic cheilitis

▶ Actinic keratosis on lips

▷ Lips dry, cracked, scaly, pale or white

▷ Mainly affect lower lip (more sun than upper lip)

▶ Leukoplakia

▷ White patches on tongue or inside mouth

▷ Squamous cell carcinoma could develop

▶ Bowen's disease

▷ Superficial squamous cell cancer, does not spread

▷   Persistent red-brown, scaly psoriasis, or eczema patch

▷   If untreated, may invade deeper structures

Management

►   Cryosurgery

►   Curettage and desiccation

►   Topical medications such as 5-FU (5 fluorouracil 0.5–5 percent)

►   Chemical peeling

►   Photodynamic therapy

REFERENCES

Centers for Disease Control and Prevention. 2016. "Overview." Shingles (Herpes Zoster). https://www.cdc.gov/shingles/about/overview.html.

Dunphy, L., J. Winland-Brown, B. Porter, and D. Thomas, eds. 2015. *Primary Care: The Art and Science of Advanced Practice Nursing.* 4th ed. Philadelphia: F. A. Davis.

MedlinePlus. 2017. "Seborrheic Dermatitis." Medical Encyclopedia.https://medlineplus.gov/ency/article/000963.htm.

Miller, J. L. 2017. "Nummular Dermatitis: Background, Pathophysiology, Epidemiology." *Medscape: Dermatology.* http://emedicine.medscape.com/article/1123605-overview#a5.

Melanoma Research Foundation. 2017. "The ABCDEs of Melanoma." http://www.melanoma.org/understand-melanoma/diagnosing-melanoma/detection-screening/abcdes-melanoma.

World Health Organization. 2017. "Herpes Simplex Virus." http://www.who.int/mediacentre/factsheets/fs400/en/.

CHAPTER 7

HEAD, EYES, EARS, NOSE, AND THROAT

LEARNING OBJECTIVES

► Recognize common head, eye, ear, nose, and throat disorders.
  ▷ Risk factors
  ▷ Signs and symptoms
  ▷ Diagnostic tests
  ▷ Differential diagnoses
► Describe treatment and management of the disorders of these systems.
  ▷ Management
  ▷ Prevention

EYES

► Assess vision acuity (Snellen chart).
► Attempt funduscopic exam.
► Refer for cataract evaluation if unable to see eye grounds.
► Many eye disorders present similarly.
► Refer immediately for sudden, painless vision loss.
► Monitor medication effects.
  ▷ Local reaction
  ▷ Systemic effects
  ▷ To avoid damage to contacts, eye drops should not be used with contacts in.

Symptoms of Acute Eye Disorders

▶ Blurred vision that does not clear with blinking

▶ Sudden vision loss or decrease

▶ Halos around lights

▶ Flashing lights

▶ Sudden floating spots or cobwebs

▶ Photophobia

▶ Periocular headache

▶ Ocular pain

▶ Ciliary flush

▶ Corneal damage (trauma)

▶ Abnormal pupils

▶ Increased intraocular pressure

▶ Appearance of cells in anterior chamber

▶ Proptosis

▶ Acute-onset limited ocular movement

▶ Facial cellulitis

Emergency Referral Conditions

▶ Keratitis

▶ Uveitis

▶ Corneal abrasion

▶ Acute angle glaucoma

▶ Retinal tear or detachment

▶ Retinal artery occlusion

▶ Retinal venous occlusion

Hordeolum (Stye)

▶ Common upper or lower eyelid staphylococcal abscess involving the Zeis and Moll glands on lid margin (external) or the meibomian gland abscess on conjunctival surface (internal)

Risk Factors

▶ Poor hygiene

▶ Chronic illness

▶ Chronic blepharitis

▶ Meibomian gland dysfunction

TABLE 7–1.
COMMON NONURGENT EYE PROBLEMS

PROBLEM	SIGNS AND SYMPTOMS	MANAGEMENT
Dry eyes	Sensation of dryness, burning, foreign body	Artificial tears
Subconjunctival hemorrhage	Blood beneath conjunctiva; rule out hyphema	Resolves spontaneously
Foreign body	Sudden, sharp pain because of irritation to epithelium of cornea	Saline irrigation for 10 min. Evert eyelid. *No patch*. Check in 24 h.
Xanthelasma	Yellow plaque along nasal aspect of lid; occurs in diabetes mellitus (DM) and lipid disorders	Cosmetic removal
Ectropion	Eyelid turns out from decreased muscle tone	Artificial tears; surgery
Entropion	Eyelid turns in to eyeball	Artificial tears; surgery
Blepharitis	Inflammation of sebum glands on lid margins	Warm compress and baby shampoo; eyelid scrubs; antibiotic drops p.r.n.
Pingueculae	Thickened conjunctiva near corneal limbus	Very common; no treatment
Chalazion	Inflamed meibomian gland on inner aspect of lid; firm, painful nodule	Warm compresses and ophthalmic antibiotics
Hordeolum (sty)	Infection of glands that lubricate lashes and outer lid	Warm compresses and ophthalmic antibiotics
Pterygium	Triangular growth of conjunctival tissue from inner canthus to pupil	Surgery if vision is obstructed; may recur
Conjunctivitis	Virus, bacteria, or allergy causing dilation of the blood vessels of bulbar and palpebral conjunctiva	Cool or warm compresses; antibiotic or other drops

TABLE 7–2.
AGE-RELATED EYE CHANGES

SYMPTOM	AGE-RELATED CHANGES
Arcus senilis	Lipid deposits in corneal margins
Presbyopia	Lens flattens with muscular weakness
Loss of peripheral vision	Decreased elasticity of lens
Altered color perception (blue, green, violet); iris fades with irregular pigmentation	Yellowing of the lens
Loss of visual acuity	Reduced blood flow
"Floaters"	Liquefying of vitreous humor
Dry eyes	Decreased tear production because of lacrimal gland atrophy

▶ Ocular rosacea

▶ Previous hordeolum; often recur in the same eyelid

Signs and Symptoms

▶ Localized edema

▶ Acutely tender lid

▶ Pain proportional to edema

▶ Erythema

▶ Painful to palpation

Diagnostic Tests

▶ No laboratory or diagnostic tests

▶ Clinical evaluation

Differential Diagnoses

▶ Conjunctivitis

▶ Chalazion

▶ Blepharitis

▶ Dacryocystitis

Management

▶ Warm compresses

▶ ▪ Bacitracin or erythromycin ophthalmic ointment q3h

▶ Incision and drainage (I&D) if no resolution in 48 hours

Prevention

▶ Avoid touching eyes.

▶ Avoid old or contaminated makeup.

▶ Change contacts as recommended.

▶ Hand hygiene.

Chalazion

▶ Noninfectious granulomatous reaction that causes inflammation because of swelling that blocks sebum release from the meibomian gland; often evolves from internal hordeolum.

Risk Factors

▶ History of chalazion

▶ Unclean hands

Signs and Symptoms

▶ May be none

▶ Visual distortion if large enough to impress

▶ Corneal itching

▶ Hard, nontender cyst

▶ Reddened conjunctiva

Diagnostic Tests

▶ No laboratory or diagnostic tests

▶ Clinical evaluation

Differential Diagnoses

▶ Tumor

▶ Hordeolum

Management

▶ Incision and curettage by ophthalmologist

Prevention

▶ Avoid touching eyes.

▶ Avoid old or contaminated makeup.

▶ Change contacts as recommended.

▶ Hand hygiene.

Blepharitis

▶ Chronic bilateral inflamed lid margin that involves eyelid skin, lashes, and associated glands (anterior) or dysfunction of meibomian glands (posterior); associated with bacterial eye infection (usually staph), symptoms of dry eyes, or skin conditions such as acne rosacea

Risk Factors

▶ Seborrheic dermatitis

▶ Psoriasis

▶ Poor hygiene or nutritional status

▶ Immune suppression

▶ Exposure to chemical or environmental irritants

Signs and Symptoms

▶ Irritation

▶ Burning or itching

▶ Redness

▶ Crusting of lid margins

Diagnostic Tests

▶ No laboratory or diagnostic tests

▶ Clinical evaluation

Differential Diagnoses

▶ Conjunctivitis

▶ Hordeolum

▶ Dacryocystitis

▶ Chemical irritation

Management

▶ Keep scalp and brows clean.

▶ Daily removal of scales with baby shampoo.

▶ Regular expression of meibomian gland.

▶ Corneal or conjunctival involvement.

▶ Bacitracin or erythromycin ophthalmic ointment daily.

▶ Tetracycline 250 mg oral b.i.d.

▶ Erythromycin 250 mg oral t.i.d.

▶ Topical steroids.

Prevention

▶ Avoid touching eyes.

▶ Avoid old or contaminated makeup.

▶ Change contacts as recommended.

▶ Hand hygiene.

Conjunctivitis

▶ Conjunctivitis is an inflammation of the conjunctiva caused by bacteria, viruses, allergens, or irritants. It is the most common treatable eye disorder among adults and children. Bacterial and viral conjunctivitis may affect one or both eyes. Allergic conjunctivitis affects both eyes and occurs primarily in spring and summer.

Risk Factors

▶ Poor hygiene

▶ Contaminated cosmetics

▶ Crowded living or social conditions

▶ Recent ocular surgery, exposed sutures, or ocular foreign bodies

- ▶ Chronic use of topical medications
- ▶ Immunocompromised
- ▶ **Bacterial**
    - ▷ Exposure to bacteria (staph, strep, gonorrhea, Neisseria, chlamydia)
- ▶ **Viral**
    - ▷ Adenovirus
    - ▷ Herpes
- ▶ **Allergic conjunctivitis**
    - ▷ Exposure to environmental allergens

        (Center for Disease Control and Prevention [CDC], 2016)

Signs and Symptoms

- ▶ Conjunctiva inflamed, reddened, and irritated over posterior surface of lids, sclera to cornea
- ▶ **Bacterial**
    - ▷ Discharge: Copious, purulent, stringy, watery
    - ▷ Gonorrhea: Copious, purulent discharge
- ▶ **Viral**
    - ▷ Clear, watery discharge
- ▶ **Allergic**
    - ▷ Bilateral copious, watery, tearing, and stringy discharge
    - ▷ Mild discomfort
    - ▷ Blurred vision

Diagnostic Tests

- ▶ History
- ▶ Eye exam
- ▶ Gram stain or culture if suspect gonococcal infection
- ▶ Conjunctival scrapings for bacterial conjunctivitis
    - ▷ Giemsa stain for chlamydia

Differential Diagnoses

- ▶ Iritis
- ▶ Keratoconjunctivitis
- ▶ Blepharitis
- ▶ Pterygium
- ▶ Subconjunctival hemorrhage
- ▶ Herpes zoster ophthalmicus
- ▶ Corneal abrasion

Management

▶ Bacterial conjunctivitis

▷ Self-limiting, lasting 10–14 days untreated

▷ ◢ If treated, sulfacetamide 10 percent ophthalmic solution t.i.d. × 2–3 days

▶ Gonococcal conjunctivitis is an ophthalmic emergency

▷ • Hospitalize: Ceftriaxone (Rocephin) 25–50 mg/kg or cefotaxime (Claforan) 25–50 mg/kg intravenously (IV) or intramuscularly (IM) q12h × 7 days

▶ Viral conjunctivitis

▷ Treat symptoms with sulfacetamide (decrease risk of secondary infection)

▶ Herpes simplex

▷ Refer to ophthalmologist

▶ Allergic conjunctivitis

▷ Can be treated with short-term topical steroids and antihistamines

Prevention

▶ Good hand hygiene.

▶ Avoid touching eyes.

▶ Do not share personal items, such as pillows, washcloths, towels, eye drops, eye makeup, face makeup, makeup brushes, contact lenses and contact lens containers, or eyeglasses.

▶ Stop wearing contact lenses.

Glaucoma

▶ Increased intraocular pressure causing progressive peripheral vision loss by irreversibly damaging the optic nerve

▶ Causes 9–12 percent of cases of blindness in United States; leading cause of irreversible blindness worldwide (Glaucoma Research Foundation [GRF] 2016a).

▶ Main types

▷ **Acute closed-angle glaucoma (ACG)**

▶ Narrow anterior chamber suddenly blocked and intraocular pressure (IOP) abruptly rises

▶ More common in Asian American and Inuit people

▷ **Open-angle glaucoma (OAG)**: 90 percent of cases; chronic (GRF 2016b)

▶ Resistance to outflow of aqueous humor causes a slow rise in IOP

▷ **Secondary glaucoma**

▶ Obstruction of outflow tracts because of complications of other disease states (DM, hypertension [HTN], eye injury, medications, eye conditions)

▷ Both ACG and OCG can be *secondary* when there is a known cause.

Risk Factors

▶ ACG

▷ Family history

▷ Age > 40–50 years

▷ Female

▷ Hyperopia because of shape of eyeball, with narrow angle

▷ Anticholinergic use

▷ Anatomically small eye with shallow anterior chamber

▷ Eye pathology: Cysts of iris or ciliary bodies, cataracts, intraocular tumor

▶ OAG

▷ Elevated IOP

▷ Advanced age

▷ More common in African American people

▷ Family history

▷ Corticosteroid use: Topical, oral, inhaled

▷ Systemic hypertension, diabetes, cardiovascular disease

▶ Secondary glaucoma

▷ Other disease states (DM, HTN, eye injury, medications, eye conditions) that can obstruct outflow tracts

Differential Diagnoses

▶ Conjunctivitis

▶ Uveitis

▶ Medication-induced intraocular pressure increase

Prevention

▶ Regular eye exams

Diabetic Retinopathy

▶ A microvascular disease of the eyes that is a complication of diabetes related to prolonged elevation of serum glucose levels that affect vision because of damage to blood vessels of the retina. Diabetic retinopathy usually affects both eyes.

▶ Leading cause of new-onset blindness in persons aged 25–74 years.

▶ Third leading cause of blindness.

▶ Nonproliferative

▷ Microaneurysms occur early.

▷ Eye vessels weaken, allowing fluids to leak into retina.

TABLE 7–3.
GLAUCOMA SIGNS, SYMPTOMS, AND DIAGNOSTIC TESTS

SIGNS AND SYMPTOMS	ACUTE CLOSED-ANGLE GLAUCOMA (ACG) DIAGNOSTICS	OPEN-ANGLE GLAUCOMA (OAG) DIAGNOSTIC TESTS
IOP	40–80 mm Hg	Up to 22 mm Hg
Pain	Severe	No early symptoms
Visual loss	Profound	Progressive
Exam	Hard, red eye, ciliary flush, steamy cornea, dilated pupil	Optic nerve head pale, increased cup-to-disc ratio
Management	Immediate referral	Less urgent referral

TABLE 7–4.
GLAUCOMA MANAGEMENT

MEDICATION CLASS	EXAMPLE	METHOD OF ACTION	LOCAL EFFECTS	SYSTEMIC EFFECTS
Beta blocker	Timolol	Decrease aqueous production	Transient discomfort, tearing, blurred vision	Congestive heart failure (CHF), asthma, bradycardia
Parasympathetic	Pilocarpine	Increase aqueous outflow	Constricted pupil	Diarrhea, sweating, bronchospasm
Adrenergic	Epinephrine	Decrease inflow and increase outflow	Allergic lid reaction and eye irritation	Increased heart rate, palpitations
Prostaglandin agonist	Xalatan	Increase outflow	Eye pigment change, local irritation	Rare
Carbonic anhydrase inhibitors	Trusopt	Decrease aqueous production	Conjunctivitis	Side effects of sulfonamides: dizziness, headache (HA), lethargy, diarrhea, anorexia, vomiting, nausea, skin rashes

▷ Well-demarcated, small, red spots around optic nerve and macula; exudates and dilated capillaries.

▷ Dilated vessels steal circulation from retinal surface; aneurysms leak and bleed.

▶ Proliferative (wet)

▷ Neovascularization.

▷ Fragile new vessels form to repair circulation; support tissues can cause retinal detachment.

Risk Factors

▶ Diabetes

▶ Poor control of glucose levels

▶ • Proteinuria

▶ Hyperlipidemia

▶ Hypertension

Signs and Symptoms

▶ Blurred vision

▶ Fluctuating vision, vision loss

▶ Impaired color vision

▶ Dark or empty areas in vision

▶ Floaters, cloudy vision, or "curtain over eye" if retina detaches

Diagnostic Tests

▶ Blood glucose

▶ Hemoglobin A1C

▶ Routine ophthalmology exams and good control of blood sugar may delay onset.

▶ Visual acuity test

▶ Dilated eye exam

▷ Examination for retina and optic nerve damage, macular edema

▶ Tonometry

▷ Measures pressure inside eye

Differential Diagnoses

▶ Hypertensive retinopathy

▶ Retinal detachment

▶ Glaucoma

▶ Macular degeneration

Management

▶ Refer all patients with diabetes to ophthalmologist for evaluation and monitoring.

▶ Optimal blood sugar control.

▶ Ophthalmologic exam annually (also preventive).

▶ Laser photocoagulation:

▷ Scatter laser treatment to shrink abnormal vessels

▷ Focal laser treatment for macular edema

▶ Vitrectomy for vitreous hemorrhage and tractional retinal detachment

Prevention

▶ Regular eye exams that include glaucoma screening

Age-Related Macular Degeneration (AMD)

▶ Progressive deterioration of central vision because of damage to the macula and affecting central vision

▶ Leading cause of blindness in older adults; one third of patients develop depression

▶ Two types:

▷ • Wet AMD (10–15 percent; American Macular Degeneration Foundation [AMDF], n.d.)

▶ Neovascularization with hemorrhage or exudation of fluid between retinal pigment epithelium and retina

▶ Examination reveals neovascularization, retinal pigment change, fluid exudation, and hemorrhage

▷ • Dry AMD (85–90 percent; AMDF, n.d.)

▶ Atrophy of retinal pigment epithelium and photoreceptor cells

▶ Examination reveals drusen and macular pigmentary changes

▶ May progress to wet AMD

Risk Factors

▶ Smoking

▶ High-fat diet

▶ Cardiovascular disease

▶ Family history

Signs and Symptoms

▶ Asymptomatic in early disease

▶ Loss of central vision in one or both eyes, sudden or gradual

▶ Vision alterations

▷ Straight lines appear blurry, wavy, or missing segments

▷ Patchy, blurry vision, distorted central field

Diagnostic Tests

▶ Dilated exam with slit lamp (biomicroscopy)

▶ Fluorescein angiography

▶ Optic coherence therapy

Differential Diagnoses

▶ Diabetic retinopathy

▶ Hypertensive retinopathy

Management

▶ Dry AMD

▷ No effective treatment

► Wet AMD

▷ Vascular endothelial growth factor

▷ Thermolaser photocoagulation

Prevention

► • Antioxidants and minerals

Cataracts

► Abnormal, uniform, progressive opacity (clouding) of eye lens that reduces visual acuity

► Leading and most common cause of vision loss after age 40 years; by 75 years, most have cataracts

► Senile cataracts most common

Risk Factors

► Systemic disease

► Heavy alcohol use

► Congenital

► Age

► Cigarette smoking

► Ultraviolet B (UVB) light exposure

► Diabetes

► Corticosteroid use (inhaled or oral)

► Trauma

Signs and Symptoms

► Loss of red reflex

► Enhanced glare

► Generalized vision decrease

Diagnostic Tests

► Funduscopic exam shows lens opacity

Differential Diagnoses

► Corneal scar

► Macular degeneration

► Retinal tear

Management

► Magnification glasses.

▶ Contact lenses.

▶ Cataract removal.

▶ Intraocular lens implant.

▶ Optimal vision is critical to maintain function across the lifespan. Cataract removal may be appropriate even for persons with moderate dementia to decrease misinterpretation of environmental cues.

Prevention

▶ Regular eye exams.

▶ Antioxidants and minerals.

▶ Protect eyes from the sun.

▶ Avoid using corticosteroid medications for extended periods.

▶ Quit smoking.

▶ Reduce alcohol intake.

EARS

Hearing Loss

▶ Diminished ability to detect pure tones ≥30 decibels may be conductive or sensorineural.

Risk Factors

▶ Exposure to loud noises

▶ Ototoxic drugs

▶ Eustachian tube obstruction

▶ Chronic middle ear infections

Signs and Symptoms

▶ **Conductive loss**

▷ Decreased ability to conduct sound from external to inner ear

▷ Causes

▶ Impacted wax

▶ Infection

▶ Foreign object

▶ Perforated TM

▶ Bony growth or tumor in middle ear

▶ **Sensorineural loss**

▷ Decreased ability to hear faint sounds because of damage to nerve pathways from inner ear to brain

TABLE 7–5.
AUDITORY SYSTEM AND HEARING LOSS

SYMPTOM	AGE-RELATED CHANGES
Hearing loss with sound distortion	Reduced blood flow leading to cochlear deterioration
Gradual loss of hearing	Cilia and neuronal decrease
	Eardrum thickens, reducing sound transmission

TABLE 7–6.
TYPES OF HEARING LOSS

TYPE OF LOSS	HISTORY	PATTERN OF LOSS	DIAGNOSTIC TESTS
Conductive	Unilateral loss of low tones; may have tinnitus; gradual or acute	Good speech discrimination; understands when loud enough	Air conduction (AC) < bone conduction (BC) Weber test lateralized to affected ear; fluid, cerumen, or foreign body may be in canal or fluid behind tympanic membrane (TM)
Sensorineural	Slow onset, usually bilateral; high frequency loss; may have tinnitus or vertigo	Loss of tone and discrimination; can hear but not understand	No abnormalities seen AC $\geq$ BC Weber lateralizes to better ear
Mixed	Bilateral sensorineural and unilateral conductive loss; slow onset with acute worsening	Loss of both volume and discrimination	Weber and Rinne tests nonconclusive; same as conductive

▷ Causes

▶ Exposure to loud noises

▶ Ototoxic meds

▶ Cranial nerve VIII dysfunction

▶ Multiple sclerosis

▶ Syphilis

▶ Ménière's disease

Diagnostic Tests

▶ See table 7–6 above.

Differential Diagnosis

▶ Cerumen impaction

▶ Foreign body obstruction

Management

- ▶ Treat cause if possible.
- ▶ Refer for hearing aid evaluation.
- ▶ Educate family regarding improving communication.
- ▶ Refer to otorhinolaryngologist (ENT) for acute-onset loss.
- ▶ Be alert for decreased function, depression, and social isolation.

Prevention

- ▶ Avoid loud noises
- ▶ Hearing protection such as ear plugs
- ▶ Buy quieter home products
- ▶ Turn down TV or radio

Cerumen Impaction

Management

- ▶ Soften with 1–2 drops baby or mineral oil daily × 5–7 days.
- ▶ Irrigate with 10:1 solution of hydrogen peroxide (avoid excessive pressure).
- ▶ Can develop otitis externa after wax removal.
- ▶ Educate regarding no foreign bodies in ear.
- ▶ Prophylactic oil may decrease recurrence.

Tinnitus

- ▶ Ringing, buzzing, hissing, roaring, or whistling sound in the ears from a number of factors
- ▶ Pulsatile tinnitus
  - ▷ Often muscle movements near ear, changes in ear canal, or vascular problems in face or neck
- ▶ Nonpulsatile tinnitus
  - ▷ Problems in nerves involved with hearing
  - ▷ Sometimes described as coming from inside the head

Risk Factors

- ▶ Cerumen impaction
- ▶ Hearing loss
- ▶ Perforated tympanic membrane
- ▶ Caffeine
- ▶ Alcohol
- ▶ Anemia

- ▶ Ménière's disease
- ▶ Hyperthyroid
- ▶ Multiple sclerosis
- ▶ Acoustic neuroma
- ▶ Vascular disorders
- ▶ Communicating cardiac murmurs

Signs and Symptoms

- ▶ Intermittent or continuous ringing, buzzing, hissing, roaring, or whistling

Diagnostic Tests

- ▶ Computed tomography (CT) scan, contrast magnetic resonance imaging (MRI), or angiography for pulsatile tinnitus
- ▶ Audiometric testing
- ▶ Lab work to rule out other etiologies

Differential Diagnoses

- ▶ Cerumen impaction
- ▶ Perforated tympanic membrane
- ▶ Caffeine
- ▶ Alcohol
- ▶ Anemia
- ▶ Ménière's disease
- ▶ Hyperthyroid
- ▶ Multiple sclerosis
- ▶ Acoustic neuroma
- ▶ Vascular disorders
- ▶ Communicating cardiac murmurs
- ▶ Medications
  - ▷ Aspirin and other nonsteroidal anti-inflammatory drugs (NSAIDs); tricyclic antidepressants (TCAs); antineoplastic drugs; aminoglycosides; loop diuretics; oral contraceptives

Management

- ▶ Treat cause if possible.
- ▶ Hearing aids.
- ▶ Biofeedback.
- ▶ Antidepressants.
- ▶ Gingko biloba (bleeding risk).

▶ Exercise regularly.

▶ Cut back on alcohol and caffeine.

▶ Stop smoking and use of smokeless tobacco products; nicotine reduces blood flow to structures of the ear.

Prevention

▶ Avoid loud noises.

▶ Wear protective earplugs if loud noises cannot be avoided.

▶ Avoid aspirin and other nonsteroidal anti-inflammatory drugs (NSAIDs); tricyclic anti-depressants (TCAs); aminoglycosides; loop diuretics; oral contraceptives.

▶ Decrease alcohol intake.

Otitis Externa

▶ Inflammation or infection of external auditory canal, auricle, or both, often after water activities or ear trauma (forceful ear cleaning, cotton swab use, or water in ear canal)

Risk Factors

▶ Ear trauma

▶ Water sports or activities

▶ Submersion in water

Signs and Symptoms

▶ Otalgia progressing over 1–2 days

▶ Ear fullness or pressure, hearing loss

▶ Tinnitus

▶ Fever (occasionally)

▶ Itching, especially fungal or chronic

▶ Severe, deep pain

▶ Cellulitis of face or neck

▶ Ear canal erythema, edema, discharge—initially clear, then purulent and foul-smelling

▶ Pain on auricular manipulation

▶ Erythema on lateral surface tympanic membrane (TM)

Diagnostic Tests

▶ Pneumatic otoscopy demonstrates normal mobility

Differential Diagnoses

▶ Acute otitis media

▶ Ruptured tympanic membrane

▶ Mastoiditis

▶ Bullous myringitis

▶ Foreign bodies

▶ Neoplasms

▶ Chronic suppurative otitis media

Management

▶ Remove purulent debris.

▶ •Surgical debridement.

  ▷ For necrotizing complications such as canal stenosis

  ▷ Often necessary with copious discharge in ear

  ▷ Mainstay for fungal infections

▶ Incision and drainage of abscess.

▶ Protect from moisture and injury.

▶ Avoid swimming while infected.

▶ Topical medications:

  ▷ Place wick or gauze in canal to draw in otic drops

  ▷ 2 percent acetic acid, 1–2 drops after swimming

  ▷ Acetic acid in aluminum acetate, hydrocortisone, and acetic acid otic solution, alcohol-vinegar otic mix

  ▷ Antibiotics: otic hydrocortisone-neomycin-polymyxin B, ofloxacin, ciprofloxacin

  ▷ Combinations: Gentamicin 0.3 percent prednisolone 1 percent ophthalmic, dexamethasone-tobramycin, otic ciprofloxacin-dexamethasone, otic ciprofloxacin-hydrocortisone suspension

  ▷ Antifungal agents: Otic clotrimazole 1 percent solution, nystatin powder

▶ Oral medications

  ▷ Antibiotic: Ciprofloxacin

▶ Pain management

  ▷ Analgesics: Acetaminophen, acetaminophen with codeine (Tylenol 3)

  ▷ Local heat to outer ear

Otitis Media

▶ **Acute Otitis Media (AOM)**

  ▷ Bacterial or viral infection of mucus-lined spaces of temporal bone (*Streptococcus, Haemophilus influenzae, Moraxella catarrhalis*)

  ▷ Frequently precipitated by viral upper respiratory infection (URI)

  ▷ More common in males

- ▶ **Serous Otitis Media (SOM)**
  - ▷ Also known as chronic otitis media with effusion
  - ▷ Blocked Eustachian tube unable to equalize pressure, possibly precipitated by allergy, subacute infection, neoplasms, or barotrauma

Risk Factors

- ▶ Eustachian tube dysfunction
- ▶ Recent URI, allergies
- ▶ Anatomic anomaly (adenoid hypertrophy, cleft palate)
- ▶ Cigarette smoking or secondhand smoke
- ▶ Family history of AOM
- ▶ Day care attendance, under age 2 years

Signs and Symptoms

- ▶ Acute
  - ▷ Decreased hearing
  - ▷ Otalgia or aural pressure
  - ▷ Fever, vertigo, nausea, vomiting
  - ▷ TM rarely bulges
  - ▷ TM erythema bullae
- ▶ Serous
  - ▷ Hearing loss
  - ▷ Popping sensation when pressure altered
  - ▷ Fullness in the ear
  - ▷ Air bubbles behind TM
  - ▷ Decreased TM mobility

Diagnostic Tests

- ▶ Usually clinical diagnosis
- ▶ Impaired TM mobility
- ▶ Weber and Rinne tests suggest conductive loss in serous otitis media
- ▶ Tympanocentesis and culture (special circumstances)

Differential Diagnoses

- ▶ Otitis externa
- ▶ Barotrauma
- ▶ Tonsillitis, sinusitis, mumps, mastoiditis, dental abscess
- ▶ Anatomic abnormalities

▶ Foreign body

▶ Temporomandibular (TMJ) dysfunction

▶ Trauma

▶ Nasopharyngeal carcinoma

Management

▶ Acute otitis media

▷ • Amoxicillin 500 mg q8h × 5–7 days

▷ If ineffective

▶ Amoxicillin-clavulanate (Augmentin) 875 mg q12h × 5–7 days

▶ Azithromycin (Zithromax) 125 mg first day, then 250 mg days 2–5

▶ Cefaclor (Ceclor) 250–500 mg q8h × 5–7 days

▷ Nasal decongestants

▶ Serous otitis media

▷ Topical or oral decongestants and antihistamines.

▶ Use sparingly in older adults

▷ Oral decongestants (phenylephrine, pseudoephedrine) may elevate blood pressure and cause palpitations.

▷ Intranasal anticholinergic (ipratropium bromide 0.03 percent) may cause nasal dryness epistaxis.

▷ Intranasal glucocorticoids (fluticasone, budesonide) decrease rhinorrhea and congestion.

Prevention

▶ Smoking cessation

Cholesteatoma

▶ Type of chronic otitis media in which chronic negative middle ear pressure draws TM inward from prolonged auditory tube dysfunction. Squamous epithelium–lined sac is created and filled with chronically infected desquamated keratin. Over time, bone, inner ear, or facial nerve erodes.

▶ Three types

▷ Congenital cholesteatoma

▶ Squamous epithelium becomes trapped in temporal bone during embryogenesis.

▷ Primary acquired cholesteatoma

▶ Chronic negative middle-ear pressure because of Eustachian tube dysfunction

     ▷   Secondary acquired cholesteatoma

       ▶   TM perforation because of acute otitis media, trauma, or surgical manipulation of TM

Risk Factors

▶   Birth defect of middle ear

▶   Chronic ear infections

▶   Trauma

▶   Surgical manipulation of TM

Signs and Symptoms

▶ • Hallmark: Painless otorrhea

▶   Conductive hearing loss in affected ear

▶   Dizziness

▶   Ear drainage

▶   Other signs or symptoms dependent on degree of bone erosion

▶   Epitympanic retraction pocket

▶   TM perforation marginal

Diagnostic Tests

▶   CT scan

▶   Electronystagmography

Differential Diagnoses

▶   Chronic suppurative otitis media

▶   Myringosclerosis

     ▷   Thickening and calcification of the tympanic membrane secondary to inflammation

▶   Myospherulosis

     ▷   Rare foreign body reaction to oil-based ointments used in packing after surgery

Management

▶   ENT consult

▶   Surgical removal or marsupialization of sac

Prevention

▶   Prompt and thorough treatment of chronic ear infection

NOSE

Epistaxis (Nosebleed)

▶ Most nosebleeds are benign, self-limiting, and spontaneous, but can be recurrent.

▶ They are classified based on origin of bleed, anterior or posterior.

▶ Located most often on the anterosuperior portion of the nasal septum known as Little's area (Kiesselbach's triangle or Kiesselbach's plexus).

▶ More than 90 percent of nosebleeds result from local irritation related to trauma or inflammation, without any anatomical abnormality (Dunphy et al. 2015).

Risk Factors

▶ Trauma (falls)

▶ Mucosal irritations

　▷ Nasal sprays, nasal cannula oxygen

　▷ Dry air

　▷ Allergies or common cold

▶ Hypertension

▶ Aspirin or blood thinners

▶ Septal abnormality

▶ Inflammatory diseases

▶ Tumors

▶ Systemic causes

　▷ Blood dyscrasias, arteriosclerosis, hereditary hemorrhagic telangiectasia

Signs and Symptoms

▶ Bleeding usually occurs in one nostril.

▶ Blood can also drip into the back of the throat or down into the stomach, causing spitting up or vomiting blood.

Diagnostic Tests

▶ None

▶ Based on history

Differential Diagnoses

▶ Chronic sinusitis

▶ Allergic rhinitis

▶ Cocaine abuse

▶ Nasal foreign body

▶ Hemophilia

▶ Von Willebrand disease

▶ Warfarin toxicity

Management

▶ Direct pressure (pinch fleshy part of nose).

▶ Topical vasoconstrictors (Neo-Synephrine).

▶ Cautery or packing (rarely).

▶ Topical antibiotic ointment to nares can prevent recurrent nosebleeds.

▶ Use nasal saline spray.

▶ Avoid hard nose-blowing or sneezing.

▶ Sneeze with the mouth open.

▶ Avoid nasal digital manipulation.

▶ Avoid hot and spicy foods.

▶ Avoid hot showers.

▶ Avoid aspirin and other NSAIDs.

Prevention

▶ Use saline nasal spray.

▶ Avoid forceful nose-blowing.

▶ Limit aspirin and NSAID use.

▶ Use a humidifier.

Sinusitis

▶ Inflammation or infection of paranasal sinus cavities. Drainage of sinus is blocked. Secretions accumulate and provide bacterial media.

▶ Dental infections may be the cause.

▶ Often affects maxillary sinus.

▶ Change in quality of secretions.

▶ Majority are viral.

▶ Three categories:

▷ Acute: Infection in one or more paranasal cavities with symptoms that resolve with treatment within 3–4 weeks; considered recurrent infections if more than three episodes per year

▷ Subacute: Ongoing symptoms of purulent nasal discharge and sinus inflammation that resolve within 3 months

▷ Chronic: Prolonged sinus inflammation with or without infection for more than 3 months

▶ May be bacterial, viral, or fungal.

▷ **Bacterial:** *S. pneumoniae, H. influenzae, S. aureus, M. catarrhalis*

    ▷ **Viral**: Adenovirus, coronavirus, rhinovirus

    ▷ **Fungal:** Especially seen in immunocompromised persons; *Aspergillus*

► The following clinical presentations (any of three) are recommended for identifying patients with acute bacterial versus viral rhinosinusitis:

    ▷ Onset with persistent symptoms or signs compatible with acute rhinosinusitis, lasting for 10 or more days without any evidence of clinical improvement

    ▷ Onset with severe symptoms or signs of high fever ($\geq$102°F) and purulent nasal discharge or facial pain lasting for at least 3–4 consecutive days at the beginning of illness

    ▷ Onset with worsening symptoms or signs characterized by the new onset of fever, headache, or increase in nasal discharge following a typical viral upper respiratory infection (URI) that lasted 5–6 days and was initially improving (Chow et al. 2012)

Risk Factors

► Dental or upper respiratory infections

► Anatomic anomalies: Hypertrophied tonsils and adenoids, deviated septum, nasal polyps, cleft palate

Signs and Symptoms

► Pain or pressure over cheeks

► Headache; throbbing worsens when head dependent

► Discolored, yellow or greenish nose or throat discharge

► Postnasal drip and cough

► Halitosis

► Stuffy nose

► Fever

► Toothache

► Reduced sense of taste or smell

► External facial edema, erythema, or cellulitis over an involved sinus; vision changes (diplopia); difficulty moving eyes; proptosis; neurological signs; or severe pain indicative of serious complications requiring urgent referral and treatment

Diagnostic Tests

► Often via clinical presentation

► Transillumination

    ▷ Not particularly helpful

► CT scan preferred

    ▷ More sensitive

► May culture nasal discharge

▶ Maxillary sinus puncture or aspiration lavage culture when atypical pathogen suspected

▶ CBC if severely ill

Differential Diagnoses

▶ Nasopharyngeal tumor

▶ Wegener's syndrome

▶ Immotile cilia syndrome

▶ Nasal polyps

▶ Deviated septum

▶ Cystic fibrosis

▶ Granuloma

▶ Viral URI

Management

▶ Steam inhalation.

▶ Saline nasal spray.

▶ Neti pot nasal irrigation.

▶ Pseudoephedrine 60–120 mg t.i.d.

▶ Oxymetazoline 0.05 percent 1–2 sprays per nostril q6–8h × 3 days.

▶ Amoxicillin-clavulanate (500 mg/125 mg p.o. t.i.d. or 875 mg/125 mg p.o. b.i.d.) × 5–10 days or doxycycline 100 mg PO twice daily × 5–10 days.

▶ **Patients with risk factors for resistance:** High-dose amoxicillin-clavulanate (2 g/125 mg extended-release tablets orally twice daily × 5–10 days).

▶ **For penicillin-allergic patients:** Clindamycin 150 mg or 300 mg every 6 hours plus a third-generation oral cephalosporin (cefixime 400 mg daily or cefpodoxime 200 mg twice daily × 5–10 days).

▶ Improvement should be seen within 72 hours of treatment and resolution should occur within 10 days.

▶ If not resolved or if complicated, refer to ENT for surgical evaluation.

Prevention

▶ Good hand hygiene.

▶ Avoid sick contacts.

▶ Smoking cessation.

▶ Obtain flu vaccine.

Rhinitis

▶ Hyperfunction and tissue inflammation of the nasal mucosa categorized by the infectious, allergic, and nonallergic (vasomotor rhinitis) causes.

- ▶ Allergic rhinitis

- ▶ IgE-mediated hypersensitivity reaction, most often related to seasonal (pollens, grass, mold) or perennial (pet dander, dust mites, cigarette smoke, pollutants, cockroaches) allergens that cause inflammation of nasal membranes

- ▶ Characterized by nasal congestion, itching, rhinorrhea and sneezing

- ▶ Nonallergic

- ▶ **Infectious rhinitis (common cold)**

  - ▷ Most often a self-limiting upper respiratory tract infection (URI) caused by rhinovirus, coronavirus, adenovirus, parainfluenza, and sometimes bacteria

  - ▷ Incidence decreases with age

- ▶ **Vasomotor rhinitis**

  - ▷ Chronic, noninfectious process of unknown etiology without accompanying eosinophilia, characterized by periods of abnormal autonomic responsiveness and vascular engorgement unrelated to specific allergens (Dunphy et al. 2015)

  - ▷ Fluctuations and reductions in estrogen associated with menses, hormonal birth control preparations, pregnancy, and menopause may predispose to nonallergic rhinitis (Dunphy et al. 2015)

  - ▷ May be caused by medications

- ▶ **Atrophic rhinitis**

  - ▷ The nasal epithelia and bones progressively atrophy, resulting in distinct morphological changes

Signs and Symptoms

See Table 7-7. Signs and Symptoms of Rhinitis

Risk Factors

- ▶ Exposure to irritants

- ▶ Exposure to viruses

- ▶ Medications

Diagnostic Tests

- ▶ Clinical presentation

- ▶ Throat culture if strep infection suspected

- ▶ Allergic rhinitis

  - ▷ Allergy skin tests

  - ▷ Total serum IgE

  - ▷ White blood count (WBC): Elevated eosinophil count supports the diagnosis of allergic rhinitis, but it is not sensitive or specific for diagnosis

  - ▷ Nasal cytology: Nasal scrapings show eosinophils

- ▶ X-ray, CT scan, MRI will show presence of sinusitis

TABLE 7–7.
SIGNS AND SYMPTOMS OF RHINITIS

TYPES	ALLERGIC RHINITIS	INFECTIOUS RHINITIS	VASOMOTOR RHINITIS	ATROPHIC RHINITIS
Onset	Ages 5–40 years	Anytime	Adulthood	Older adulthood
Common Primary Symptoms	Sneezing Nasal congestion Rhinorrhea (clear or colored) may exist Itching of nose, eyes, palate Postnasal drip Frequent throat clearing Cough Malaise Fatigue	Nasal congestion Sneezing Scratchy sore throat Obstruction Nasal crusting Cloudy or colored drainage	Abrupt onset congestion and pronounced watery postnasal drip Sneezing	Nasal congestion Thick postnasal drip Repeated clearing of throat Bad smell from nose
Associated Symptoms	Cough, sore throat, itching, puffy eyes	Cough Malaise Fever > 100°F Possible facial or sinus tenderness	Watery eyes	None
Physical Findings	Pale, boggy nasal mucosa Enlarged turbinates "Allergic shiners" Nasal salute Mouth-breathing	Edema or hyperemia of mucous membranes Throat erythema without edema Postnasal drainage Cervical lymph node tenderness and enlargement Lungs clear	Pale, edematous turbinates	Dry, nonedematous nasal mucosa Airway patent

Differential Diagnoses

▶ URI

▶ Foreign body

▶ Hormonal: Oral contraceptive or pregnancy

▶ Sinusitis

▶ Nasal polyps or overgrowths

▶ Adenoid hypertrophy

▶ Otitis media

▶ Endocrine disease (hypothyroidism)

Management

▶ Rest, hydration, humidification (except for allergic), intranasal saline solution irrigation.

▶ Avoid triggers.

▶ Warm saline gargles.

▶ Decongestant or saline spray for congestion.

▶ Over-the-counter (OTC) analgesics.

▶ Aspirin or acetaminophen for headache or fever.

▶ Topical antihistamine azelastine HCl 0.1 percent.

▶ Oral antihistamines (nonsedating are best).

   ▷ First generation (diphenhydramine) causes drowsiness; use cautiously

   ▷ Second generation (fexofenadine, loratadine, cetirizine) preferred for regular use

▶ Oral decongestants.

   ▷ Cause vasoconstriction, decrease blood supply to nasal mucosa, decreased mucosal edema; can be used with antihistamines (phenylephrine, pseudoephedrine)

▶ Topical steroids are not fully effective until several days after start.

   ▷ Beclomethasone, fluticasone, triamcinolone preparations

   ▷ Refer to package for age-related dosage

▶ Intranasal anticholinergic: Ipratropium bromide 0.03 percent.

▶ Intranasal glucocorticoids: Fluticasone, budesonide.

▶ Intranasal cromolyn sodium.

▶ Leukotriene modifiers: Singulair.

▶ Severe symptoms may require combination treatment.

▶ If no relief, refer to allergist.

▶ Immunotherapy for those not responsive to pharmacologic therapy.

Prevention

▶ Rest, hydration, humidification (except for allergic), intranasal saline solution irrigation.

▶ Avoid triggers.

▶ Decongestant or saline spray for congestion.

MOUTH AND NOSE

Pharyngitis (Sore Throat)

▶ Inflammation of the pharynx frequently caused by acute infection of virus, bacteria (e.g., *Staphylococcus aureus*), or fungi.

▶ Droplet transmission via oral, respiratory, and nasal secretions.

▶ Viruses are the most common cause of infectious pharyngitis, accounting for 30–50 percent of cases (Dunphy et al. 2015).

Risk Factors

▶ Exposure to Group A beta-hemolytic streptococcus, virus, or causative agent

▶ Communal living (e.g., dormitories, barracks, nursing homes)

▶ Immunocompromised, diabetes (for fungal infections)

▶ Recent illness, fatigue, exposure to smoke, excessive alcohol intake

Signs and Symptoms

▶ Dysphagia, mild to severe

▶ Pharyngeal erythema

▶ Exudate (bacterial)

▶ Rhinorrhea (viral)

▶ Malaise

▶ Fever (more pronounced in bacterial)

▶ Anterior cervical adenopathy (bacterial)

Diagnostic Tests

▶ Rapid strep antigen screen: 50 percent sensitivity, 95 percent specificity.

  ▷ If positive, do not perform a culture

  ▷ If strep screen is negative in case of high probability of strep, perform a culture to confirm.

TABLE 7–8.
AGE-RELATED CHANGES OF THE MOUTH AND OLFACTORY SYSTEMS

SYMPTOM	AGE-RELATED CHANGES
Diminished sense of smell	Olfactory fibers decrease
Xerostomia (dry mouth), halitosis; diminished taste	Saliva production decreases and becomes more alkaline
Pale gums	Capillary blood supply to teeth decreases
Missing vermillion border of mouth (lips)	Loss of skin elasticity
Loose or missing teeth	Bone resorption increases Vitamin absorption diminishes
Elongated teeth; bleeding gums	Gingiva migrate toward apex of mouth
Discolored teeth; dysphagia	Decreased saliva production; poor oral care

TABLE 7–9.
CAUSATIVE ORGANISMS

VIRUSES	BACTERIA	FUNGI
Coxsackievirus, echovirus, respiratory syncytial virus, influenza A and B, Epstein-Barr virus, adenovirus, coronavirus, herpes simplex, human immunodeficiency virus (HIV)	*Streptococcus pyogenes**; Group A , C, G streptococcus*; *Arcanobacterium haemolyticum**; *Neisseria gonorrhoeae; Mycoplasma pneumoniae; Chlamydia pneumoniae; Corynebacterium; H. influenzae; Staphylococcus aureus;* Group A beta-hemolytic streptococcus**	*Candida albicans*

Notes: *Most common bacterial agents. **Group A beta-hemolytic streptococcus is concerning because of its potential to cause complications of scarlet fever, rheumatic fever, and glomerulonephritis. Early detection and treatment can avoid such complications.

▶ Throat culture is the gold standard for diagnosing Group A beta-hemolytic streptococcus.

▶ Monospot if suspicion of mononucleosis.

▶ CBC with differential; increased in bacterial infection, decreased in viral.

▶ KOH 10–20 percent wet mount for candidiasis.

▶ The Modified Centor Score can be used to predict group A beta-hemolytic streptococcal (GABHS) pharyngitis in adults (>14 years of age) presenting with sore throat symptoms (McIsaac et al. 2004).

　▷ Patients receive a point for the presence or absence of signs and symptoms:

　　▶ Tonsillar exudate or erythema

　　▶ Anterior cervical adenopathy

　　▶ Cough absent

　　▶ Fever present

　　▶ Age under 15

　　▶ Age over 44 (subtract 1 point)

　▷ Each patient is assigned a score between 0 and 5:

　　▶ –1, 0, or 1 point: No antibiotic or throat culture necessary.

　　▶ 2 or 3 points: Should receive a throat culture and treat with an antibiotic if culture is positive (risk of strep infection 32 percent if three criteria, 15 percent if two).

　　▶ 4 or 5 points: Consider rapid strep testing and or culture.

Differential Diagnoses

▶ Epiglottitis

▶ Tonsillitis

▶ Abscess

▶ Thyroiditis

▶ Postnasal drip from rhinitis or sinusitis

Management

▶ Peritonsillar abscess requires immediate referral to otolaryngologist for possible I&D, IV antibiotics, and surgical intervention.

▶ General

 ▷ Treat symptoms.

 ▷ Hydration, warm saline gargles.

 ▷ OTC analgesics (acetominophen, NSAIDs), throat lozenges.

 ▷ Cool mist humidifier.

 ▷ Rest.

▶ Viral

 ▷ OTC analgesics

 ▷ Warm saline gargles

 ▷ Hydration

▶ Bacterial

 ▷ Strep *(choose one)*

  ▶ Benzathine penicillin 1.2 mil units IM once

  ▶ Penicillin VK 250 mg p.o. q.i.d. or 500 mg b.i.d. × 10 days

  ▶ Amoxicillin 50 mg per kg (maximum = 1,000 mg) daily or 25 mg per kg b.i.d. (maximum = 500 mg) × 10 days

  ▶ Cephalexin (Keflex) 20 mg per kg per dose b.i.d. (maximum = 500 mg per dose) × 10 days

  ▶ Clindamycin 7 mg per kg per dose t.i.d. (maximum = 300 mg per dose) × 10 days

  ▶ Azithromycin (Zithromax) 12 mg per kg daily (maximum = 500 mg) × 5 days

  ▶ Clarithromycin (Biaxin) 7.5 mg per kg per dose b.i.d. (maximum = 250 mg per dose)

 ▷ Gonococcal

  ▶ Ceftriaxone 250 mg IM in a single dose and

  ▶ Azithromycin 1 g p.o. in a single dose

 ▷ Chlamydia

  ▶ Doxycycline 100 mg b.i.d. × 10 days or

  ▶ Azithromycin 1 g in a single dose

 ▷ Candidiasis

  ▶ Nystatin 100,000 U/mL oral suspension 4–6 cc q.i.d.

Prevention

▶ Hand hygiene.

▶ Smoking cessation.

▶ Avoid contact with sick people.

▶ Do not share eating utensils and drinking glasses.

REFERENCES

American Macular Degeneration Foundation. N.d. "What Is Macular Degeneration?" https://www.macular.org/what-macular-degeneration.

Centers for Disease Control and Prevention. 2016."For Clinicians." Conjunctivitis (Pink Eye). https://www.cdc.gov/conjunctivitis/clinical.html.

Chow, A., M. Benninger, I. Brook, J. Brozek, E. Goldstein, L. Hicks, G. A. Pankey, et al. 2012. "IDSA Clinical Practice Guideline for Acute Bacterial Rhinosinusitis in Children and Adults." *Clinical Infectious Disease*s 54 (8): 1041–45. http://dx.doi.org/10.1093/cid/cir1043.

Dunphy, L., J. Winland-Brown, B. Porter, and D. Thomas, eds. 2015. *Primary Care: The Art and Science of Advanced Practice Nursing*. 4th ed. Philadelphia: F. A. Davis

Glaucoma Research Foundation. 2016a. "Glaucoma Facts and Stats." http://www.glaucoma.org/glaucoma/glaucoma-facts-and-stats.php.

———. 2016b. "Types of Glaucoma." http://www.glaucoma.org/glaucoma/types-of-glaucoma.php.

McIsaac, W., J. D. Kellner, P. Aufricht, A. Vanjaka, and D. E. Low. 2004. "Empirical Validation of Guidelines for the Management of Pharyngitis in Children and Adults." *Journal of the American Medical Association* 291 (13): 1587–95. http://dx.doi.org/10.1001/jama.291.13.1587.

CHAPTER 8

CARDIOVASCULAR SYSTEM DISORDERS

LEARNING OBJECTIVES

▶ Recognize common cardiovascular system disorders.

  ▷ Risk factors

  ▷ Signs and symptom

  ▷ Diagnostic tests

  ▷ Differential diagnoses

▶ Describe the treatment and management of cardiovascular disorders.

  ▷ Management

  ▷ Prevention

ARTERIOSCLEROTIC HEART DISEASE (ASHD)

▶ Cardiac condition in which plaques form in the intimal lining of an artery. Plaque first forms as a fatty streak in the lining, then foam cells form as plaque develops. Foam cells necrose and rupture. The fibrous cap tears and bleeds. The artery blockage prevents adequate oxygen supply, causing angina. Ruptured plaque causes acute coronary syndrome (either unstable angina or acute myocardial infarction [MI]).

▶ Heart disease is the leading cause of death for both men and women in the United States. Coronary heart disease is the most common heart disease. About 610,000 Americans die from heart disease each year—that's *one in every four* deaths or 193.3 deaths per 100,000. Coronary heart disease is the most common type of heart disease, killing about 365,000 people in 2014 (Mozafarian et al. 2015).

▶ Costs to treat heart disease exceed $207 billion in health care, medications, and lost productivity annually (Centers for Disease Control and Prevention [CDC] 2016).

▶ Family genes, behaviors, lifestyles, and environments influence health and disease risk. A positive family history of disease (cancer, coronary artery disease [CAD], diabetes, hypertension [HTN], hyperlipidemia) places family members at higher risk of developing such diseases.

Risk Factors

▶ Nonmodifiable risk factors

▷ Increasing age

▷ Male

▷ Family history

▶ Modifiable risk factors

▷ Cigarette smoking

▷ Sedentary lifestyle

▷ High dietary saturated fat

▷ Hypertension

▷ Obesity

▷ Hyperglycemia

▷ Elevated low-density lipoprotein (LDL) cholesterol; elevated triglycerides (TG); decreased high-density lipoproteinc (HDL) cholesterol

Signs and Symptoms

▶ Chest pain

▶ Shortness of breath

▶ Fatigue

▶ Palpitations

Diagnostic Tests

▶ Electrocardiogram (ECG)

▶ Stress testing

▶ Cardiac enzymes

▶ Echocardiogram

▶ Cardiac catheterization

▶ Cardiac computed tomography (CT) scan

Differential Diagnoses

▶ Gastroesophageal reflux disease

▶ Esophageal spasm

- ▶ Biliary colic
- ▶ Anxiety
- ▶ Costochondritis
- ▶ Pericarditis
- ▶ Pulmonary embolism
- ▶ Aortic dissection
- ▶ Pneumonia

Management

- ▶ Reduce risk factors.
- ▶ Lifestyle changes.
- ▶ Medication compliance.
- ▶ Stress management.
- ▶ Encourage exercise.
- ▶ Monitor drug side effects.
- ▶ Education
  - ▷ Sublingual nitroglycerin
  - ▷ Signs and symptoms of acute coronary syndrome

Prevention

- ▶ Smoking cessation, blood pressure control, diabetes management, lipid management, physical activity, weight management, improved nutrition
- ▶ Medications
  - ▷ • Beta blockers; antiplatelet agents
  - ▷ • Supplements (e.g., stanol or sterol ester margarines, soluble fiber, soy protein)
  - ▷ • Lipid modification therapy

ANGINA

- ▶ Chest pain or discomfort because of coronary heart disease caused by reduced blood flow to the heart muscle
- ▶ Typical angina
  - ▷ 1) Substernal chest discomfort with a characteristic quality and duration that is 2) provoked by exertion or emotional stress and 3) relieved by rest or nitroglycerin
- ▶ Unstable angina
  - ▷ New onset, increasing (in frequency, intensity, or duration), or occurring at rest (Fihn et al. 2012)

Risk Factors

▶ Nonmodifiable risk factors

▷ Increasing age

▷ Male

▷ Family history

▶ Modifiable risk factors

▷ Cigarette smoking

▷ Sedentary lifestyle

▷ High dietary saturated fat

▷ Hypertension

▷ Obesity

▷ Hyperglycemia

▷ Elevated LDL cholesterol (LDL-C); elevated TG; decreased HDL

Signs and Symptoms

▶ Chest pain

▶ Jaw pain

▶ Neck pain

▶ Dyspnea

▶ Fatigue

▶ Elevated blood pressure (BP), pulse, respirations

Diagnostic Tests

▶ ECG

▶ Cardiac enzymes

▶ Cardiac catheterization

Differential Diagnoses

▶ Gastroesophageal reflux disease

▶ Esophageal spasm

▶ Biliary colic

▶ Anxiety

▶ Costochondritis

▶ Pericarditis

▶ Pulmonary embolism

▶ Aortic dissection

▶ Pneumonia

Management

▶ Risk factor modification: Physical activity, maintain healthy weight, stop smoking, optimal blood pressure and glucose control and lipid levels.

▶ Slow down or take rest breaks if physical exertion triggers angina.

▶ Avoid large, heavy meals and rich foods that leave a stuffed feeling if these trigger angina.

▶ Try to avoid situations that are upsetting or stressful if emotional stress triggers angina.

▶ Medications: Beta blockers, calcium channel blockers, nitroglycerin, anticoagulants.

▶ Take all medicines as prescribed.

▶ Cardiac procedures:

▷ Angioplasty

▷ Stents

▷ Bypass

▶ Cardiac rehabilitation.

▶ Depression screening.

▶ Immunizations.

Prevention

▶ Risk factor modification

▷ Smoking cessation, blood pressure control, diabetes management, lipid management

▷ Physical activity, weight management, improved nutrition

▶ Medications

▷ Beta blockers, antiplatelet agents, nitroglycerin

▷ Lipid modification therapy

MYOCARDIAL INFARCTION

▶ Death of cardiac muscle because of extended reduced blood flow to the myocardium

Risk Factors

▶ Male

▶ HTN

▶ Hyperlipidemia

▶ Tobacco use

▶ Family history of cardiac death before age 35 years

▶ Menopausal women using long-term estrogen-plus-progesterone hormone replacement therapy (National Institutes of Health [NIH] 2012)

▶ Cocaine use

▶ Advanced age

▶ Obesity

Signs and Symptoms

▶ Chest or substernal pain or discomfort, pressure, or heaviness; may radiate to back, jaw, throat, or arm.

▶ Indigestion, nausea, vomiting.

▶ Sweating, dizziness, weakness, anxiety.

▶ Shortness of breath.

▶ Rapid or irregular heartbeats.

▶ ● Women may have different symptoms than men, including shortness of breath, abdominal pain, dizziness, anxiety, diaphoresis (WomenHeart 2016).

Diagnostic Tests

▶ ECG

▶ Cardiac enzymes

▶ Echocardiogram

▶ Cardiac catheterization

TABLE 8–1.
MYOCARDIAL INFARCTION DIFFERENTIAL DIAGNOSES

CARDIAC	GI	RESPIRATORY	MUSCULOSKELETAL	PSYCHOLOGICAL
MI	Gastroesophageal reflux (GERD)	Pneumothorax	Chest wall syndrome	Anxiety
Congestive heart failure	Cholecystitis	Costochondral pain	Shoulder arthropathy	Depression
Pericarditis	Esophageal spasm	Pulmonary emboli		Panic disorders
Aortic dissection	Peptic ulcer	Pneumonia		
		Pleurisy		
		Asthma		

Management

- ▶ Bed rest
- ▶ Aspirin (325 mg chewed) at first sign of MI
- ▶ Oxygen
- ▶ Nitroglycerin
- ▶ Narcotics
- ▶ Beta blockers
- ▶ Angiotensin-converting enzyme inhibitors (ACEIs)
- ▶ HTN monitoring
- ▶ Percutaneous transluminal coronary angioplasty (PTCA) with or without stenting or coronary artery bypass graft (CABG)

Prevention

- ▶ Risk factor modification
  - ▷ Smoking cessation, blood pressure control, diabetes management, lipid management
  - ▷ Physical activity, weight management, improved nutrition
- ▶ Medications
  - ▷ Beta blockers, antiplatelet agents, ACEIs, statins

MURMURS

- ▶ Heart murmurs are caused by turbulent blood flow through the valve, heart wall, or great vessel (Dunphy et al. 2015). A stenotic heart valve cannot open completely, restricting forward flow of blood, while an incompetent valve does not close completely, allowing regurgitant blood to flow backward.
- ▶ A benign murmur is one in which there is no cardiac structural change or anomaly.
- ▶ Congenital defects, pregnancy, fever, thyrotoxicosis, and anemia are also causes of murmurs.
- ▶ Murmur grading (Williams 2012) 1-6
  - ▷ I/VI: Barely audible
  - ▷ II/VI: Faint but easily audible
  - ▷ III/VI: Loud murmur without a palpable thrill
  - ▷ IV/VI: Loud murmur with a palpable thrill
  - ▷ V/VI: Very loud murmur heard with stethoscope lightly on chest
  - ▷ VI/VI: Very loud murmur that can be heard without a stethoscope

► Timing of heart murmurs
  ▷ Either systolic or diastolic, never normal
    ► Systole occurs between the S1 and S2
    ► Diastole occurs between S2 and S1
► Common murmurs
  ▷ Aortic stenosis
    ► Harsh systolic, heard best at the right sternal border, second intercostal space, and may radiate into the neck
  ▷ Aortic regurgitation
    ► Blowing diastolic, heard best at the third left intercostal space
  ▷ Mitral regurgitation
    ► Systolic murmur heard best heard at the apex, with radiation into the axilla
  ▷ Mitral stenosis
    ► Rumbling, diastolic, heard at left sternal border

Risk Factors
► More common in children and older adults
► ● Fever, anemia, pregnancy
► Heart disease

Signs and Symptoms
► Shortness of breath
► Excessive perspiration with minimal or no exertion
► Chest pain
► Dizziness or fainting
► Cyanosis, especially at fingertips and lips
► Chronic cough
► Swelling or sudden weight gain
► Enlarged liver
► Enlarged neck veins

Diagnostic Tests
► Chest X-ray
► ECG
► Echocardiogram
► Stress echocardiogram

Differential Diagnoses

- ▶ Hypertrophic cardiomyopathies
- ▶ Papillary dysfunction
- ▶ Congenital heart disease
- ▶ Atrial myxomas
- ▶ Endocarditis

Management

- ▶ Education on disease progression and importance of reporting symptoms to health-care provider
- ▶ Lifestyle modifications
- ▶ Diuretics
- ▶ Antiarrhythmics
- ▶ Anticoagulants
- ▶ Surgical repair or valve replacement

Prevention

- ▶ Murmurs and valvular heart disease are not preventable.
- ▶ Comorbidity treatment is vital for symptom management.

HYPERTENSION (HTN)

- ▶ Hypertension is elevated systemic arterial pressure above 140/90 mm Hg.

Risk Factors

- ▶ Older than 60 years
- ▶ Male
- ▶ Postmenopausal women
- ▶ Family history of cardiovascular disease (CVD) in women under age 65 and men under age 55 years
- ▶ African American
- ▶ CAD
- ▶ Left ventricular hypertrophy
- ▶ Cerebrovascular disease
- ▶ Sleep apnea
- ▶ Medications
  - ▷ • Oral contraceptives, corticosteroids, NSAIDs, sympathomimetics

- ► Primary HTN (most common)
  - ▷ Genetic predisposition
  - ▷ African American
  - ▷ Increased weight
  - ▷ Smoking
  - ▷ Decreased physical activity
  - ▷ Decreased vessel wall compliance and atherosclerosis
  - ▷ Decreased renal mass and function
  - ▷ Increased plasma renin levels
- ► Secondary cause of HTN
  - ▷ Renal artery stenosis
  - ▷ Diabetes or glomerulonephritis
  - ▷ Chronic kidney infections
  - ▷ Obstructions (stones, tumors, stenosis)
  - ▷ Autoimmune (lupus, scleroderma)
  - ▷ Pheochromocytoma
  - ▷ Renin-producing tumors
  - ▷ Alcohol, decongestants, salt, corticosteroids, NSAIDs

Signs and Symptoms

- ► Usually asymptomatic
- ► Severe headache, dizziness
- ► Pounding in chest, neck, and/or ears
- ► Epistaxis (rare)
- ► Fatigue, somnolence
- ► Confusion, vision problems
- ► Hematuria
- ► S4 gallop, displaced point of maximal impulse (PMI) from ventricular hypertrophy
- ► Renal artery bruit, carotid bruit, hepatosplenomegaly
- ► Edema, decreased peripheral pulses
- ► Arteriovenous (AV) nicking

Diagnostic Tests

- ► Complete blood count (CBC), blood chemistry: potassium, sodium, creatinine, fasting glucose
- ► 12-lead ECG

▶ ◦Urinalysis, urine protein, urinary albumin (microalbumin), BUN (blood urea nitrogen) and/or creatinine, cortisol, catecholamines

▶ Echocardiogram

Differential Diagnoses

▶ Amphetamine or cocaine use

▶ Hyperthyroidism

▶ MI

▶ Anxiety

▶ Aortic coarctation

Management

▶ Lifestyle modifications:

▷ Cease smoking; lose weight if overweight; reduce dietary saturated fat and cholesterol; limit alcohol intake; increase physical activity; reduce sodium intake; maintain adequate intake of dietary potassium; manage stress; obtain annual eye exam.

▶ ◦According to the Eighth Joint National Committee (JNC 8), the main objective of hypertension treatment is to attain and maintain goal BP.

▶ JNC 8 treatment guidelines (James et al. 2014)

▷ General population:

▶ Aged 60 or older

▷ Initiate pharmacological treatment at systolic blood pressure (SBP) ≥ 150 mm Hg or diastolic blood pressure (DBP) ≥ 90 mm Hg

▷ Goal: SBP < 150 mm Hg and DBP < 90 mm Hg

▶ Younger than 60

▷ Initiate pharmacological treatment at SBP ≥ 140 mm Hg or DPB ≥ 90 mm Hg

▷ Goal: SBP < 140 mm Hg and DBP < 90 mm Hg

▶ ◦Nonblack population: Include thiazide diuretic, calcium channel blocker, ACEI, or ARB with initial therapy

▶ ◦African American population: Include thiazide diuretic or calcium channel blocker (CCB) with initial therapy

▷ Adults with chronic kidney disease (CKD):

▶ Initiate pharmacological treatment at SBP ≥ 140 mm Hg or DPB ≥ 90 mm Hg

▶ Goal: SBP < 140 mm Hg and DBP < 90 mm Hg

▶ Include ACEI or ARB as initial or add-on therapy

▷ Adults with diabetes:

- ▶ Initiate pharmacological treatment at SBP ≥ 140 mm Hg or DPB ≥ 90 mm Hg

- ▶ Goal: SBP < 140 mm Hg and DBP < 90 mm Hg

- ▶ Nonblack population: Include thiazide diuretic, CCB, ACEI, or ARB with initial therapy

- ▶ Black population: Include thiazide diuretic or CCB with initial therapy

▷ ⬤ If goal BP is not reached within a month of treatment, increase the dose of the initial drug or add a second drug from one of these classes: thiazide-type diuretic, CCB, ACEI, or ARB.

▷ The clinician should continue to assess BP and adjust the treatment regimen until goal BP is reached.

▷ If goal BP cannot be reached with two drugs, add and titrate a third drug from the list provided (thiazide-type diuretic, CCB, ACEI, or ARB).

▷ Do not use an ACEI and an ARB together in the same patient.

▷ If goal BP cannot be reached using only thiazide-type diuretics, CCBs, ACEIs, and ARBs because of a contraindication or the need to use more than three drugs to reach goal BP, antihypertensive drugs from other classes can be used.

▷ Referral to a hypertension specialist may be indicated for patients in whom goal BP cannot be attained using the above strategy or for the management of complicated patients for whom additional clinical consultation is needed.

Prevention

- ▶ Eating a healthy diet, including low sodium
- ▶ Maintaining a healthy weight
- ▶ Physical activity
- ▶ Not smoking
- ▶ Limiting alcohol use

DYSLIPIDEMIA

- ▶ Term used to describe a variety of lipid abnormalities that deviate from normal ranges and increase the risk of cardiovascular disease

- ▶ Primary

  ▷ Genetically based, but defects are known for only a minority of patients

- ▶ Secondary

  ▷ Diabetes, thyroid disease, renal disorders, liver disorders, Cushing's syndrome, obesity, alcohol, estrogen administration, and other drug-associated changes in lipid metabolism

Risk Factors

▶ Cigarette smoking.

▶ Family history of premature CAD.

▶ HTN (or on medication for HTN).

▶ Diet high in saturated fat.

▶ Diabetes mellitus, kidney disease, hypothyroidism (hypertriglyceridemia).

▶ Age: Men over 45 years and women over 55 years.

▶ Low HDL cholesterol.

▶ High HDL (>60 mg/dL) is cardioprotective and is a negative risk factor for cardiovascular disease.

Signs and Symptoms

▶ Corneal arcus

▶ Tendinous xanthomas

▶ Tuberous and tuberoeruptive xanthomas

▶ Planar xanthomas

▶ Eruptive xanthomas

Diagnostic Tests

▶ Total cholesterol (mg/dL)

  ▷ <200 = desirable

  ▷ 200–239 = borderline high

  ▷ ≥240 = high

▶ TG (mg/dL; Morris 2014; Chen 2016)

  ▷ <150 mg/dL = desirable

  ▷ 50 to 199 mg/dL = borderline high

  ▷ 200 to 499 mg/dL = high

  ▷ ≥500 mg/dL = very high

▶ HDL (mg/dL; Devkota 2014)

  ▷ ≥60 = high, cardioprotective

  ▷ 40–50 mg/dL in men = optimal

  ▷ 50–60 mg/dL in women = optimal

  ▷ <40 = low, major heart disease (HD) risk factor

▶ LDL (mg/dL; NIH 2012)

  ▷ <100 = optimal

  ▷ 100–129 = near optimal

    ▷   130–159 = borderline high

    ▷   160–189 = high

    ▷   ≥190 = very high

Management

▶ Heart-healthy lifestyle habits (i.e., adhering to a heart healthy diet, regular exercise habits, avoidance of tobacco products, and maintenance of a healthy weight).

▶ Treatment of blood cholesterol to reduce atherosclerotic cardiovascular disease (ASCVD) risk.

▶ Risk assessment for 10-year and lifetime risk is recommended using an updated ASCVD risk calculator: http://my.americanheart.org/cvriskcalculator.

▶ ❾ If patient is age 40–75 years without clinical ASCVD or diabetes and with LDL-C 70–189 mg/dL, recalculate estimated 10-year ASCVD risk every 4–6 years (Stone et al. 2014).

▶ Diet (Department of Health and Human Services [DHHS] and Department of Agriculture [USDA] 2015)

    ▷   Plant stanols or sterols 2 g/day.

    ▷   Soluble fiber 10–25 g/day.

    ▷   A variety of vegetables from all of the subgroups— dark green, red and orange, legumes (beans and peas), starchy, and other.

    ▷   Fruits, especially whole fruits.

    ▷   Grains, at least half of which are whole grains.

    ▷   Fat-free or low-fat dairy, including milk, yogurt, cheese, and fortified soy beverages.

    ▷   A variety of protein foods, including seafood, lean meats and poultry, eggs, legumes (beans and peas), and nuts, seeds, and soy products.

    ▷   Oils: extracted from plants like canola, corn, olive, peanut, safflower, soybean, and sunflower oils. Oils also are naturally present in nuts, seeds, seafood, olives, and avocados

    ▷ ❸ Consume less than 2,300 milligrams (mg) per day of sodium.

    ▷   Limit alcohol consumption.

         ▶ One drink per day for women

         ▶ Two drinks per day for men

    ▷   Limit trans fatty acids.

         ▶ Found in partially hydrogenated vegetable oils and foods (e.g., commercially prepared fried foods, some margarines, prepackaged cookies and crackers, baked goods)

    ▷   Consume less than 10 percent of calories per day from added sugars.

    ▷   Consume less than 10 percent of calories per day from saturated fats.

▶ Exercise

▷ For overall cardiovascular health (Office of Disease Prevention and Health Promotion [ODPHP] 2008):

▶ At least 30 minutes of moderate-intensity aerobic activity at least 5 days per week for a total of 150 minutes

or

▶ At least 25 minutes of vigorous aerobic activity at least 3 days per week for a total of 75 minutes; or a combination of moderate- and vigorous-intensity aerobic activity

and

▶ Moderate- to high-intensity muscle-strengthening activity at least 2 days per week for additional health benefits

▷ For lowering blood pressure and cholesterol (Physical Activity Guidelines Advisory Committee 2008):

▶ An average 40 minutes of moderate- to vigorous-intensity aerobic activity three or four times per week

▶ Pharmacological interventions

▷ Statins: See table 8–2 for identification of four groups in which the potential for an ASCVD risk reduction benefit clearly exceeds the potential for adverse effects and table 8–3 for description of low-, moderate-, and high-intensity statin treatment.

▶ Check baseline lipids, liver and renal function, and creatine phosphokinase (CK).

▶ Adherence to medication and lifestyle, therapeutic response to statin therapy, and safety should be regularly assessed. Assessment should include a fasting lipid panel performed within 4–12 weeks after initiation or dose adjustment, and every 3–12 months thereafter (Stone et al. 2014).

▶ Statin contraindications

▷ Liver disease

▷ Pregnancy

▷ Statin intolerance

▶ Relative contraindication

▷ Concomitant use of Cy P-450 inhibitors

▷ Caution with concomitant use of fibrates or nicotinic acid

▶ Adverse reactions

▷ Muscle pain

▷ Rhabdomyolysis

▷ Elevated liver function tests

▷ Dyspepsia

TABLE 8–2.
CHOLESTEROL MANAGEMENT GUIDELINES

BENEFIT GROUPS	STATIN RECOMMENDATION
Persons with clinical ASCVD >21 years old Age < 75 years	High-intensity statin (Moderate-intensity statin if not candidate for high-intensity statin)
Age > 75 years *or* if not candidate for high-intensity statin	Moderate-intensity statin
Persons with primary elevations of LDL ≥ 190 mg/dL	High-intensity statin (Moderate-intensity statin if not candidate for high-intensity statin)
Persons 40–75 years of age *with diabetes* with LDL-C 70–189 mg/dL	Moderate-intensity statin
If estimated 10-year ASCVD risk ≥ 7.5 percent	High-intensity statin
Persons *without* clinical ASCVD or diabetes who are 40–75 years of age with LDL 70–189 mg/dL and an estimated 10-year ASCVD risk of 7.5 percent or higher	Moderate- to high-intensity statin

Source: Stone et al. 2013

▷ Bile acid sequestrants (BAS)

　▶ Very few able to tolerate because of unpalatability

　▶ ⬥ A fasting lipid panel should be obtained before BAS is initiated, 3 months after initiation, and every 6–12 months thereafter

　▶ Contraindications

　　▷ Triglycerides > 300mg/dL

　　▷ Adverse drug reactions

　　▷ ● Constipation

　　▷ Gastrointestinal (GI) distress

　　▷ Absorption of other drugs

▷ Nicotinic acid

　▶ Lowers LDL and TG and raises HDL

　▶ Absolute contraindications (Stone et al. 2014)

　　▷ ● Chronic liver disease, severe gout

　　▷ Hepatic transaminase elevations higher than two to three times upper limit of normal (ULN)

　　▷ ● Persistent severe cutaneous symptoms, persistent hyperglycemia, acute gout, unexplained abdominal pain, or gastrointestinal symptoms

　　▷ ● New-onset atrial fibrillation or weight loss

　▶ Relative contraindications

　　▷ ● Hyperuricemia, diabetes, peptic ulcer disease (PUD)

TABLE 8–3.
STATIN THERAPY INTENSITIES

HIGH-INTENSITY STATIN	MODERATE-INTENSITY STATIN	LOW-INTENSITY STATIN
Daily dose lowers LDL on average by approximately 50 percent or more	Daily dose lowers LDL on average by approximately 30 percent to <50 percent	Daily dose lowers LDL on average by <30 percent
Atorvastatin 40–80 mg or Rosuvastatin 20–40 mg	Atorvastatin 10–20mg Rosuvastatin 5–10 mg Pravastatin 40–80 mg Simvastatin 20–40 mg	Simvastatin 10 mg Pravastatin 10–20 mg Lovastatin 20 mg

Source: Stone et al. 2013

▶ Adverse drug reactions(Stone et al. 2014)

▷ ● Liver toxicity

▷ Flushing

▷ Upper GI distress

▷ ● Elevated glucose, uric acid

▷ ● To reduce the frequency and severity of adverse cutaneous symptoms,

    ▶ Start nicotinic acid at a low dose and titrate to a higher dose over a period of weeks as tolerated;

    ▶ ● Take nicotinic acid with food or premedicate with aspirin 325 mg 30 minutes before niacin dosing to alleviate flushing symptoms;

    ▶ If an extended-release preparation is used, increase the dose of extended-release nicotinic acid from 500 mg to a maximum of 2,000 mg per day over 4–8 weeks, with the dose of extended-release niacin increasing not more than weekly; and

    ▶ If immediate-release nicotinic acid is chosen, start at a dose of 100 mg 3 times daily and up-titrate to 3 g per day, divided into 2 or 3 doses.

▷ Fibric acids

    ▶ Lower TG and raise HDL

    ▶ Work at gut wall to prevent absorption of cholesterol

    ▶ Contraindications

      ▷ Severe liver or renal disease.

      ▷ ● Gemfibrozil should not be initiated in patients on statin therapy because of an increased risk for muscle symptoms and rhabdomyolysis.

    ▶ Relative contraindications (Stone et al. 2014)

      ▷ Fenofibrate may be considered concomitantly with a low- or moderate-intensity statin only if the benefits from ASCVD risk reduction or triglyceride-lowering when triglycerides are >500 mg/dL are judged to outweigh the potential risk for adverse effects.

▷ • Renal status should be evaluated before fenofibrate initiation, within 3 months after initiation, and every 6 months thereafter. Assess renal safety with both a serum creatinine level and an estimated glomerular filtration rate (eGFR) based on creatinine.

▷ ❧ Fenofibrate should not be used if moderate or severe renal impairment (defined as eGFR < 30 mL/min per 1.73 m²) is present.

▷ If eGFR is between 30 and 59 mL/min per 1.73 m², the dose of fenofibrate should not exceed 54 mg per day.

▷ If, during follow-up, the eGFR decreases persistently to ≤30 mL/min per 1.73 m², fenofibrate should be discontinued.

▶ Adverse drug reactions

  ▷ • Dyspepsia, gallstones, myopathy

  ▷ Cholesterol absorption inhibitor

  ▷ Major side effects

  ▷ GI = 4 percent

  ▷ Adding to a statin slightly increases HDL

▷ Cholesterol absorption inhibitors

  ▶ Prevent absorption of cholesterol from the intestine

  ▶ ❧ When coadministered with a statin, monitor transaminase levels as clinically indicated, and discontinue ezetimibe if persistent alanine aminotransferase (ALT) elevations over three times ULN occur

  ▶ Lower LDL and TG and raises HDL

▷ PCSK9 inhibitors

  ▶ Newer class of drug that can lower LDL cholesterol levels

▷ Nutritional supplements

  ▶ Fish oil reduces TGs.

  ▶ Plant stanols and sterols block the absorption of cholesterol in the intestine.

  ▶ Soy protein may lower LDL.

Prevention

▶ Heart-healthy lifestyle habits: Heart-healthy diet, regular exercise, avoidance of tobacco products, and healthy weight maintenance

ATRIAL FIBRILLATION

▶ Atrial fibrillation (AF) is a common arrhythmia that occurs because the heart's electrical signals don't begin in the sinoatrial node, but in another part of the atria or pulmonary veins. This causes the electrical impulse to travel throughout the atria in a rapid, disorganized way, causing the atria to fibrillate, which in turn can cause the ventricles to also beat very fast (National Heart, Lung, and Blood Institute [NHLBI] 2014).

▶ The classifications of atrial fibrillation are as follows: (January et al. 2014)

  ▷ Paroxysmal: Terminates spontaneously or with intervention within 7 days of onset and episodes may recur with variable frequency

  ▷ Persistent: Continuous and sustained for more than 7 days

  ▷ Long-standing persistent: Continuous for more than 12 months in duration

  ▷ Permanent AF: Term used when the patient and clinician make a joint decision to stop further attempts to restore or maintain sinus rhythm

  ▷ Nonvalvular: AF in the absence of rheumatic mitral stenosis, a mechanical or bioprosthetic heart valve, or mitral valve repair

▶ Risk of thromboembolism, cerebrovascular accident (CVA), heart failure.

Risk Factors

▶ Increasing age

▶ Hypertension

▶ Diabetes mellitus

▶ Valvular heart disease

▶ Obstructive sleep apnea

▶ Heart surgery

▶ Hyperthyroidism

▶ Alcohol use

▶ Obesity

▶ Left ventricular hypertrophy

  (January et al., 2014)

Signs and Symptoms

▶ General fatigue

▶ Rapid or irregular heartbeat or palpitations

▶ Dizziness, weakness, faintness, confusion

▶ Shortness of breath

▶ Anxiety

▶ Heart failure

Diagnostic Tests

▶ ECG

▶ Holter monitor

▶ Event recorder

▶ Labs: Serum electrolytes, thyroid panel

▶ Transthoracic echocardiogram

Differential Diagnoses

▶ Supraventricular tachycardia

▶ Premature atrial and ventricular contractions

▶ Atrial flutter

▶ Atrial tachycardia

▶ Wolff-Parkinson-White Syndrome

Management

▶ Stratify risk for stroke and thromboembolism with the CHA_2DS_2-VASc score (Lane and Lip 2012):

▷ Congestive heart failure (1 pt.)

▷ Hypertension (1 pt.)

▷ Age 75 or greater (2 pt.)

▷ Diabetes (1 pt.)

▷ Stroke: Prior episode (2 pt.)

▷ Vascular disease: Prior heart attack, peripheral artery disease, or aortic plaque (1 pt.)

▷ Age 65–74 (1 pt.)

▷ Female (1pt)

▶ • Oral anticoagulants are recommended (warfarin, dabigatran, rivaroxaban, or apixaban) for nonvalvular AF with prior stroke, transient ischemic attack, or a CHA_2DS_2-VASc score of 2 or higher. (January et al. 2014)

▶ • Left atrial appendage occlusion or excision

▷ Cardioversion if atrial fibrillation less than 48 hours or properly anticoagulated

▶ • Rate control medications: Beta blocker or nondihydropyridine calcium channel antagonist is recommended with paroxysmal, persistent, or permanent AF.

▶ • Rhythm control medications: amiodarone, dofetilide, dronedarone, flecainide, propafenone, sotalol.

▶ • Catheter ablation.

▶ • Surgery: Maze procedure.

▶ Complications:

▷ Congestive heart failure (CHF)

▷ Stroke

▷ Peripheral arterial embolism

▷ Medications: Bradycardia, torsades de pointes

▷ Anticoagulants: Uncontrolled bleeding

Prevention

▶ Blood pressure control

▶ Limited alcohol

▶ Heart-healthy lifestyle habits: Heart-healthy diet, regular exercise, avoidance of tobacco products, and healthy weight maintenance

HEART FAILURE (HF)

▶ Impaired ability of ventricle to fill or eject blood, rendering cardiac output inadequate to meet metabolic demands

▶ Most common and costly hospital Medicare diagnosis-related group (DRG)

▶ US prevalence: 5 million annually

▶ • Heart failure with reduced ejection fraction (HFrEF)

▷ Inadequate pump

▷ Ejection fraction < 40 percent

▶ • Heart failure with preserved ejection fraction (HFpEF)

▷ Ineffective relaxation

▷ Ejection fraction > 50 percent

▷ Inadequate filling and low stroke volume

▶ HFpEF, borderline

▷ Ejection fraction 41–49 percent

Risk Factors

▶ HTN

▶ Diabetes mellitus (DM)

▶ Metabolic syndrome

▶ Atherosclerosis

▶ Obesity

▶ Cardiomyopathies

▶ Thyroid disease

Signs and Symptoms

▶ Weight gain

▶ Pallor or fatigue

TABLE 8–4.
HF STAGES AND CLASSIFICATION

ACCF/AHA STAGES OF HF (HUNT ET AL. 2009)		NYHA FUNCTIONAL CLASSIFICATION (DOLGIN 1994)	
A	At high risk for HF but without structural heart disease or symptoms of HF	None	
B	Structural heart disease but without signs or symptoms of HF	I	No limitation of physical activity. Ordinary physical activity does not cause symptoms of HF.
C	Structural heart disease with prior or current symptoms of HF	I	No limitation of physical activity. Ordinary physical activity does not cause symptoms of HF.
		II	Slight limitation of physical activity. Comfortable at rest, but ordinary physical activity results in symptoms of HF.
		III	Marked limitation of physical activity. Comfortable at rest, but less than ordinary activity causes symptoms of HF.
D	Refractory HF requiring specialized interventions	IV	Unable to carry on any physical activity without symptoms of HF, or symptoms of HF at rest.

Sources: Hunt et al. 2009; Dolgin 1994

- ▶ Shortness of breath (SOB), orthopnea, cough
- ▶ Basilar rales, wheezes
- ▶ Tachycardia or S3 gallop
- ▶ Anxiety or mental status changes
- ▶ Edema
- ▶ Jugular venous distention
- ▶ Nausea or anorexia
- ▶ Hepatomegaly

Diagnostic Tests

- ▶ Chest X-ray (CXR)
- ▶ ECG
- ▶ Echocardiogram
- ▶ CBC, urinalysis, serum electrolytes (including calcium and magnesium), blood urea nitrogen, serum creatinine, glucose, fasting lipid profile, liver function tests, and thyroid-stimulating hormone
- ▶ Noninvasive imaging

Differential Diagnoses

► COPD

► Acute respiratory distress syndrome

► Pneumonia

► MI

Management

► Identify and treat underlying disease.

► Control precipitating factors.

► Sodium and fluid restriction as needed.

► Limit alcohol; stop smoking.

► Heart-healthy diet.

► Daily weights.

► ❂ Optimal treatment: Multidrug regimen

▷ Diuretics or aldosterone antagonists

▷ ACEIs, ARBs, beta blockers, aldosterone receptor antagonists, and angiotensin-receptor/neprilysin inhibitor (ARNI)

▷ Digoxin

▷ ❂ Hydralazine and isosorbide dinitrate for African Americans

▷ Anticoagulants

▷ Omega-3 fatty acids

► May require cardioversion, ablation.

► Cardiac resynchronization (CRT)

▷ NYHA Class II, III, or ambulatory IV, reduced ejection fraction (EF), and prolonged QRS >150 msec, normal sinus rhythm (NSR)

► Implantable cardioverter defibrillator (ICD)

▷ Primary prevention of sudden cardiac death (SCD) in selected patients with HFrEF at least 40 d post-MI with left ventricular ejection fraction (LVEF) ≤ 35 percent and NYHA class II or III symptoms on chronic, guideline-determined medical therapy (GDMT), who are expected to live longer than 1 year

► Self-care education: Symptom and weight monitoring, sodium restriction, medication compliance, and staying physically active.

Prevention

► Blood pressure control

► Limited alcohol

► Heart-healthy lifestyle habits: Heart-healthy diet, regular exercise, avoidance of tobacco products, and healthy weight maintenance

PERIPHERAL ARTERY DISEASE (PAD)

▶ Circulatory problem in which narrowed arteries reduce blood flow to extremities because of an acute thrombus, embolus, or atherosclerosis (Gerhard-Herman et al. 2016)

Risk Factors

▶ Smoking

▶ Obesity

▶ Hyperlipidemia

▶ HTN

▶ DM

▶ Family history

▶ Elevated homocysteine

▶ Coronary artery disease

▶ Cardiac arrhythmias

Signs and Symptoms

▶ Acute: Six Ps

  ▷ Pain, pallor, paraesthesia, pulselessness, polar (cool), paralysis

▶ Chronic intermittent claudication

▶ Lower extremity aching, fatigue

▶ Tiredness with activity or relief by activity cessation

▶ Abdominal or femoral bruit if in aorta, back or abdominal pain

Diagnostic Tests

▶ The resting ankle-brachial index (ABI) should be used to establish the diagnosis in patients with suspected lower extremity PAD, defined as persons with one or more of the following (Rooke et al. 2011):

  ▷ Exertional leg symptoms

  ▷ Nonhealing wounds

  ▷ Age 65 years and older, or 50 years and older with a history of smoking or diabetes

▶ ABI $< .5$ to 1

  ▷ 1.0 = normal

  ▷ 0.9 = minimal

  ▷ 0.5–<0.9 = moderate disease, arterial claudication typical

  ▷ <0.5 = severe disease, rest pain common

Management

- ▶ Smoking cessation
- ▶ Pharmacology: Antiplatelet therapy
  - ▷ Aspirin
  - ▷ Cilostazol (Pletal)—contraindicated in CHF
  - ▷ Clopidogrel (Plavix)
  - ▷ Pentoxifylline (Trental)
  - ▷ Antihypertensives
  - ▷ Cholesterol lowering
- ▶ Surgery or procedures
  - ▷ Bypass grafting
  - ▷ Endovascular repair
  - ▷ Angioplasty and stent placement
  - ▷ Atherectomy
- ▶ Exercise program
- ▶ Risk factor management

Prevention

- ▶ Heart-healthy lifestyle habits: Heart-healthy diet, regular exercise, avoidance of tobacco products, and healthy weight maintenance

DEEP VEIN THROMBOSIS (DVT)

- ▶ Acute blood clot formed in the deep veins of lower extremity or pelvic veins with ambiguous presenting signs and symptoms
- ▶ Three primary predisposing factors:
  1. Venous stasis
  2. Hypercoagulability
  3. Injury to intimal wall of vein

Risk Factors

- ▶ Orthopedic surgery
- ▶ Immobility
- ▶ Carcinoma
- ▶ Venous catheters
- ▶ Rheumatoid disease, lupus
- ▶ High altitude

▶ Coagulation defects

▶ Polycythemia vera

Signs and Symptoms

▶ Sometimes no presenting symptoms

▶ • Pain, swelling, tenderness, heavy ache in affected area

▶ Warmth at clot site

▶ Skin redness

▶ Visible veins

Diagnostic Tests

▶ Venous Doppler

▶ D-dimer assay

▶ Spiral CT (if pulmonary embolism [PE] is suspected)

Differential Diagnoses

▶ Heart failure

▶ Lymphedema

▶ Venous insufficiency

▶ Cellulitis

Management

▶ • Refer for acute therapy with low molecular weight heparin (LMWH) or intravenous (IV) unfractionated heparin

▶ Transition to oral anticoagulants

▶ Maintain INR 2.0–3.0 if on warfarin

▶ Duration of treatment dependent on source, occurrence, risk factors

▶ Thrombolytics

▶ Vena cava filter

▶ Compression stockings

Prevention

▶ Avoid prolonged bed rest or sitting

▶ Heparin prophylaxis

▶ Compression stockings

▶ Loose-fitting clothes

▶ Exercise

▶ Maintain healthy weight

VENOUS INSUFFICIENCY

▶ Chronic, noninflammatory venous valve incompetency with venous engorgement and edema of the lower leg

Risk Factors

▶ Prior history of pregnancy

▶ Deep vein thrombosis

▶ Prolonged immobility, particularly standing

▶ Family tendency

▶ Varicose veins

▶ Advanced age

▶ Obesity

▶ Prior injury

Signs and Symptoms

▶ ● Fatigue, aching, heaviness in lower extremities

▶ ● Hyperpigmentation of distal extremity

▷ Dark (brown, sometimes red), brawny, thickened skin

▶ ● Urticaria; papular rash

▶ ● Stasis ulcers

▷ Lower extremity edema worsens with prolonged standing

▶ ● Pedal pulses intact

Diagnostic Tests

▶ History and physical exam

▶ Duplex ultrasound

▶ Venogram

▶ Doppler studies if DVT suspected

Differential Diagnoses

▶ Lymphedema

▶ Heart failure

▶ Cellulitis

Management

▶ Elastic compression stockings

▶ Leg elevation

▶ Low-sodium diet

▶ Diuretics of limited value

▶ Skin protection

Prevention

▶ Avoid prolonged standing or sitting

▶ Compression stockings

▶ Exercise

▶ Maintain healthy weight

REFERENCES

Centers for Disease Control and Prevention. 2016. "Heart Disease Fact Sheet." Division for Heart Disease and Stroke Prevention. https://www.cdc.gov/dhdsp/data_statistics/fact_sheets/fs_heart_disease.htm.

Chen, M. A. 2016. "Triglyceride Level." Medical Encyclopedia, MedlinePlus.gov. https://medlineplus.gov/ency/article/003493.htm.

Department of Health and Human Services and Department of Agriculture. 2015. *Dietary Guidelines for Americans 2015–2020*. 8th ed. http://health.gov/dietaryguidelines/2015/guidelines/.

Devkota, B. P. 2014. "HDL Cholesterol." *Medscape*. http://emedicine.medscape.com/article/2087757-overview.

Dolgin, M. 1994. *Nomenclature and Criteria for Diagnosis of Diseases of the Heart and Great Vessels*. Boston: Little, Brown, and Co.

Dunphy, L., J. Winland-Brown, B. Porter, and D. Thomas, eds. 2015. *Primary Care: The Art and Science of Advanced Practice Nursing*. 4th ed. Philadelphia: F. A. Davis Company.

Fihn, S., J. Gardin, J. Abrams, K. Berra, J. Blankenship, A. Dallas, P. S. Douglas, et al. 2012. "2012 ACCF/AHA/ACP/AATS/PCNA/SCAI/STS Guideline for the Diagnosis and Management of Patients with Stable Ischemic Heart Disease: Executive Summary." *Circulation* 126 (25): 3097–137. http://dx.doi.org/10.1161/cir.0b013e3182776f83.

Gerhard-Herman, M., H. Gornik, C. Barrett, N. Barshes, M. Corriere, D. Drachman, L. A. Fleisher, et al. 2016. "2016 AHA/ACC Guideline on the Management of Patients with Lower Extremity Peripheral Artery Disease: Executive Summary." *Journal of the American College of Cardiology* 69 (11): 1465–508. http://dx.doi.org/10.1016/j.jacc.2016.11.008.

Hunt, S., W. Abraham, M. Chin, A. Feldman, G. Francis, T. Ganiats, M. Jessup, et al. 2009. "2009 Focused Update Incorporated into the ACC/AHA 2005 Guidelines for the Diagnosis and Management of Heart Failure in Adults." *Circulation* 119 (14): e391–e479. http://dx.doi.org/10.1161/circulationaha.109.192065.

James, P., S. Oparil, B. Carter, W. C. Cushman, C. Dennison-Himmelfarb, J. Handler, D. T. Lackland, et al. 2014. "2014 Evidence-Based Guideline for the Management of High Blood Pressure in Adults: Report from the Panel Members Appointed to the Eighth Joint National Committee (JNC 8)." *Journal of the American Medical Association* 311 (5): 507–20. http://dx.doi.org/10.1001/JAMA.2013.284427.

January, C. T., L. S. Wann, J. S. Alpert, H. Calkins, J. E. Cigarroa, J. C. Cleveland, J. B. Conti, et al. 2014. "2014 AHA/ACC/HRS Guideline for the Management of Patients with Atrial Fibrillation: Executive Summary." Circulation 130 (23): 2071–104. http://dx.doi.org/10.1161/cir.0000000000000040.

Lane, D. A., and G. Y. H. Lip. 2012. "Use of the CHA2DS2-VASc and HAS-BLED Scores to Aid Decision Making for Thromboprophylaxis in Nonvalvular Atrial Fibrillation." *Circulation* 126 (7): 860–65. http://doi.org/10.1161/CIRCULATIONAHA.111.060061.

Morris, B. 2014. "Lipid Profile (Triglycerides)." Medscape. http://emedicine.medscape.com/article/2074115-overview.

Mozafarian, D., E. J. Benjamin, A. S. Go, D. K. Arnett, M. J. Blaha, M. Cushman, S. de Ferranti, et al. 2015. "Heart Disease and Stroke Statistics—2015 Update: A Report from the American Heart Association." *Circulation* 131 (4): e29–e322. https://doi.org/10.1161/CIR.0000000000000152.

National Heart, Lung, and Blood Institute. 2012. "Lower Heart Disease Risk: Menopausal Hormone Therapy and Heart Disease." https://www.nhlbi.nih.gov/health/educational/hearttruth/lower-risk/hormone-therapy.htm.

———. 2014. "What Is Atrial Fibrillation?" http://www.nhlbi.nih.gov/health/health-topics/topics/af/.

National Institutes of Health. 2012. "Cholesterol Levels: What You Need to Know." *Medline Plus* 7 (2): 6–7. https://medlineplus.gov/magazine/issues/summer12/articles/summer12pg6-7.html.

Office of Disease Prevention and Health Promotion. 2008. "Active Older Adults." In *Physical Activity Guidelines for Americans,* 29–34. ODPHP Publication No. U0036. Washington, DC: Department of Health and Human Services. https://health.gov/paguidelines/guidelines/chapter5.aspx.

Physical Activity Guidelines Advisory Committee. 2008. "Cardiorespiratory Health." In *Physical Activity Guidelines Advisory Committee Report, 2008*, G2-1–G2-41. ODPHP Publication No. U0049. Washington, DC: Department of Health and Human Services. https://health.gov/paguidelines/report/g2_cardio.aspx#_Toc199847829.

Rooke, T., A. Hirsch, S. Misra, A. Sidawy, J. Beckman, L. K. Findeiss, J. Golzarian, et al. 2011. "2011 ACCF/AHA Focused Update of the Guideline for the Management of Patients with Peripheral Artery Disease (Updating the 2005 Guideline)." *Circulation* 124 (18): 2020–45. http://dx.doi.org/10.1161/cir.0b013e31822e80c3.

Slawson, D. 2014. "JNC 8 Report on Prevention, Evaluation, and Treatment of Hypertension." *American Family Physician* 89 (7): 574–76.

Stone, N., J. Robinson, A. Lichtenstein, D. C. Goff Jr., D. M. Lloyd-Jones, S. C. Smith Jr., C. Blum, and J. S. Schwartz . 2014. "Treatment of Blood Cholesterol to Reduce Atherosclerotic Cardiovascular Disease Risk in Adults: Synopsis of the 2013 American College of Cardiology/American Heart Association Cholesterol Guideline." *Annals of Internal Medicine* 160 (5): 339–43. http://dx.doi.org/10.7326/m14-0126.

Stone, N. J., J. Robinson, A. Lichtenstein, C. N. B. Merz, C. Blum, R. H. Eckel, A. C. Goldberg, et al. 2013. "2013 ACC/AHA Guideline on Treatment of Blood Cholesterol to Reduce Atherosclerotic Cardiovascular Risk in Adults." *Circulation* 136 (S3): S1–S45. https://doi.org/10.1161/01.cir.0000437738.63853.7a.

Williams, M. E. 2012. "Cardiac Auscultation in the Older Adult." Medscape. http://www.medscape.com/viewarticle/756829.

WomenHeart: The National Coalition for Women with Heart Disease. 2016. "Symptoms of Heart Attack in Women." https://womenheart.site-ym.com/page/Support_Symptoms.

CHAPTER 9

RESPIRATORY SYSTEM DISORDERS

LEARNING OBJECTIVES

▶ Recognize common respiratory system disorders.

  ▷ Risk factors

  ▷ Signs and symptoms

  ▷ Diagnostic tests

  ▷ Differential diagnoses

▶ Describe treatment and management of respiratory disorders.

  ▷ Management

  ▷ Prevention

TABLE 9–1.
PULMONARY SYSTEM AGE-RELATED CHANGES

SYMPTOM	AGE-RELATED CHANGES
Fatigue	PO_2 (partial pressure of oxygen) reduced 15 percent between ages 20 and 80
Dyspnea; shortness of breath (SOB)	Weaker musculature
Upper respiratory infections (URIs) increase	Fewer alveoli; decreased ciliary action
Barrel chest	Increased anterior-posterior (AP) diameter
Flu and pneumonia risk	Calcification of costal cartilage

ASTHMA

▶ A complex disorder characterized by variable and recurring symptoms, airflow obstruction, bronchial hyperresponsiveness, and an underlying inflammation (National Heart, Lung, and Blood Institute [NHLBI] 2012).

▶ ● To establish a diagnosis of asthma, the clinician should determine that symptoms of recurrent episodes of airflow obstruction or airway hyperresponsiveness are present; airflow obstruction is at least partially reversible; and alternative diagnoses are excluded (NHLBI 2007).

Risk Factors

▶ Smoking

▶ Respiratory infections

▶ Allergies

▶ Air pollution

▶ Occupational exposures

Signs and Symptoms

▶ Episodic acute-onset wheezing

▶ Chest tightness, dyspnea, cyanosis

▶ Chronic dry or nonproductive cough

▶ Diaphoresis

▶ Tachycardia

▶ ● Tachypnea, decreased breath sounds, prolonged expiration, hyperresonance

▶ ● In older persons, cough is most common presentation

Diagnostic Tests

▶ Routine monitoring with peak flow meter

▶ 80–100 percent of "personal best" = good control

▶ 50–80 percent = acute exacerbation

▶ <50 percent = severe exacerbation, emergency treatment needed

Differential Diagnoses

▶ Chronic obstructive pulmonary disease (COPD)

▶ Congestive heart failure (CHF)

▶ Vocal cord dysfunction

▶ Respiratory infection

▶ Allergic rhinitis

▶ Airway obstruction

▶ Pulmonary embolism

Management

▶ Four components of asthma care

   1. Assessing and monitoring asthma severity (see table 9–2) and asthma control

   2. Education for a partnership in care

   3. Control of environmental factors and comorbid conditions that affect asthma

   4. Medications

▶ Stepwise approach (table 9–3)

▶ Patient education

▶ Environmental control

▶ Avoid triggers

▶ Pneumococcal vaccination

▶ Annual flu vaccines

▶ Air filters or air conditioners

▶ Treat URIs

▶ ⚬ Pharmacologic treatment

  ▷ Long-term medications

  ▷ Inhaled corticosteroids

  ▷ Mast cell stabilizers

    ▶ Cromolyn sodium (Intal) inhalation

  ▷ Leukotriene receptor antagonists

    ▶ Zafirlukast (Accolate)

    ▶ Zileuton (Zyflo)

    ▶ Montelukast (Singulair)

  ▷ Long-acting beta-2 agonists

    ▶ Salmeterol (Serevent)

  ▷ Methylxanthines

    ▶ Theophylline (Theo-Dur, Slo-bid)

      ▷ Use with caution

    ▶ Drug interactions and side effects

      ▷ Arrhythmias.

      ▷ Seizures.

      ▷ Increased gastric ulcers.

TABLE 9–2.
ASTHMA SEVERITY

COMPONENTS OF SEVERITY		CLASSIFICATION OF ASTHMA SEVERITY ≥12 YEARS OF AGE			
		INTERMITTENT	PERSISTENT		
			MILD	MODERATE	SEVERE
Impairment Normal FEV1/FVC: 8–9 yr 85 percent 20–39 yr 80 percent 40–59 yr 75 percent 60–80 yr 70 percent	Symptoms	≤2 days/week	>2 days/week but not daily	Daily	Throughout the day
	Nighttime awakenings	≤2 times/month	2–4 times/month	>Once/week but not nightly	Often 7 times/week
	Short-acting beta2-agonist use for symptom control (not prevention of EIB)	≤2 days/week	>2 days/week but not daily, and not more than once on any day	Daily	Several times per day
	Interference with normal activity	None	Minor limitation	Some limitation	Extremely limited
	Lung function	• Normal FEV1 between exacerbations • FEV1 > 80 percent predicted • FEV1/FVC normal	• FEV1 > 80 percent predicted • FEV1/FVC normal	• FEV1 > 60 percent but < 80 percent predicted • FEV1/FVC reduced 5 percent	• FEV1 < 60 percent predicted • FEV1/FVC reduced > 5 percent
Risk	Exacerbations requiring oral systemic corticosteroids	0–1/year	≥2/year		
		Consider severity and interval since last exacerbation. Frequency and severity may fluctuate over time for patients in any severity category. Relative annual risk of exacerbations may be related to FEV1.			
Recommended Step for Initial Treatment (See Table 9–3. Stepwise Approach to Managing Asthma Form treatment steps.)		Step 1	Step 2	Step 3 Consider short course of oral systemic corticosteroids	Step 4 or 5 Consider short course of oral systemic corticosteroids
		In 2–6 weeks, evaluate level of asthma control that is achieved and adjust therapy accordingly.			

Note: FEV1 = forced expiratory volume in 1 second.

Source: NHLBI 2012

TABLE 9–3.
STEPWISE APPROACH TO MANAGING ASTHMA

INTERMITTENT ASTHMA	PERSISTENT ASTHMA: DAILY MEDICATION CONSULT WITH ASTHMA SPECIALIST IF STEP 4 CARE OR HIGHER IS REQUIRED CONSIDER CONSULTATION AT STEP 3					
Step 1	**Step 2**	**Step 3**	**Step 4**	**Step 5**	**Step 6**	
Preferred: SABA PRN	*Preferred:* Low-dose ICS *Alternative:* Cromolyn, LTRA, Nedocromil, or Theophylline	*Preferred:* Low-dose ICS + LABA, or Medium-dose ICS *Alternative:* Low-dose ICS + either LTRA, Theophylline, or Zileuton	*Preferred:* Medium-dose ICS + LABA *Alternative:* Medium-dose ICS + either LTRA, Theophylline, or Zileuton	*Preferred:* High-dose ICS + LABA *And:* Consider Omalizumab for patients who have allergies	*Preferred:* High-dose ICS + LABA + oral corticosteroid *And:* Consider Omalizumab for patients who have allergies	

Step up if needed (first, check adherence, environmental control, and comorbid conditions)

Access control

Step down if possible (and asthma is well controlled for at least 3 months)

Each step: Patient education, environmental control, and management of comorbidities.

Steps 2–4: Consider subcutaneous allergen immunotherapy for patients who have allergic asthma (see notes).

Quick-Relief Medication for All Patients

- SABA as needed for symptoms. Intensity of treatment depends on severity of symptoms: up to 3 months at 20-minute intervals as needed. Short course of oral systemic corticosteroids may be needed.
- Use of SABA >2 days a week for symptom relief (not prevention of EIB) generally indicates inadequate control and the need to step up treatment.

Note: SABA = short-acting beta agonist; ICS = inhaled corticosteroids; LABA = long-acting beta agonist

Source: NHLBI 2007

▷ Side effects of methylxanthines include nausea and vomiting, heartburn (especially in asthma), insomnia, headache, nervousness, tachycardia, tachypnea, arrhythmias, and seizures.

▷ Drug interactions: Caffeine (caffeine derivative), ciprofloxacin, cimetidine, and erythromycin increase methylxanthine levels; carbamazepine and phenytoin decrease methylxanthine levels.

▷ Quick-relief medications

▶ • Short-acting beta agonists

▷ Albuterol (Proventil, Ventolin)

▶ • Anticholinergics

▷ Ipratropium bromide (Atrovent)

▶ • Systemic corticosteroids

▷ Prednisone or prednisolone

Prevention

▶ Instruct patient to

▷ Avoid known asthma triggers,

▷ Take medications as prescribed,

▷ Obtain flu vaccine, and

▷ Not smoke.

BRONCHITIS

▶ Irritation and inflammation of mucosal lining of tracheobronchial tree

▶ • Increased airway swelling

▶ Increased mucus secretion
(Hart 2014)

▶ • Inhaled bronchodilators

▷ Albuterol or metaproterenol: 1–2 puffs q 4–6 hrs

▷ Fluticasone or budesonide: 1–2 puffs b.i.d.

▷ Ipratropium: 2–4 puffs three to four times per day

▶ • Inhaled steroids and combination drugs (Alangari 2014)

▷ Beclomethasone dipropionate (Qvar)

▷ Budesonide (Pulmicort)

▷ Budesonide/Formoterol (Symbicort): A combination drug that includes a steroid and a long-acting bronchodilator drug

▷ Fluticasone (Flovent)

▷ Fluticasone/Salmeterol (Advair): A combination drug that includes a steroid and a long-acting bronchodilator drug

TABLE 9–4.
ACUTE AND CHRONIC BRONCHITIS

	ACUTE	CHRONIC
	Self-limiting infection with cough as the primary symptom Difficult to distinguish from other illnesses that cause cough Usually viral	Long-term disorder lasting at least 3 consecutive months for 2 years in a row Associated with smoking Induces right-sided heart failure
Risk Factors	Smoking, air pollution, sick contacts, allergies, compromised immune system	
Signs and Symptoms	Productive mucoid or purulent cough, usually accentuated on inspiration, lasting 10–20 days; wheezing; low-grade fever	Productive mucoid cough, usually accentuated on inspiration; wheezing; chest discomfort Increased expiratory resistance Excess mucus Predisposition for superimposed respiratory infections
Physical Findings	Appearance not acute Rhinitis, harsh cough Normal breath sounds, rhonchi, expiratory wheeze, resonance, hyperresonance, tachycardia	SOB greater when speaking Pedal edema, pallor, grey or cyanotic Rhonchi, resonance, hyperresonance, long expiration with wheeze, frequent productive cough, jugular venous distention, S_3
Diagnostic Tests	By exception Unclear presentation: CBC, ECG, CXR	Peak expiratory flow rate (PEFR), airway reactivity, CBC, ECG, CXR
Differential Diagnoses	Asthma, pneumonia, pertussis, CHF, common cold, malignancy, GERD, sinusitis	Asthma, pneumonia, pertussis, CHF, common cold, malignancy, GERD
Management	Cough suppressants or expectorants Analgesics or antipyretics, hydration Smoking cessation, bronchodilators Humidifier or steam to loosen mucus and relieve wheezing No antibiotics if otherwise healthy	Cough suppressants or expectorants Bronchodilators, analgesics, hydration, smoking cessation Humidifier or steam to loosen mucus and relieve wheezing No antibiotics if otherwise healthy
Prevention	Stop smoking; avoid allergens, air pollution, irritants Hand hygiene, updated immunizations	

Note: S_3 = ventricular gallop; CBC = complete blood count; ECG = electrocardiogram; CXR = chest X-ray; CHF = congestive heart failure; GERD = gastroesophageal reflux disease

▷   Mometasone (Asmanex)

▷   Mometasone/formoterol (Dulera): A combination drug that also includes a long-acting bronchodilator drug

▷   Fluticasone inhalation powder (Arnuity Ellipta)

▶   Anticholinergics

▷   Aclidinium (Tudorza Pressair; long-acting)

▷   Ipratropium (Atrovent; short-acting)

▷   Tiotropium (Spiriva; long-acting)

▶   Xanthines

▷   Theophylline

▶   Corticosteroids

▷   Prednisone

CHRONIC OBSTRUCTIVE PULMONARY DISEASE (COPD)

▶   A common preventable and treatable disease characterized by persistent airflow limitation that is usually progressive and associated with an enhanced chronic inflammatory response in the airways and the lung to noxious particles or gases.

▶   Often asymptomatic in early phases.

Risk Factors

▶   Smoking

▶   Environmental or occupational exposure

▶   Allergies

▶   Medications

Signs and Symptoms

▶   Cough with sputum production

▶   Dyspnea or airflow limitation

▶   Frequent infections

▶   Impaired gas exchange

▶   Shortness of breath

▶   Tachycardia (sometimes)

▶   Accessory muscle use

▶   Decreased breath sounds

▶   Prolonged expiratory phase

▶   Adventitious lung sounds

▶ ◦ Barrel chest

▶ ●Decreased diaphragm movement

Diagnostic Tests

▶   Chest radiographs

▶ ●Pulmonary function tests (PFTs)

▶   Pulse oximetry

▶   Blood gases

▶   CBC, electrolytes, blood urea nitrogen (BUN), creatinine

▶   12-lead ECG

▶ ◦ Spirometry required to make a clinical diagnosis of COPD; presence of a postbron-chodilator FEV1/FVC (forced vital capacity) < 0.70 confirms persistent airflow limita-tion and thus COPD (see table 9–5)

▶   GOLD guideline

▶   The goals of COPD assessment are to determine the severity of the disease, its im-pact on patient's health status, and the risk of future events (exacerbations, hospital admissions, death) to guide therapy.

▶   Assess the following aspects of the disease separately:

▷   Symptoms

▷ ● Degree of airflow limitation (using spirometry)

▷   Risk of exacerbations

▷   Comorbidities

Differential Diagnoses

▶   Bronchitis

▶   Asthma

▶   Congestive heart failure

TABLE 9–5.
GLOBAL INITIATIVE FOR CHRONIC OBSTRUCTIVE LUNG DISEASE (GOLD) CRITERIA CLASSIFICATION IN PATIENTS WITH FEV1/FVC < 0.70

CLASSIFICATION	SEVERITY	POST-BRONCHODILATOR FEV$_1$
GOLD 1	Mild	FEV1 ≥ 80% predicted
GOLD 2	Moderate	50% ≤ FEV < 80% predicted
GOLD 3	Severe	30% ≤ FEV < 50% predicted
GOLD 4	Very Severe	FEV1 < 30% predicted

Source: Global Initiative for Chronic Obstructive Lung Disease 2017

Management

- ▶ Bronchodilators
  - ▷ Beta agonist: Albuterol (Proventil, Ventolin)
- ▶ Methylxanthines
  - ▷ Theophylline (Theo-Dur, Slo-bid)
- ▶ Corticosteroids, inhaled or oral
- ▶ Anticholinergics
  - ▷ Ipratropium bromide (Atrovent)
  - ▷ Tiotropium (Spiriva)
- ▶ Phosphodiesterase-4 inhibitors
- ▶ Mucolytics
- ▶ Oxygen
- ▶ Pulmonary rehabilitation

Prevention

- ▶ Smoking cessation

PNEUMONIA

- ▶ Infection or inflammation of the lungs caused by bacteria, viruses, or fungi
- ▶ Causative organisms
  - ▷ Community-acquired pneumonia (CAP)
    - ▶ *Streptococcus pneumoniae*, respiratory viruses, *Mycoplasma pneumoniae*, *Haemophilus influenzae*, gram-negative bacteria, *Chlamydia pneumoniae*, *Moraxella catarrhalis*, *Legionella pneumophilia*
  - ▷ Nursing home–acquired pneumonia
    - ▶ *S. pneumoniae*, gram-negative bacteria, *Staphylococcus aureus,* anaerobes, *H. influenzae, Chlamydia pneumoniae*
  - ▷ Hospital-acquired pneumonia (HAP)
    - ▶ Fungi, gram-negative bacteria, anaerobes

Risk Factors

- ▶ Smoking
- ▶ Viral respiratory infections
- ▶ COPD
- ▶ Advanced age
- ▶ Immunocompromised states
- ▶ Alcoholism

Signs and Symptoms

▶ Tachypnea or tachycardia

▶ Hypotension

▶ Often afebrile, absent, or blunted fever in the elderly (Norman 2000)

▶ Abnormal breath sounds

▶ Poor chest expansion

▶ ○ Dullness to percussion over area of consolidation

▶ ● Fatigue, falls, anorexia, lethargy

▶ Classic presentation

▷ ● Fever, chills, sweats, rigors

▷ ○ Cough and dyspnea are classic but often not present

Diagnostic Tests

▶ CXR

▷ ● May be negative if dehydrated

▶ CBC, BUN, creatinine, electrolytes, glucose, blood culture

▶ Arterial blood gasses (ABGs) or pulse oximetry

▶ Sputum Gram stain and culture not common in outpatient setting

▶ ○ Pneumonia severity assessment

▷ CURB-65 score

▷ Pneumonia severity index (PSI)

▷ Decision to hospitalize based on objective measures such as CURB-65 or PSI score

Differential Diagnoses

▶ Bronchitis

▶ Heart failure

▶ COPD

▶ Tuberculosis (TB)

Management

▶ Patients with CAP (Mandell et al. 2007)

▷ ● Should be treated for a minimum of five days (level I evidence),

▷ ○ Should be afebrile for 48–72 hours, *and*

▷ ○ Should have no more than one CAP-associated sign of clinical instability before discontinuation of therapy.

▶ Guidelines vary for calculating creatinine clearance and altering dose. (See table 9–6.)

  ▷ ● Chest percussion

  ▷ Inhaled beta agonists

  ▷ Oxygen and rehydration

  ▷ Bilevel positive airway pressure (BiPAP) or mechanical ventilation

▶ Nursing home–acquired

  ▷ "Pneumonia in nonambulatory residents of nursing homes and other long-term care facilities epidemiologically mirrors hospital-acquired pneumonia and should be treated according to the healthcare–associated pneumonia (HCAP) guidelines" (Mandell et al. 2007, S27).

  ▷ Treat intravenously first with (American Thoracic Society 2005)

    ▶ ● Antipseudomonal cephalosporins or antipseudomonal carbapenems or beta-lactam inhibitor *plus* antipseudomonal fluoroquinolone or

    ▶ ● Aminoglycoside *plus* linezolid or vancomycin.

  ▷ Sputum culture should be obtained to identify pathogen.

  ▷ Decisions to withhold antimicrobial therapy and promote comfort may be appropriate in many frail older adults, especially with end-stage dementia.

Prevention

▶ Pneumococcal and influenza immunizations

▶ Smoking cessation

PRIMARY LUNG MALIGNANCIES

▶ Two classes of bronchogenic cancer.

▶ Two main cellular types (Dunphy et al. 2015):

  ▷ ● Small cell (15 percent)

  ▷ ● Non-small cell (85 percent)

▶ The most frequent cause of cancer death in men and women in North America.

▶ Accounts for 28 percent of all cancer deaths.

▶ 86 percent of patients die within 5 years.

▶ The death rate for women is now higher than from any other cancer because of increased cigarette smoking by women and because they may be more susceptible than men to the carcinogenic effects of tobacco smoke (Dunphy et al. 2015).

▶ ● Metastasis in 50 percent at diagnosis.

  ▷ ● Most to brain, bone, liver

Risk Factors

▶ Cigarette smoking and secondhand smoke

▶ Radon or other toxic substances

▶ Environmental and occupational exposure

▶ Genetics

TABLE 9–6.
EMPIRIC THERAPY FOR OUTPATIENT CAP OR INPATIENT TREATMENT

CIRCUMSTANCES	RECOMMENDED TREATMENT
Previously healthy and no risk factors for drug-resistant *S. pneumoniae*	A macrolide (azithromycin, clarithromycin, or erythromycin) or Doxycycline (weaker recommendation)
Presence of comorbidities, such as chronic heart, lung, liver, or renal disease; diabetes mellitus; alcoholism; malignancies; asplenia; immunosuppressing conditions or use of immunosuppressing drugs; use of antimicrobials within the previous 3 months (in which case an alternative from a different class should be selected)	A respiratory fluoroquinolone (moxifloxacin, gemifloxacin, or levofloxacin [750 mg]) or A beta-lactam *plus* a macrolide (high-dose amoxicillin [e.g., 1 g t.i.d.] or amoxicillin-clavulanate [2 g b.i.d.] is preferred; alternatives include ceftriaxone, cefpodoxime, and cefuroxime [500 mg b.i.d.]; doxycycline
In regions with a high rate (>25 percent) of infection with high-level (MIC ≥ 16 mcg/mL) macrolide-resistant *S. pneumoniae*	A respiratory fluoroquinolone (moxifloxacin, gemifloxacin, or levofloxacin [750 mg]) or A beta-lactam *plus* a macrolide
Inpatient, non-ICU treatment	A respiratory fluoroquinolone or A beta-lactam *plus* a macrolide
Inpatient, ICU treatment For penicillin-allergic patients	A beta-lactam (cefotaxime, ceftriaxone, or ampicillin-sulbactam) *plus* either azithromycin or a respiratory fluoroquinolone A respiratory fluoroquinolone and aztreonam
If *Pseudomonas* is a consideration For penicillin-allergic patients	An antipneumococcal, antipseudomonal beta-lactam (piperacillin-tazobactam, cefepime, imipenem, or meropenem) *plus* either ciprofloxacin or levofloxacin (750 mg) *or* The above beta-lactam plus an aminoglycoside and azithromycin *or* The above beta-lactam plus an aminoglycoside and an antipneumococcal fluoroquinolone Substitute aztreonam for above beta-lactam
If CA-MRSA is a consideration	Add vancomycin or linezolid

Note: MIC = minimal inhibitory concentration; ICU = intensive care unit; CA-MRSA = methicillin-resistant *S. aureus*.

Source: Mandell et al. 2007

Signs and Symptoms

▶ Physical findings vary

▶ Initial: Persistent cough longer than 1 month

  ▷ Later: Chest pain, weight loss, dyspnea

  ▷ Metastasis (bone pain)

  ▷ Hemoptysis (not common)

Diagnostic Tests

▶ Chest radiographs

▶ Computed tomography (CT) scan

▶ Refer for bronchoscopy

▶ Histologic confirmation essential

▶ Refer to pulmonologist

Differential Diagnoses

▶ Lung abscess

▶ Infections

▶ Pneumonia

▶ TB

Management

▶ Surgical resection

▶ Radiation and chemotherapy

▶ Supportive care

  ▷ Pain management

  ▷ Manage side effects

  ▷ Oxygen

  ▷ Home medical equipment

  ▷ Hospice, if appropriate

Prevention

▶ Patient education:

  ▷ Stop smoking and avoid secondhand smoke.

  ▷ Healthy lifestyle.

  ▷ Avoid environmental carcinogens such as asbestos.

TUBERCULOSIS (TB)

▶ ● Infection caused by *Mycobacterium tuberculosis* that primarily affects the lungs but can attack kidney, spine, and brain

▶ If not treated properly, can be fatal

Risk Factors

▶ Chronic institutionalization

▶ Corticosteroid use

▶ Diabetes mellitus

▶ Malignancy

▶ Malnutrition

▶ Renal failure

▶ HIV

▶ ● Gastrectomy

▶ Resistant TB risk factors

  ▷ HIV infection

  ▷ Homelessness

  ▷ Intravenous drug use

  ▷ Previous TB, history of failed treatment

  ▷ Positive AFB (acid-fast bacilli) after 2 months' treatment

  ▷ Positive cultures after 4 months' treatment

  ▷ New infection from geographic areas with high rates of resistant organisms (New York, Mexico, Southeast Asia)

Signs and Symptoms

▶ Chronic, productive cough

▶ Fatigue, malaise, weight loss

▶ Night sweats, appears chronically ill

▶ History of HIV infection or AIDS

Diagnostic Tests

▶ Chest exam:

  ▷ ● Small, homogeneous infiltrate in upper lobes

  ▷ ● Hilar and paratracheal lymph nodes enlarged

▶ Sputum for AFB.

  ▷ ● AFB smear presumptive of active TB

▶ Tuberculin skin tests (TSTs; see table 9–7).

▶ Mantoux (purified protein derivative [PPD] of tuberculin).

▶ • Two-step PPD recommended for older adults.

▶ Screening recommendations (Centers for Disease Control and Prevention [CDC] 2016f; Dunphy et al. 2015):

  ▷ Persons with signs or symptoms of current TB

  ▷ Persons with HIV infection

  ▷ Persons who inject illicit drugs

  ▷ Persons from medically underserved or high-risk minority populations

  ▷ Residents or employees in prisons or long-term care facilities

  ▷ Infants, children, and adolescents exposed to adults in high-risk categories (use of interferon-gamma release assays [IGRAs] is not established for children younger than 5 years old)

  ▷ Foreign-born persons arriving within 5 years from countries that have high TB incidence or prevalence

  ▷ Persons on long-term high-dose corticosteroid therapy (use TST rather than IGRA)

  ▷ Persons on immunosuppressive therapy (use TST rather than IGRA)

  ▷ Persons with medical conditions that increase the risk of TB: chronic renal failure, diabetes, hematological disorders, cancer of the head or neck, body weight 10 percent or more less than the ideal body weight, silicosis, gastrectomy, jejunal bypass

  ▷ People who have spent time with someone who has TB disease

  ▷ People from a country where TB disease is common (most countries in Latin America, the Caribbean, Africa, Asia, Eastern Europe, and Russia)

  ▷ People who live or work in high-risk settings (for example, correctional facilities, long-term care facilities or nursing homes, homeless shelters)

  ▷ Healthcare workers who care for patients at increased risk for TB disease

  ▷ Infants, children, and adolescents exposed to adults who are at increased risk for latent tuberculosis infection or TB disease

▶ Factors contributing to a decreased response to TST (Dunphy et al. 2015):

  ▷ Infections

    ▶ Viral: Measles, mumps, chickenpox, HIV infection

    ▶ Bacterial: Typhoid fever, brucellosis, typhus, leprosy, pertussis, recent or overwhelming *M. tuberculosis* infection

    ▶ Fungal: South American blastomycosis

    ▶ Live virus vaccinations: Measles, mumps, polio

  ▷ Nutritional factors: Severe protein depletion

  ▷ Diseases affecting lymphoid organs: Hodgkin lymphoma, chronic lymphocytic leukemia

TABLE 9–7.
INTERPRETATION OF PPD SKIN TEST RESULTS

CLASSIFICATION OF THE TST REACTION		
Induration of 5 mm or more is considered positive in	**Induration of 10 mm or more** is considered positive in	**Induration of 15 mm or more** is considered positive in
• HIV-infected persons	• Recent immigrants (<5 years) from high-prevalence countries	• Any person, including persons with no known risk factors for TB
• Recent contacts of a person with TB disease	• Persons who inject illicit drugs	• However, targeted skin testing programs should only be conducted among high-risk groups
• Persons with fibrotic changes on chest radiograph consistent with prior TB	• Residents and employees of high-risk congregate settings	
• Patients with organ transplants	• Mycobacteriology laboratory personnel	
• Persons who are immunosuppressed for other reasons (e.g., taking the equivalent of >15 mg/day of prednisone for 1 month or longer, taking TNF-α antagonists)	• Persons with clinical conditions that place them at high risk	
	• Children <4 years of age	
	• Infants, children, and adolescents exposed to adults in high-risk categories	

Source: CDC 2016c

> ▷ Drugs: Corticosteroids and other immunosuppressive agents

> ▷ Age: Newborns, older adults

> ▷ Stress: Surgery, burns, mental illness, graft-versus-host reactions

▶ In older adults or in persons who are being tested for the first time, the reaction to the Mantoux test may develop more slowly and may not peak until after 72 hours. Older adults should be checked initially at 72 hours, and then 1 and 2 days later (Dunphy et al. 2015).

▶ CXR with infiltrates, sputum smears with acid-fast bacilli.

> ▷ Any sputum smear suspicious for mycobacteria should be cultured, and the culture should be checked weekly during weeks 3–6 to confirm tuberculosis (Dunphy et al. 2015).

▶ Definitive diagnosis

> ▷ Culture of *M. tuberculosis* × 3

Differential Diagnoses

▶ Acute respiratory distress syndrome (ARDS)

▶ URI

► Lymphangitic spread of cancer

► Pneumonia

► Sarcoidosis

► Silicosis

► Coal workers' pneumoconiosis (black lung disease)

Management

► Notify local and state health agencies

► Refer to infectious disease department for treatment

► Direct observation of therapy (DOT)

▷ TB drugs given to patient while watching that they are taken (see table 9–8)

▷ Preferred core management strategy for all patients with TB

► Chemoprophylaxis for recent converters

▷ Positive skin test

▷ INH (isoniazid) recommended for 6 months

► Rifampin and isoniazid for resistant TB strains

► In the United States, a positive TST without clinical TB infection (negative CXR findings and no symptoms) should be treated to minimize the possibility of reactivation (secondary) TB (Dunphy et al. 2015)

► Standard regimen to prevent TB reactivation is INH for 9 months (least hepatotoxic regimen), rifampin for 4 months, or rifampin plus pyrazinamide for 2 months (most hepatotoxic regimen; Dunphy et al. 2015)

Prevention

► Avoid close contact with persons with TB.

► TB screening.

► Patient education on cough hygiene (cover mouth).

► Encourage patient medication adherence.

► Healthcare workers should use respiratory protective equipment when warranted.

► Prophylactic latent TB infection treatment.

PULMONARY EMBOLISM (PE)

► Obstruction of pulmonary vessels by a thrombus or other embolic material that can be large or small.

► Cannot be confirmed or ruled out based on clinical presentation alone; no individual risk factor, patient symptom, or clinical sign can definitively diagnose or exclude (Raja et al. 2015).

TABLE 9–8.
TB MEDICATION REGIMENS

DRUG-SUSCEPTIBLE TB DISEASE TREATMENT REGIMENS. REGIMENS FOR TREATING TB DISEASE HAVE AN INTENSIVE PHASE OF 2 MONTHS, FOLLOWED BY A CONTINUATION PHASE OF EITHER 4 OR 7 MONTHS.

	INTENSIVE PHASE	CONTINUATION PHASE
Preferred regimen for patients with newly diagnosed pulmonary TB	Daily INH 300 mg, RIF 600 mg, PZA 100–200 mg, *and* EMB* 800–1,600 mg × 56 doses	Daily INH 300 mg, RIF 600 mg × 126 doses, or Five times per week INH 900 mg and RIF × 90 doses
Preferred alternative regimen in situations in which more frequent DOT during continuation phase is difficult to achieve	Daily INH 300 mg, RIF 600 mg, PZA 2,000–4,000 mg, and EMB* 2,000–4,000 mg × 40 doses (8 weeks)	Three times per week INH 900 mg, RIF 600 mg × 18 weeks
Use regimen with caution in patients with HIV and/or cavitary disease; missed doses can lead to treatment failure, relapse, and acquired drug resistance	INH 300 mg, RIF 600 mg, PZA 100–200 mg, and EMB* 800–1,600 mg three times weekly for 24 doses (8 weeks)	Three times weekly for 54 doses (18 weeks) INH 900 mg, RIF 600 mg
	May give • Streptomycin 15 mg/kg IM daily initially • Vitamin B6 50 mg p.o. daily For HIV, liver disorders, <3 months postpartum, regular alcohol use, older adults on meds for chronic diseases: • Baseline LFTs, CBC, serum creatinine, and platelet count. • Hepatitis B and C screening for patients with risk factors such as injection drug use, foreign birth, and HIV infection. • Susceptibility testing for INH, RIF, ethambutol (EMB), and pyrazin-amide (PZA) should be performed on any initial culture that is positive. • NH, RIF, and EMB susceptibility tests for positive initial culture. • Sputum cultures at a minimum of monthly intervals until two consecutive specimens are negative on culture. It is critical to obtain a sputum specimen at the end of the intensive phase (2 months) to determine if the continuation phase should be extended.	Routine measurements not necessary during treatment unless baseline abnormal or risk for hepatotoxicity Continued symptoms or positive cultures after 3 months raise drug resistance suspicion Minimum of monthly clinical evaluations to identify possible adverse effects of medications and to assess adherence Visual acuity and red-green color discrimination for EMB treatment HIV testing and counseling for all with TB

Note: RIF = rifampin, PZA = pyrazinamide, EMB = ethambutol, IM = intramuscularly, LFT = liver function tests. *EMB can be discontinued if drug susceptibility studies demonstrate susceptibility to first-line drugs.

Sources: CDC 2016e; Sia and Wieland 2011

Risk Factors

▶ Cancer

▶ Obesity

▶ Immobility

▶ Hypercoagulable states

▶ Smoking

▶ Heart failure

▶ Previous deep vein thrombosis (DVT)

▶ Pregnancy

▶ Surgery

Signs and Symptoms

▶ Shortness of breath (SOB)

▶ Pleuritic chest pain

▶ ● Cough, hemoptysis

▶ Apprehension, diaphoresis

▶ Restlessness, confusion

▶ Leg pain or swelling

▶ Arrhythmias, tachycardia, S3 or S4 gallop

▶ CHF, tachypnea

▶ Crackles, pleural friction rub, decreased O_2 saturation

▶ Low-grade fever

▶ Tachycardia

Diagnostic Tests

▶ The first step when evaluating a patient with suspected acute PE is to establish their pretest probability of PE by using a validated tool.

   ▷ ●The Wells and Geneva rules have been validated and are considered equally accurate in predicting the probability of PE.

   ▷ ● The pulmonary embolism rule-out criteria (PERC) were specifically developed to help clinicians identify patients with low pretest probabilities of PE in whom the risks of any testing outweigh the risk for PE (Kline et al. 2004).

      ▶ Age younger than 50 years

      ▶ Heart rate (HR) less than 100 beats per minute (BPM)

      ▶ Arterial oxygen saturation (SaO2) on room air greater than 94 percent

      ▶ No history of venous thromboembolism

      ▶ No recent (<28 days) trauma or surgery

  ▶ No unilateral leg swelling

  ▶ No hemoptysis

  ▶ No oral hormone use

▶ ◦ D-dimer testing

  ▷ Do not obtain D-dimer measurements or imaging studies in patients with a low pretest probability of PE and who meet all PERC.

  ▷ ◦Obtain a high-sensitivity D-dimer measurement as the initial diagnostic test in patients who have an intermediate pretest probability of PE or in patients with low pretest probability of PE who do not meet all PERC.

  ▷ ◦ Do not obtain a D-dimer measurement in patients with high pretest probability of PE.

▶ Imaging

  ▷ Do not use imaging studies as the initial test in patients who have a low or intermediate pretest probability of PE.

  ▷ ◦ Do not obtain any imaging studies in patients with a D-dimer level below the age-adjusted cutoff.

  ▷ ◦Obtain imaging with CT pulmonary angiography (CTPA) in patients with high pretest probability of PE.

  ▷ Clinicians should reserve ventilation-perfusion (VQ) scans for patients who have a contraindication to CTPA or if CTPA is not available.

  ▷ ◦ The predominant test a is spiral CT.

  ▷ CXR

  ▷ ABGs

  ▷ Transesophageal echocardiogram (TEE)

Differential Diagnoses

  ▶ Pulmonary edema

  ▶ Heart failure

  ▶ ARDS

  ▶ Anxiety

  ▶ Fat embolism

  ▶ Acute coronary syndrome

  ▶ Pneumonia

  ▶ COPD

Management

  ▶ O_2 monitor

  ▶ ◦ Anticoagulation

  ▷ Heparin, warfarin

▶ Surgical

▷ Embolectomy

▷ Vena cava filter (not routine)

Prevention

▶ Patient education:

▷ Limit immobility.

▷ DVT prevention and prophylaxis.

▷ No smoking.

▷ Exercise.

▷ Maintain a healthy weight.

▷ Compression stockings.

REFERENCES

Alangari, A. 2014. "Corticosteroids in the Treatment of Acute Asthma." *Annals of Thoracic Medicine* 9 (4): 187–192. http://dx.doi.org/10.4103/1817-1737.140120.

American Thoracic Society. 2005. "Guidelines for the Management of Adults with Hospital-Acquired, Ventilator-Associated, and Healthcare-Associated Pneumonia." *American Journal of Respiratory and Critical Care Medicine* 171 (4): 388–416. http://dx.doi.org/10.1164/rccm.200405-644st.

Centers for Disease Control and Prevention. 2003. "Treatment of Tuberculosis," supplement, *Morbidity and Mortality Weekly Report* 52 (RR-11). http://www.cdc.gov/mmwr/PDF/rr/rr5211.pdf.

———. 2016a. "Fast Facts." Smoking and Tobacco Use. http://www.cdc.gov/tobacco/data_statistics/fact_sheets/fast_facts/.

———. 2016b. "TB Elimination: Treatment of Latent Tuberculosis Infection; Maximizing Adherence." https://www.cdc.gov/tb/publications/factsheets/treatment/adherence_revised.pdf.

———. 2016c. "TB Elimination: Tuberculin Skin Testing." https://www.cdc.gov/tb/publications/factsheets/testing/skintesting.pdf.

———. 2016d. "Testing and Diagnosis." Tuberculosis (TB). http://www.cdc.gov/tb/topic/testing/.

———. 2016e. "Treatment for TB Disease." Tuberculosis (TB). http://www.cdc.gov/tb/topic/treatment/tbdisease.htm.

———. 2016f. "Who Should Be Tested." Tuberculosis (TB). http://www.cdc.gov/tb/topic/testing/whobetested.htm.

Dunphy, L., J. Winland-Brown, B. Porter, and D. Thomas, eds. 2015. *Primary Care: The Art and Science of Advanced Practice Nursing*. 4th ed. Philadelphia: F. A. Davis.

Fiore, A., A. Fry, D. Shay, L. Gubareva, J. Bresee, and T. Uyeki. 2011. "Antiviral Agents for the Treatment and Chemoprophylaxis of Influenza: Recommendations of the Advisory Committee on Immunization Practices (ACIP)." *Morbidity and Mortality Weekly Report* 60 (RR01): 1–24. http://www.cdc.gov/mmwr/preview/mmwrhtml/rr6001a1.htm.

Global Initiative for Chronic Obstructive Lung Disease. 2017. *Pocket Guide to COPD Diagnosis, Management, and Prevention: A Guide for Health Care Professionals.* N.p.: Global Initiative for Chronic Obstructive Lung Disease, Inc. http://goldcopd.org/wp-content/uploads/2016/12/wms-GOLD-2017-Pocket-Guide.pdf.

Hart, A. 2014. "Evidence-Based Diagnosis and Management of Acute Bronchitis." *Nurse Practitioner* 39 (9): 32–39. http://dx.doi.org/10.1097/01.npr.0000452978.99676.2b.

Kline, J., A. Mitchell, C. Kabrhel, P. Richman, and D. Courtney. 2004. "Clinical Criteria to Prevent Unnecessary Diagnostic Testing in Emergency Department Patients with Suspected Pulmonary Embolism." *Journal of Thrombosis and Haemostasis* 2 (8): 1247–55. http://dx.doi.org/10.1111/j.1538-7836.2004.00790.x.

Mandell, L., Wunderink, R., Anzueto, A., Bartlett, J., Campbell, G., N. Dean, S. F. Dowell, et al. 2007. "Infectious Diseases Society of America/American Thoracic Society Consensus Guidelines on the Management of Community-Acquired Pneumonia in Adults." *Clinical Infectious Diseases* 44 (Supplement 2): S27–S72. http://dx.doi.org/10.1086/511159.

National Heart, Lung, and Blood Institute. 2007. *Expert Panel Report 3: Guidelines for the Diagnosis and Management of Asthma.* Full report. Washington, DC: National Institutes of Health.

———. 2012. "Asthma Care Quick Reference: Diagnosing and Managing Asthma." https://www.nhlbi.nih.gov/files/docs/guidelines/asthma_qrg.pdf.

Norman, D. 2000. "Fever in the Elderly." *Clinical Infectious Diseases* 31 (1): 148–51. http://dx.doi.org/10.1086/313896.

Raja, A. S., J. O. Greenberg, A. Qaseem, T. D. Denberg, N. Fitterman, and J. D. Schuur. 2015. "Evaluation of Patients with Suspected Acute Pulmonary Embolism: Best Practice Advice from the Clinical Guidelines Committee of the American College of Physicians." *Annals of Internal Medicine* 163 (9): 701–11. http://dx.doi.org/10.7326/m14-1772.

Sia, I. G., and M. L. Wieland. 2011. "Current Concepts in the Management of Tuberculosis." *Mayo Clinic Proceedings* 86 (4): 348–61. http://doi.org/10.4065/mcp.2010.0820.

CHAPTER 10

GASTROINTESTINAL (GI) SYSTEM DISORDERS

LEARNING OBJECTIVES

▶ Recognize common disorders and then analyze processes useful to providing differential diagnosis among gastrointestinal conditions.

▷ Risk factors

▷ Signs and symptoms

▷ Diagnostic tests

▷ Differential diagnoses

▶ Describe treatment and management of gastrointestinal disorders.

▷ Management

▷ Prevention

CONSTIPATION

▶ Difficult defecation or excessive straining to defecate and infrequent stools, hard stools, a feeling of incomplete evacuation, abdominal discomfort, bloating and distention, a sense of anorectal blockage during defecation, and the need for manual maneuvers during defecation (Bharucha et al. 2013).

▶ Multifactorial causes that include decreased colonic motility because of aging, poor dietary intake of fiber and fluids, behavioral habits, decreased activity, immobility, cognitive impairment, and psychogenic issues.

▶ More women refer to themselves as constipated.

▶ Prevalence rises with age.

▶ Treatment for constipation accounts for more than 2.5 million visits to doctors' offices each year, with at least $800 million spent annually for laxatives (Harvard Health Publications 2014).

Risk Factors

- ▶ Female
- ▶ Advanced age
- ▶ Dehydration, poor fluid intake
- ▶ Diet low in fiber
- ▶ Sedentary lifestyle
- ▶ Medications
- ▶ • Sedatives, narcotics, antihypertensives

Signs and Symptoms

- ▶ Change in pattern, character, and color of stool.
- ▶ Distention, abdominal tenderness.
- ▶ • Palpable stool in colon, decreased bowel sounds.
- ▶ Anorectal pain.
- ▶ • Frail older adults may present with fever, delirium, urinary retention or incontinence, arrhythmia, tachypnea, or weight loss.

Diagnostic Tests

- ▶ • Digital rectal exam: Assess sphincter tone, masses, impaction, hemorrhoids, fissures, rectal prolapse
- ▶ Stool for occult blood
- ▶ CBC, electrolytes (calcium, blood urea nitrogen [BUN]), creatinine, glucose, thyroid function tests
- ▶ • Flat plate and upright abdominal X-ray to look for obstruction

Differential Diagnoses

- ▶ Neurologic dysfunction
- ▶ Diabetes
- ▶ Multiple sclerosis
- ▶ Metabolic disorders
- ▶ Hypothyroidism
- ▶ Hypercalcemia
- ▶ Obstruction
- ▶ Medications
- ▶ Irritable bowel syndrome (IBS)
- ▶ Anorectal pain, fissures, hemorrhoids

Management

- ▶ • Fiber: 25–30 grams per day.
- ▶ Hydrophilic colloids or bulk-forming agents.
- ▶ Osmotic laxatives (sorbitol or lactulose).
- ▶ Stimulant laxatives may cause dependency.
- ▶ Fluids: Must stay well hydrated, especially when increasing fiber.
- ▶ Exercise.
- ▶ Bowel training program.
- ▶ Avoid constipating medications.
   - ▷ Persons on opioids are usually dependent on these agents; do not use if obstruction suspected.
- ▶ • Initial or mild:
   - ▷ Hydrophilic colloids or bulk-forming agents
- ▶ • Severe:
   - ▷ Osmotic or stimulant laxatives
- ▶ Enemas.
- ▶ Surfactants (stool softeners).
- ▶ Peripherally acting mu opioid receptor antagonists (PAMORA): Movantik (naloxegol).
- ▶ Guanylate cyclase-C agonists: Linzess (linaclotide).

Prevention

- ▶ Avoid processed food.
- ▶ Increase fruits and vegetables.
- ▶ Increase fiber.
- ▶ Drink eight 8-ounce glasses of water a day.
- ▶ Exercise.

ACUTE DIARRHEA

- ▶ An increase in the frequency, volume, or fluid content of bowel movements over what is normal for the person (Dunphy et al. 2015).
- ▶ May be caused by viral, bacterial, protozoal, or parasitic gastroenteritis infections, food allergies, or certain types of medications.
- ▶ Usually has an abrupt onset and lasts for less than 1 week; nausea, vomiting, or fever may be associated with acute types of diarrhea (Dunphy et al. 2015).
- ▶ Most common cause for acute diarrhea in a healthy person is infection (Dunphy et al. 2015).

► Types of diarrhea:

▷ Osmotic: Seen in patients with injury to the small intestine that results in malabsorption or maldigestion

▷ Secretory: Produces voluminous watery diarrhea, primarily caused by bacterial enterotoxins, laxative abuse, bile salt malabsorption, and endocrine tumors that stimulate pancreatic or intestinal secretion

▷ Can result from morphological changes within intestinal wall that occur with inflammatory conditions of the intestines, and these changes can result in acute or chronic diarrhea

▷ Can also result from altered intestinal motility secondary to diabetic neuropathy, dumping syndrome, or irritable bowel syndrome (IBS)

► Some medications, such as antibiotics, can induce diarrhea by disrupting the normal balance of bacteria (Dunphy et al. 2015).

Risk Factors

► Travel outside United States
► Contaminated food, water
► Antibiotic use
► Lactose intolerance
► Food allergies
► Ulcerative colitis
► IBS

Signs and Symptoms

► Frequent, loose, watery stools.
► Abdominal cramps, pain, bloating.
► Fever; weight loss may be present.
► • Possible signs of dehydration: Tachycardia, orthostatic hypotension, poor skin turgor, decreased urine output.
► Hyperactive bowel sounds, generalized tenderness.
► Stool test for guaiac may be positive.

Diagnostic Tests

► • None for diarrhea of less than 48 hours' duration
► Stool culture
► *C. difficile* toxin (recent antibiotics)
► Stool for
▷ Ova and parasites, leukocytes, occult blood
▷ CBC, electrolytes

Differential Diagnoses

▶ Drug-induced diarrhea

▶ Abdominal disorders

Management

▶ Antidiarrheal agent use is controversial.

▶ • Empiric therapy if suspect inflammatory bacterial pathogen.

▶ Monitor blood pressure, BUN, creatinine.

▶ Adequate hydration.

▶ • Questran (cholestyramine resin) may help absorb toxins.

▶ Maintain a healthy diet.

▶ • Avoid caffeine.

▶ Educate about handwashing, food handling.

Prevention

▶ Hand hygiene.

▶ Cook food thoroughly.

▶ Avoid contaminated water.

CHRONIC DIARRHEA

▶ • Lasts for more than 2 weeks or recurs over months or years.

▶ • The most frequent causes of chronic diarrhea are IBS, medications, dietary factors, inflammatory bowel disease (IBD), and colon cancer (Dunphy et al. 2015).

Risk Factors

▶ Pancreatic disease

▶ Colitis, Crohn's disease, IBS

▶ Medications

▷ Antibiotics, laxatives

▶ Food allergies

▷ Soy protein, cow's milk, sorbitol, fructose, olestra

▶ Hyperthyroidism

▶ Previous surgery or radiation of abdomen or gastrointestinal tract

▶ Tumors

▶ Reduced blood flow to the intestine

▶ Altered immune function

▶ Hereditary disorders

▷ Cystic fibrosis

▷ Enzyme deficiencies

Signs and Symptoms

▶ Fever; weight loss may be present.

▶ • Possible signs of dehydration: Tachycardia, orthostatic hypotension, poor skin turgor, decreased urine output.

▶ Hyperactive bowel sounds, generalized tenderness.

▶ Stool test for guaiac may be positive.

Diagnostic Tests

▶ • Sigmoidoscopy or colonoscopy to diagnose colitis

▶ • For malabsorption: Vitamin B12, D levels; folate; albumin; cholesterol; prothrombin time (PT); iron; total iron-binding capacity (TIBC)

▶ • For steatorrhea:

▷ 24-hour stool test for fecal fat

▶ Stool test for guaiac may be positive

Differential Diagnoses

▶ Drug-induced diarrhea

▶ Abdominal disorders

Management

▶ Anti-tumor necrosis factor therapy infliximab, adalimumab, certolizumab pegol.

▶ Integrin inhibitors (vedolizumab and natalizumab).

▶ Antidiarrheal agent.

▶ Empiric therapy if suspect inflammatory bacterial pathogen.

▶ Questran (cholestyramine resin) may help absorb toxins.

▶ Maintain a healthy diet and hydration.

▶ Avoid caffeine.

Prevention

▶ Maintain a healthy diet and hydration.

▶ Avoid caffeine.

DYSPHAGIA

▶ Difficulty swallowing and passing food from mouth to esophagus to stomach

Risk Factors

▶ Oropharyngeal disorders

▶ Neurologic disorders

▶ Muscular disorders

▶ Motility disorders

▶ Structural disorders

▶ Esophageal disorder

▶ Mechanical obstruction

Signs and Symptoms

▶ Difficulty chewing or swallowing

▶ Coughing during or after eating or drinking

▶ Gurgling, wet-sounding voice during or after eating or drinking

▶ Food or liquid leaking from the mouth or getting stuck in the mouth

▶ Recurring pneumonia or chest congestion after eating

Diagnostic Tests

▶ Observe eating

▷ Positioning, utensil use, feeding technique

▶ Swallowing evaluation by speech therapist

▶ Barium swallow

Differential Diagnoses

▶ Esophageal cancer

▶ Gastroesophageal reflux disease (GERD)

▶ Multiple sclerosis

▶ Hiatal hernia

▶ Achalasia

Management

▶ Position upright at 90-degree angle during meals

▶ Position upright for 30 minutes after meals

▶ Frequent cueing

▶ • Small bites, chin tuck

▶ • Thicken liquids

▶ Wear dentures

▶ Mouth care

Prevention

▶ Eat slowly.

▶ Chew food thoroughly.

▶ Sit upright when eating.

ACUTE ABDOMEN

▶ Sudden, severe abdominal pain of unclear etiology for less than 24 hours.

▶ Identifying the location, duration, type, precipitating and relieving factors, and pain intensity, and differentiating abdominal pain from chest pain, narrow differential diagnoses.

Risk Factors

▶ • Gallstones

▶ Hypertension out of control

▶ Hypotension

▶ • Bowel obstruction

▶ Previous abdominal surgery

Signs and Symptoms

▶ Pain

▶ • Rebound tenderness (seen in peritonitis and appendicitis)

▶ • Cardiac pain can extend from jaw to epigastric area

▶ • Nitroglycerin

▷ May relieve some GI pain as a result of decreasing tone of esophageal muscles

▶ • Shock

▷ Often seen in pancreatitis or hemorrhage

▶ • Vomiting

▷ Often means obstruction of bowel or biliary duct

▶ • Muscular rigidity

▷ Seen with perforated viscous or mucosal ulceration

▶ Abdominal distension

▷ Seen in large-bowel obstruction

Diagnostic Tests

▶ CBC, electrolytes, amylase, lipase, liver function tests (LFTs)

▶ Urinalysis

▶ Stool for occult blood

▶ Electrocardiogram (ECG)

▶ Chest X-ray (CXR)

▶ Flat plate and upright abdominal film to test for obstruction, ileus, perforation, biliary or renal stones

▶ US and/or CT scans

Differential Diagnoses

▶ Cholecystitis

▶ Ischemic bowel

▶ Abdominal trauma

▶ Aortic aneurysm

▶ Celiac disease

▶ Peptic ulcer

▶ Diverticulitis

▶ Abdominal compartment syndrome

Management

▶ Depends on etiology.

▶ Signs and symptoms may be subtle in older adults.

▷ Absence of fever

▷ Altered pain perception from chronic pain medications

▷ Comorbidities

▷ Localized tenderness diminished

▷ Reduced rebound and guarding

▶ Refer for surgical evaluation in acute situation.

▶ Can refer to gastroenterologist for less acute cases.

Prevention

▶ No known prevention

GASTROESOPHAGEAL REFLUX DISEASE (GERD)

▶ Lower esophageal sphincter dysfunction with transient, spontaneous relaxation in lower esophageal sphincter (LES) tone allows reflux of acid that irritates mucosa

Risk Factors

▶ Factors that decrease LES tone

▶ Delayed gastric emptying

▶ Sliding hiatal hernia

▶ Decreased saliva and esophageal peristalsis at night

▶ Eating large meals or lying down within 3 hours after eating

▶ Wearing tight clothing

▶ Obesity

▶ Anxiety

▶ Smoking, opioid or alcohol consumption

Signs and Symptoms

▶ • Heartburn; retrosternal burning discomfort 30–60 minutes after meals exacerbated by lying supine or bending over

▶ Dysphagia, odynophagia, nausea

▶ Chest pain, asthma

▶ Hoarseness, sore throat, cough

Diagnostic Tests

▶ • pH monitoring to measure acid over 24–48 hours

▶ • Endoscopy

▶ • Manometry for LES motility and pressure

Differential Diagnoses

▶ Achalasia

▶ Gastritis

▶ Cholelithiasis

▶ Coronary artery disease (CAD)

▶ Esophageal cancer

▶ Esophageal or intestinal motility disorders

▶ Esophageal spasm, esophagitis

▶ *H. pylori* infection

▶ Hiatal hernia

▶ Intestinal malrotation

▶ Irritable bowel syndrome

▶ Peptic ulcer disease

Management

▶ Instruct patient to

▷ Maintain optimal weight;

▷ Avoid chocolate, caffeine, spicy foods, citrus, carbonated beverages;

▷ Avoid tobacco;

▷ Limit alcohol intake;

▷ Eat small, frequent meals;

▷ Refrain from lying down for 3 hours after eating; and

▷ Elevate the head of the bed when sleeping.

▶ Antacids to neutralize gastric acid

▷ Calcium carbonate (Tums, Rolaids), sodium bicarbonate (Alka-Seltzer), aluminum salts (Amphojel, Basaljel), magnesium salts (milk of magnesia, Uro-Mag, Mag-Ox)

▷ Combination products: Aluminum hydroxide and magnesium hydroxide (Maalox, Mylanta, Gelusil), alginic acid, magnesium trisilicate, calcium stearate (Gaviscon)

▶ Alginic acid derivatives (Gaviscon) to act as a barrier to keep acid below the esophagus

▶ Histamine-2 (H2) receptor antagonists

▷ Inhibit H2 receptors and decrease stomach acid

▷ Used first-line for mild to moderate symptoms

▷ Ranitidine (Zantac) 300 mg h.s., famotidine (Pepcid) 40 mg h.s., nizatidine (Axid) 300 mg h.s.

▶ Proton pump inhibitors (PPIs)

▷ Decrease stomach acid

▷ First-line therapy for erosive esophagitis or symptoms not relieved by H2 blockers

▷ Omeprazole (Prilosec) 40 mg daily or 20 mg b.i.d.; esomeprazole (Nexium) 40 mg daily; lansoprazole (Prevacid) 30 mg daily; rabeprazole (Aciphex) 20 mg daily; pantoprazole (Protonix; injectable or p.o.), normal dose 40 mg p.o.

▶ Complications

▷ Aspiration pneumonitis

▷ Asthma

▷ Laryngeal granulomas

▷ Subglottic stenosis

Prevention

▶ Avoid agents that reduce LES tone (table 10–1).

TABLE 10–1.
AGENTS THAT REDUCE LES TONE

Anticholinergics	Alcohol
Morphine	Caffeine
Theophylline	Mint
Calcium channel blockers	Chocolate
Nitrates	Citrus and spicy foods
Nicotine	High-fat foods

PEPTIC ULCER DISEASE (PUD)

▶ Ulceration in gastric or duodenal mucosa of the stomach.

▶ ● Most often occurs between ages 55 and 70 years.

▶ ● Alcohol and dietary factors do not appear to cause PUD; role of stress is uncertain.

Risk Factors

▶ ● Tobacco use

▶ Acid hypersecretory states

▶ ● Chronic *H. pylori* infection (95 percent of duodenal ulcers)

▶ ● Nonsteroidal anti-inflammatory drugs (NSAIDs; 15 percent gastric and 5 percent duodenal ulcers)

▶ Possibly stress

▶ Family history of ulcers

Signs and Symptoms

▶ ● Gnawing, rhythmic epigastric pain or dull ache

▶ ● Pain well localized to epigastrium

▶ ● Pain relieved after meals (duodenal)

▶ ● Pain worsened with meals (gastric)

▶ ● Nausea, anorexia, weight loss (gastric)

▶ Mild, localized epigastric tenderness on deep palpation

Diagnostic Tests

▶ Endoscopic: Culture, histology, rapid urease testing, polymerase chain reaction (PCR; Chey and Wong 2007).

▶ Nonendoscopic: Antibody testing, urea breath tests, fecal antigen test (Chey and Wong 2007).

▶ Indications for post *H. pylori* treatment testing:

▷ *H. pylori*–associated ulcer

▷ Persistent dyspeptic symptoms despite the test-and-treat strategy

▷ ● *H. pylori*–associated mucosa-associated lymphoid tissue (MALT) lymphoma

▷ History of resection of early gastric cancer (Chey and Wong 2007)

▶ Detect malignancy and *H. pylori* infection.

▷ For gastric ulcers: Endoscopy after 8–12 weeks of treatment

▶ Late disease or acute bleed.

▷ Anemia

▶ Leukocytosis indicates ulcer penetration or perforation.

▷ ● Elevated serum amylase with pain indicates penetration into pancreas.

▶ ● Secretin stimulation test: Serum gastrin > 200 pg/mL in 85 percent of gastrinomas.

▶ ● Serum gastrin > 150 pg/mL in hypersecretion states.

Differential Diagnoses

▶ GERD

▶ Hiatal hernia

▶ Cholecystitis

▶ Pancreatitis

▶ Biliary tract disease

▶ Gastric carcinoma

▶ Cardiovascular disease (CVD)

▶ Diverticulitis

▶ Esophagitis

▶ Irritable bowel disease

▶ Viral hepatitis
(Anand and Katz 2017)

Management

▶ Stop smoking.

▶ Stop NSAIDs.

▶ Limit alcoholic beverages.

▷ No more than two drinks daily for men and one for women.

- ▶ ● *H. pylori*–induced ulcers
    - ▷ Eradicate *H. pylori*.
    - ▷ Proton pump inhibitor (PPI) and antibiotics for 7–14 days.
    - ▷ Continue PPI or H2 blocker after eradication.
- ▶ NSAID- and corticosteroid-induced ulcers
    - ▷ Discontinue offending agent if possible.
    - ▷ ● Misoprostol 100 mcg q.i.d. or 200 mcg b.i.d.
    - ▷ ● If stopping NSAIDs is not possible, use a PPI.
    - ▷ ● H2 blockers, sucralfate, and antacids do not prevent NSAID-induced ulcers.
- ▶ Prophylactic therapy for history of ulcers or GI bleeds
    - ▷ ● PPIs (take 30 minutes before meals)
        - ▶ Omeprazole (Prilosec) 20 mg daily
        - ▶ Lansoprazole (Prevacid) 30 mg daily
        - ▶ Rabeprazole (Aciphex) 20 mg daily
        - ▶ Pantoprazole (Protonix) 40 mg daily
        - ▶ Some concern about gastric cancer with long-term use
- ▶ ● H2 receptor agonists
    - ▷ Cimetidine (Tagamet) 800 mg h.s.
    - ▷ Ranitidine (Zantac) 300 mg h.s.
    - ▷ Famotidine (Pepcid) 40 mg h.s.
    - ▷ Nizatidine (Axid)300 mg h.s.
- ▶ ● Mucosal protective agents (take 2 hours apart from other meds)
    - ▷ Sucralfate (Carafate) 1 g q.i.d
        - ▶ Helps reduce incidence of nosocomial pneumonia
- ▶ ● Bismuth (Pepto-Bismol)
- ▶ *H. pylori* eradication
    - ▷ PPI b.i.d. *and* amoxicillin 1 g b.i.d. *and* clarithromycin 500 mg b.i.d. for 10–14 days if not allergic to penicillin or has not previously received a macrolide.
    - ▷ If allergic to penicillin: PPI b.i.d. *and* clarithromycin 500 mg b.i.d. *and* metronidazole 500 mg b.i.d. for 10–14 days.
    - ▷ If patient has been exposed to a macrolide, quadruple therapy for 14 days: Bismuth subsalicylate 2 tabs (525 mg) or 30 cc q.i.d. *and* metronidazole 500 mg q.i.d. *and* tetracycline 500 mg q.i.d. *and* PPI.
    - ▷ The problem of clarithromycin resistance is growing.
    - ▷ Resistance to amoxicillin or tetracycline not developing as quickly.
- ▶ *H. pylori* combination treatment
    - ▷ Combination products available but high cost, often not covered by insurance

▷ Prevpac 14-blister cards

  ▶ Two 30 mg lansoprazole capsules

  ▶ Four 500mg amoxicillin tablets

  ▶ Two 500 mg clarithromycin tabs

TABLE 10–2.
PUD MANAGEMENT

H. PYLORI-INDUCED ULCERS	NSAID- AND CORTICOSTEROID-INDUCED ULCERS	PROPHYLACTIC THERAPY FOR HISTORY OF ULCERS OR GI BLEEDS	H2 RECEPTOR AGONISTS	MUCOSAL PROTECTIVE AGENTS
Eradicate *H. pylori*	Discontinue offending agent if possible	PPIs 30 minutes before meals • Omeprazole (Prilosec) 20 mg daily • Lansoprazole (Prevacid) 30 mg daily • Rabeprazole (Aciphex) 20 mg daily • Pantoprazole (Protonix) 40 mg daily Some concern about gastric cancer with long-term use	• Cimetidine (Tagamet) 800 mg h.s. • Ranitidine (Zantac) 300 mg h.s. • Famotidine (Pepcid) 40 mg h.s. • Nizatidine (Axid) 300 mg h.s	Take 2 hours apart from other meds • Sucralfate (Carafate) 1 g q.i.d
PPI and antibiotics for 7–14 days	Misoprostol 100 mcg q.i.d. or 200 mcg b.i.d.			• Helps reduce incidence of nosocomial pneumonia
Continue PPI or H2 blocker after eradication	If stopping NSAIDs is not possible, use a proton pump inhibitor H2 blockers, sucralfate, antacids do not prevent NSAID ulcer			

Prevention

▶ Hand hygiene.

▶ Proper food handling.

▶ Avoid contaminated water.

ZOLLINGER-ELLISON SYNDROME (ZES)

▶ • Rare condition in which gastronomas form in the duodenum or pancreas and secrete large amounts of gastrin, causing the stomach to produce excess acid

▶ Quantity of acid produced leads to gastrointestinal mucosal ulceration (duodenal ulcers between ages 30 and 55 years), diarrhea, and malabsorption

Risk Factors

▶ • Duodonal ulcer

▶ Family members with MEN 1

▶ • Multiple endocrine neoplasia type 1 (MEN 1) present a decade earlier

▶ History of endocrine disorders

Signs and Symptoms

▶ Diarrhea

▶ Abdominal pain

▶ Heartburn

▶ Nausea, vomiting

▶ Gastrointestinal bleeding

▶ Weight loss

▶ Jaundice

▶ Epigastric tenderness

▶ Hepatomegaly

Diagnostic Tests

▶ • Fasting serum gastrin level

▶ Calcium

▶ • Gastric acid secretory tests

▷ Gastric pH < 2.0 in gastric volume (>140 mL over 1 hour) is highly suggestive of ZES.

▶ Provocative tests

▷ ● Secretin stimulation test, calcium stimulation test, secretin-plus-calcium stimulation tests, bombesin test, and protein meal test

Differential Diagnoses

▶ Gastric outlet obstruction

▶ Recurrent peptic ulcers

Management

▶ Proton pump inhibitors

▶ H2 blockers

▶ Somatostatin analogs to control tumor growth

▶ Surgical intervention to remove tumors

▶ Chemotherapy in rapidly growing tumors or tumors that cannot be removed

Prevention

▶ None known

GASTRIC CANCER

▶ Malignant cells in stomach lining

Risk Factors

▶ *H. pylori* infection

▶ Chronic atrophic gastritis

▶ East Asian, South American, or eastern or central European descent

▶ Men over 40 years old

▶ Diet high in nitrites

▶ Smoking

▶ Stomach lymphoma

▶ Obesity

▶ Pernicious anemia

▶ Radiation exposure
(Karimi et al. 2014)

Signs and Symptoms

▶ ●Dyspepsia, epigastric pain, early satiety

▶ Occasional complaints of nausea and vomiting

▶ Weight loss

▶ Refer to gastroenterologist if gastric cancer suspected

Diagnostic Tests

▶ Endoscopy

▶ Biopsy

▶ Ultrasound

▶ Computed tomography (CT) scan

▷ For staging

▶ Bone scan

▶ Positron emission tomography (PET) scan

▶ Laparoscopy

Differential Diagnoses

▶ Gastritis

▶ Esophageal cancer

▶ Non-Hodgkins lymphoma

▶ Peptic ulcer disease

Management

▶ Surgery

▷ Total or partial gastrectomy and nearby lymph nodes

▶ Chemotherapy

▷ Before and after surgery or metastasis

▶ Radiation

▷ To kill cancer cells and shrink tumors

Prevention

▶ Smoking cessation

▶ Healthy diet; increased fruits and vegetables; fiber

▶ Treat GERD

CHOLELITHIASIS (GALLSTONES) AND CHOLECYSTITIS (GALLBLADDER INFLAMMATION)

▶ Blockage of bile flow through bile ducts.

▶ Over 90 percent of cases are caused by cystic duct obstruction by an impacted stone.

Risk Factors

▶ ● Genetic predisposition

▶ ● Obesity or rapid weight loss

▶ Diabetes mellitus

▶ Crohn's disease

▶ Cirrhosis

▶ Hyperlipidemia

▶ Medications that increase cholesterol saturation

▶ ● Estrogen products

▶ ● Gemfibrozil

Signs and Symptoms

▶ Cholelithiasis

▷ Frequently asymptomatic

▷ ● May have nausea or vomiting

▷ ● Right upper quadrant (RUQ) pain, usually after fatty meal

▶ Cholecystitis

▷ ● Colicky epigastric or RUQ tenderness

▷ ● Increased pain on inspiration during palpation of RUQ under costal margin

▶ Pain

▷ ● May radiate to right shoulder or scapula if phrenic nerve irritated

▶ Nausea and vomiting

▶ Fever

▶ Jaundice if biliary obstruction

▶ ● Leukocytosis, elevated ALT (alanine transaminase), AST (aspartate transaminase), GGT (gamma-glutamyl transpeptidase), alkaline phosphatase, and bilirubin

▶ Amylase elevated when bile duct obstructed

Diagnostic Tests

▶ Cholelithiasis

▷ ● Abdominal X-ray or ultrasound

▶ Cholecystitis

▷ ● CBC, electrolytes, amylase, ALT, AST, GGT, alkaline phosphatase, bilirubin,

▷ ● Magnetic resonance cholangiography

▷ ● Endoscopic retrograde cholangiopancreatography (ERCP)

▷ ● Hydroxy-iminodiacetic acid (HIDA) scan

Differential Diagnoses

▶ Acute pancreatitis or appendicitis

▶ Bile duct strictures or tumors

▶ Cholecystitis

▶ Gastroenteritis

▶ Gallbladder or pancreatic cancer

▶ Peptic ulcer disease

Management

▶ ● Low-fat diet, bile salts

▶ ● Bile salts (Actigall [ursodiol] tablets) to dissolve stones, may take years

▶ Shock wave therapy (rarely used)

▶ Cholecystectomy

Prevention

▶ Maintain optimal weight

▶ Healthy diet

▶ Exercise

IRRITABLE BOWEL SYNDROME (IBS)

▶ Chronic recurrent abdominal pain and altered bowel function of unknown etiology

▶ Abnormal intestinal motility; no organic disease

Risk Factors

▶ Young adult, late twenties

▶ Female

▶ Psychological disorders

▶ Psychological trauma

▶ Family history of IBS

Signs and Symptoms

▶ ◦ Lower abdominal pain and cramping with tenderness on palpation.

▶ ◦ Constipation, diarrhea, or both.

    ▷ Diarrhea should not wake patient from sleep.

▶ Mucus in stools is clear.

▶ ◦ Symptoms worsened with meals and stress, relieved by defecation.

Diagnostic Tests

▶ ◦ CBC, erythrocyte sedimentation rate (ESR), thyroid function tests (TFTs), fecal occult blood test (FOBT)

▶ Stool culture for bacteria, ova and parasites, *C. difficile* toxin

▶ Colonoscopy

    ▷ To rule out organic disease

    ▷ ◦ Decreased pain threshold with abdominal distention from flatus

▶ ◦ Symptom onset at least 6 months prior to diagnosis and Rome III diagnostic criteria met for the last 3 months:

    ▷ ◦ Recurrent abdominal pain or discomfort at least 3 days per month in the last 3 months associated with two or more of the following:

        ▶ ◦ Improvement with defecation

        ▶ ◦ Onset associated with a change in frequency of stool

        ▶ ◦ Onset associated with a change in form (appearance) of stool (International Foundation for Functional Gastrointestinal Disorders [IFFGD] 2016)

Differential Diagnoses

▶ Anxiety disorders

▶ Gastroenteritis

▶ Biliary disease

▶ Celiac disease (sprue)

▶ Mesenteric ischemia

▶ Colitis

▶ Cancer

▶ Lead toxicity

▶ Endometriosis

▶ Food allergies

▶ Giardiasis

▶ Hypercalcemia

▶ Thyroid disease

▶ Inflammatory bowel disease

▶ Lactose intolerance

▶ Pheochromocytoma

Management

▶ Lactose-free diet for 2 weeks to rule out lactose intolerance

▶ High-fiber diet

▶ Fiber supplement

▶ Bulk-forming agents (psyllium, methylcellulose)

   ▷ 5 HT4 receptor agonist for IBS in women with constipation-predominant disease

▶ Anticholinergic agents

   ▷ Dicyclomine, hyoscyamine

▶ Antidiarrheal agents p.r.n.

▶ Simethicone for flatus

▶ Antidepressants

Prevention

▶ Instruct patient to

   ▷ Avoid dietary triggers;

   ▷ Gradually increase dietary fiber;

   ▷ Drink eight 8-ounce glasses of water a day; and

   ▷ Eat smaller, more frequent meals.

DIVERTICULOSIS AND DIVERTICULITIS

▶ Diverticulosis: Pouches form on colon wall, resulting in hypertrophy and fibrosing of bowel wall, leading to diverticulitis from infection

▶ Diverticulitis: Caused by mechanical obstruction from retained undigested food residue and bacteria in diverticula

▶ Hypertrophy and fibrosing of bowel wall from years of moving hard stool under high intraluminal pressures; thought to be caused by low-fiber diet

Risk Factors

- ▶ Low-fiber diet
- ▶ Sedentary lifestyle
- ▶ Advanced age
- ▶ Obesity
- ▶ ● Red meat consumption

Signs and Symptoms

- ▶ Diverticulosis does not cause symptoms.
- ▶ ● Diverticulitis:
  - ▷ Diarrhea and cramping abdominal pain, bloating
  - ▷ Alternating diarrhea and constipation
  - ▷ Painful cramps
  - ▷ ● Tenderness in the lower abdomen
  - ▷ Chills or fever
  - ▷ Localized tenderness
  - ▷ Abdominal mass may be present
  - ▷ Decreased bowel sounds

Diagnostic Tests

- ▶ CBC, ESR, FOBT
- ▶ ● Flat-plate abdominal X-ray
- ▶ Endoscopy
- ▶ ● Diverticulitis
  - ▷ Mild to moderate leukocytosis; elevated ESR
  - ▷ Stool test for occult blood is often positive
  - ▷ Flat plate X-ray of abdomen to look for perforation, ileus, or obstruction
- ▶ ● Diverticulosis
  - ▷ Labs normal

Differential Diagnoses

- ▶ IBS
- ▶ Gastroenteritis
- ▶ Cholecystitis
- ▶ Appendicitis

▶ Bowel obstruction

▶ Colitis

▶ Colorectal cancer

▶ Urologic disorders

▶ Gynecological disorders

Management

▶ ▪ Diverticulosis:

  ▷ High-fiber diet

▶ ▪ Diverticulitis:

  ▷ Bowel rest: Clear liquids only.

  ▷ Low-residue diet (while acutely ill).

  ▷ Encourage fluid intake.

  ▷ Keep stools soft.

▶ Mild symptoms

  ▷ Consider no antibiotics

▶ Moderate symptoms

  ▷ Treatment duration 7–10 days, use *one* of the following treatments

    ▶ ▪ Trimethoprim with sulfamethoxazole (Bactrim DS) 160 mg/800 mg 1 tablet p.o. b.i.d. *plus* metronidazole 500 mg p.o. q.i.d.

    ▶ ▪ Ciprofloxacin 750 mg p.o. b.i.d. *plus* metronidazole 500 mg p.o. q.i.d.

    ▶ ▪ Levofloxacin 750 mg p.o. daily *plus* metronidazole 500 mg p.o. q.i.d.

    ▶ ▪ Amoxicillin/clavulanate extended release (Augmentin XR), two 1,000/62.5-mg tablets p.o. q12h

    ▶ ▪ Moxifloxacin 400 mg p.o. daily

▶ Moderate to severe symptoms

  ▷ Require hospitalization and intravenous (IV) antibiotics

Prevention

▶ Exercise

▶ Optimal weight

▶ Fiber-rich diet or fiber supplementation in patients with a history of acute diverticulitis

UNINTENTIONAL WEIGHT LOSS AND MALNUTRITION

▶ Unexplained, unintentional weight loss ≥ 5–10 percent of body weight in 3–6 months

▶ Cause not found in 25 percent of patients

▶ See table 10–3

Risk Factors

▶ Depression in 30 percent

▶ Dementia

▶ Cancer

▶ Hyperthyroidism

▶ Infection

▶ Poor dentition

▶ Gingivitis

▶ Illnesses with fatigue

▶ Anorexia

▶ Dysphagia

▶ Extreme dieting and unpalatable diets

▶ Aging changes

▷ Decreased appetite, changes in taste and smell

▶ Medications

▷ May cause dry mouth, dysgeusia, anorexia, nausea, vomiting, diarrhea, or constipation

Signs and Symptoms

▶ Fatigue, feeling cold, depression

▶ Frequent infections and extended recovery time

▶ Delayed wound-healing

▶ Poor concentration

TABLE 10–3.
ETIOLOGY OF UNINTENTIONAL WEIGHT LOSS AND MALNUTRITION

SOCIAL AND PSYCHOLOGICAL	MEDICATIONS	DIETS
Poverty	Diuretics; NSAIDs	Low salt
Bereavement	Antidepressants	Low cholesterol
Inability to get food	Parasympathetics; antineoplastics	Diabetic exchange
	Anticholinergics	

Diagnostic Tests

▶ • Cone beam computed tomography (CBCt), complete metabolic panel, calcium, albumin, TFTs, total protein, carbohydrate, prostate-specific antigen (men only), urinalysis, FOBT, chest X-ray

▶ • Body-mass index (BMI) calculation

▷ BMI 18.5–24.9: Normal

▷ BMI < 18.5: High risk of malnourishment

Differential Diagnoses

▶ Malignancy

▶ Infection

▶ Bulimia or anorexia nervosa

▶ Hyperthyroidism

▶ Diabetes mellitus

Management

▶ Drugs to stimulate appetite

▶ • Progestin (Megace) 400–800 mg daily

▷ Dosage controversial in older adults; may increase risk of DVT

▶ • Methylphenidate (Ritalin)

▷ Stimulant; use with caution

▶ • Mirtazapine (Remeron)

▶ • Nutrition consult recommended; weekly weights

▶ Gastrostomy tube (G-tube) for artificial nutrition and hydration

▷ Not recommended in terminal disease: Prolongs suffering, does not change outcome or improve quality of life

Prevention

▶ Treat underlying cause (i.e., depression, GI disorder, thyroid disorder).

▶ Dietician consult

COLORECTAL CANCER

▶ • Cancer that starts in the colon or the rectum, beginning as a noncancerous polyp on the inner lining of the colon or rectum.

▶ Third most commonly diagnosed cancer in men and women.

▶ ● Lifetime risk of developing colorectal cancer is about one in twenty (5 percent), but death rate dropping because of early identification of polyps via colonoscopy.

▶ ○ Staging is done using the American Joint Committee on Cancer (AJCC) **TNM** system (American Cancer Society 2016):

    ▷ How far the main (primary) **tumor (T)** has grown into the wall of the intestine and whether it has grown into nearby areas

    ▷ Whether the cancer has spread to nearby (regional) lymph **nodes (N)**

    ▷ Whether the cancer has spread (*metastasized*) to other organs of the body **(M)**

Risk Factors

▶ Heredity

▶ Obesity

▶ ● Red meat and processed foods

▶ ○ Polyps

▶ Smoking

▶ Sedentary lifestyle

▶ Excessive alcohol intake

Signs and Symptoms

▶ Change in bowel habits

▶ Rectal bleeding

▶ Cramping abdominal pain

▶ Weakness and fatigue

▶ Unintended weight loss

▶ Mass palpated in abdomen

▶ Rectal mass upon digital exam

▶ Liver enlargement

Diagnostic Tests

▶ Stool for occult blood

▶ CBC

▶ Carcinoembryonic antigen (CEA)

▶ Liver function tests

▶ Colonoscopy

▶ Abdominal CT

▶ FOBT and fecal immunochemical test (FIT)

Differential Diagnoses

▶ Arteriovenous malformation (AVM)

▶ Carcinoid or neuroendocrine tumors

▶ Ischemic bowel

▶ Small-intestine carcinomas

▶ Gastrointestinal lymphoma

▶ Crohn's disease

▶ Ileus

▶ Small intestinal diverticulosis

▶ Ulcerative colitis

Management

▶ Based on stages

▶ Surgical resection

▶ Chemotherapy, radiation

Prevention

▶ Colorectal cancer screening.

▶ Avoid smoking.

▶ Avoid a sedentary lifestyle.

▶ Maintain optimal weight.

▶ Follow a diet low in animal fats and high in fruits, vegetables, and whole grains.

ABDOMINAL HERNIAS

▶ Weakened abdominal wall with extrusion of abdominal organs into the fascia.

▶ Types:

▷ ● Inguinal

▶ Indirect hernias are near internal ring and often extend into scrotum.

▶ Direct hernias occur near external ring, through the inguinal floor.

▷ ● Femoral

▶ Palpable medial to femoral vessels and inferior to inguinal canal

▷ ● Umbilical

▶ Small hernias visible if patient raises their head

▷ ● Epigastric

▶ Usually a small mass between umbilicus and xiphoid

▶ All hernias are reducible or nonreducible.

  ▷ ● Reducible

    ▶ Can be pushed back into abdominal cavity

  ▷ ● Nonreducible

    ▶ Incarcerated: Cannot be pushed back into abdominal cavity.

    ▶ Strangulated: Blood supply to hernia is compromised.

Risk Factors

▶ Marked obesity

▶ Heavy lifting, coughing

▶ ● Straining with defecation and/or urination

▶ ● Ascites or peritoneal dialysis

▶ ● Chronic obstructive pulmonary disease (COPD)

▶ Family history of hernias

Signs and Symptoms

▶ May be asymptomatic

▶ ● Swelling or fullness at the hernia site

▶ Aching sensation (radiates into the area of the hernia)

▶ No true pain or tenderness upon examination if not incarcerated or strangulated

▶ ● Enlarges with increasing intra-abdominal pressure or standing

▶ Incarcerated hernias

  ▷ Painful enlargement of a previous hernia or defect

  ▷ Cannot be manipulated (either spontaneously or manually) through the fascial defect

  ▷ Nausea, vomiting, and symptoms of bowel obstruction possible

▶ Strangulated hernias

  ▷ Patients have symptoms of an incarcerated hernia.

  ▷ Systemic toxicity secondary to ischemic bowel is possible.

  ▷ ● Strangulation is probable if the pain and tenderness of an incarcerated hernia persist after reduction.

▶ Suspect alternative diagnosis in patients who have a substantial amount of pain without evidence of incarceration or strangulation

Diagnostic Tests

▶ Stain or culture of nodal tissue

▶ CBC

- ▶ Electrolytes, BUN, and creatinine
- ▶ Urinalysis
- ▶ Lactate
- ▶ Imaging studies not required but may be useful
- ▶ Ultrasonography
- ▶ Differentiate groin or abdominal wall masses, or testicular swelling
- ▶ Chest, flat plate X-ray
- ▶ CT
    - ▷ Incarcerated or strangulated hernia
    - ▷ If examination cannot be performed because of habitus, or to diagnose a spigelian or obturator hernia

Differential Diagnoses

- ▶ Constipation
- ▶ Groin abscess
- ▶ Hematoma or lipoma
- ▶ Lymphadenitis
- ▶ Obstructive uropathy
- ▶ Pseudoaneurysm
- ▶ Tumor
- ▶ Undescended or retracted testes
- ▶ Varicocele or spermatocele
- ▶ Epididymitis
- ▶ Testicular torsion

Management

- ▶ Education on proper lifting
- ▶ No straining with exertion, lifting, or bowel movement
- ▶ Trusses
- ▶ Binders or corsets
- ▶ Hernia reduction
- ▶ Topical therapy
- ▶ Compression dressings
- ▶ Surgical repair

Prevention

▶ Maintain optimal weight.

▶ Use proper body mechanics with lifting.

▶ Avoid constipation.

▶ Avoid smoking.

HEMORRHOIDS

▶ Varicosities of hemorrhoidal venous plexus classified as

▷ Internal

▶ Above pectinate line

▶ Internal hemorrhoids may prolapse and strangulate, causing thrombosis.

▷ External

▶ Below pectinate line

Risk Factors

▶ Alcoholism

▶ Anal intercourse

▶ Chronic diarrhea or constipation

▶ High-fat, low-fiber diet

▶ Obesity

▶ Long periods of sitting or standing

▶ Sedentary lifestyle

▶ Loss of pelvic floor muscle tone

▷ Due to age, pregnancy, childbirth, or surgery

▶ Severe heart disease or liver disease

▶ Straining while lifting or having a bowel movement

▶ Increased portal venous pressure

Signs and Symptoms

▶ Rectal bleeding, painless and bright red

▶ Rectal discomfort, itching, burning

▶ Constipation or straining

Diagnostic Tests

▶ ˵ Digital rectal exam

▶ ˵Anoscope, proctoscope, or sigmoidoscope exam

Differential Diagnoses

▶ IBS

▶ Acute proctitis

▶ Condyloma acuminata

▶ Rectal prolapse

▶ Ulcerative colitis

▶ Crohn's disease

▶ Pregnancy

Management

▶ Eliminate risk factors

▶ ˳ Warm sitz baths, 2–3 daily, 20 minutes each

▶ ˳ Witch hazel (Tucks) compresses t.i.d.–q.i.d., p.r.n.

▶ ˳ Bulk-forming laxatives

▶ ˳Stool softeners

▶ ˳Topical cortisone preparations

▶ Local analgesic

▶ Surgical intervention

Prevention

▶ Eat a high-fiber diet.

▶ Avoid prolonged sitting.

▶ Exercise.

▶ Drink plenty of fluids.

▶ Do not strain with bowel movements.

FLATULENCE

▶ Accumulation of gas in the alimentary canal, often caused by disaccharide (lactose, fructose) maldigestion

Risk Factors

▶   Antibiotics, laxatives, other medications

▶   Artificial sweeteners

▶   Constipation

▶   Food intolerances

▶   Diverticulitis, ulcerative colitis, or Crohn's disease

▶   Cirrhosis; bowel obstruction; or bowel, pancreatic, ovarian, or uterine cancer

Signs and Symptoms

▶   Bloating (usually)

▶   Pain

▶   Eructation

Diagnostic Tests

▶   X-ray

▶   Endoscopy

▶   Colonoscopy

▶   Tissue transglutaminase antibodies (tTG-IgA) to rule out celiac disease

Differential Diagnoses

▶   None

Management

▶   Beano as per package instructions (with food)

▶   Replace lactase enzyme

▶   Simethicone

Prevention

▶   Patient education to include

  ▷   Avoid food offenders or limit consumption;

  ▷   Eat slowly;

  ▷   Do not chew gum or use straws;

  ▷   Avoid swallowing excessive air; and

  ▷   Avoid carbonated beverages.

ERUCTATION

▶ Burping or belching to release gas from stomach

Risk Factors

▶ Air swallowing is a major source of stomach gas.

▷ Often swallowed with food.

▷ Usually functional.

Signs and Symptoms

▶ Thoracic or abdominal discomfort possible

Diagnostic Tests

▶ None

Differential Diagnoses

▶ None

Management

▶ Patient education on preventative measures

▶ ● Baclofen 10 mg three times daily

Prevention

▶ Patient education to include

▷ Avoid food offenders or limit consumption;

▷ Eat slowly;

▷ Do not chew gum or use straws;

▷ Avoid swallowing excessive air; and

▷ Avoid carbonated beverages.

GASTROENTERITIS

▶ Syndrome of acute nausea, vomiting, and diarrhea from acute gastric mucosal irritation or inflammation

▶ Etiology

▷ Viral, bacterial, or parasitic

▷ Inorganic food contents

Risk Factors

► Ingesting contaminated food or water

► Poor hand hygiene

► Immunocompromised state

► Travel to developing countries

► Attending daycare

► Nursing home residents

► Consuming raw shellfish or seafood (Dunphy et al. 2015)

Signs and Symptoms

► Nausea, vomiting, anorexia

► Watery diarrhea

► General "sick" feeling

► Crampy abdominal pain

► Febrile state (varies)

► Tachycardia, hypotension

► Neurological findings

► Hyperactive bowel sounds

► Possibly abdominal distention

Diagnostic Tests

► No diagnostics indicated unless symptoms persist longer than 72 hours or stool is bloody

► Stool guaiac and white blood count (WBC)

► Stool culture and check for ova and parasites

Differential Diagnoses

► Appendicitis

► Diverticulitis

► Cholecystitis

► Colitis

Management

► Rehydrate with clear liquids.

► Progress to bland diet.

▶ Bed rest during acute phase with progression as tolerated.

▶ Antidiarrheal drugs

  ▷ Opiates and derivatives

  ▷ Antisecretory

  ▷ Absorbents

▶ Antibiotics

  ▷ Usually not indicated, unless

    ▶ Organism isolated and symptoms not resolved;

    ▶ *Salmonella*, leukocytes, or dysentery;

    ▶ Treat for *Shigella* when more than 8–10 stools daily; or

    ▶ Immunocompromised

      ▷ • Ciprofloxacin 500 mg p.o. b.i.d. × 3 days

      ▷ • Ofloxacin 200 mg b.i.d. for up to 3 days

      ▷ • Levofloxacin 500 mg daily for up to 3 days

Prevention

▶ Safe food handling.

▶ Hand hygiene.

▶ • Prophylactic antibiotics should not be recommended for most travelers (Centers for Disease Control and Prevention [CDC] 2017).

REFERENCES

American Cancer Society. 2016. "Colorectal Cancer Stages." http://www.cancer.org/cancer/ colonandrectumcancer/detailedguide/colorectal-cancer-staged.

Anand, B. S. 2017. "Peptic Ulcer Disease Differential Diagnoses." Medscape. http://emedicine. medscape.com/article/181753-differential.

Bharucha, A., S. Dorn, A. Lembo, and A. Pressman. 2013. "American Gastroenterological Association Medical Position Statement on Constipation." *Gastroenterology* 144 (1): 211–17. http://dx.doi.org/10.1053/j.gastro.2012.10.029.

Centers for Disease Control and Prevention. 2015. "General Information." Parasites – *Giardia*. http://www.cdc.gov/parasites/giardia/general-info.html.

———. 2017. "The Pretravel Consultation." In *CDC Yellow Book 2018: Health Information for International Travel*, edited by G. W. Brunette, 16–138. Oxford: Oxford University Press. http://wwwnc.cdc.gov/travel/yellowbook/2016/the-pre-travel-consultation/travelers-diarrhea.

Chey, W., and B. Wong. 2007. "American College of Gastroenterology Guideline on the Management of *Helicobacter pylori* Infection." *American Journal of Gastroenterology* 102 (8): 1808–25. http://dx.doi.org/10.1111/j.1572-0241.2007.01393.x.

Dunphy, L., J. Winland-Brown, B. Porter, and D. Thomas, eds. 2015. *Primary Care: The Art and Science of Advanced Practice Nursing*. 4th ed. Philadelphia: F. A. Davis.

Harvard Health Publications. 2017. "Constipation and Impaction: What Is It?" Harvard Medical School. http://www.health.harvard.edu/digestive-health/constipation-and-impaction.

International Foundation for Functional Gastrointestinal Disorders. 2015. "Treatment of Gas." https://www.iffgd.org/symptoms-causes/intestinal-gas/treatment.html.

———. 2016. "Diagnosis of IBS." https://aboutibs.org/diagnosis-of-ibs.html.

———. 2017. "Newer IBS Medications." http://www.aboutibs.org/site/treatment/medications/targeted-ibs-medications.

Karimi, P., F. Islami, S. Anandasabapathy, N. Freedman, and F. Kamangar. 2014. "Gastric Cancer: Descriptive Epidemiology, Risk Factors, Screening, and Prevention." *Cancer Epidemiology Biomarkers and Prevention* 23 (5): 700–13. http://dx.doi.org/10.1158/1055-9965.epi-13-1057.

MedlinePlus. 2016. "Gas: Also Called: Belch, Burp, Eructation, Flatulence, Flatus." https://www.nlm.nih.gov/medlineplus/gas.html.

CHAPTER 11

MALE AND FEMALE REPRODUCTIVE DISORDERS

LEARNING OBJECTIVES

▶ Recognize common disorders and then analyze processes useful to providing differential diagnosis among male and female reproductive disorders.

　▷ Risk factors

　▷ Signs and symptoms

　▷ Diagnostic tests

　▷ Differential diagnoses

▶ Describe treatment and management of male and female reproductive disorders.

　▷ Management

　▷ Prevention

MEN'S HEALTH

Benign Prostatic Hypertrophy (BPH)

▶ Nonmalignant generalized increase in the number of cells that causes enlargement of the prostate gland.

▶ ⬤Normal prostate gland is approximately 3.8 × 2.5 × 3.2 centimeters, the size of a walnut or golf ball.

▶ Occurs in about half of men between the ages of 51 and 60 and up to 90 percent of men over age 80 (Urology Care Foundation [UCF] 2017).

▶ Believed to be under endocrine control.

▶ ⬤Accumulation of dihydrotestosterone and increased estrogen in aging males seems to interact in a way that causes cell proliferation.

▶ "Static constriction (buildup of prostatic tissue) and dynamic constriction (increase in prostatic muscle tone through adrenergic stimulation) are the two mechanisms that lead to constriction of the bladder neck" (Dunphy et al. 2015, 646).

Risk Factors

▶ Advanced age

  ▷ 50 percent by age 50 years

  ▷ 90 percent by age 90 years

▶ Family member with BPH

▶ ● African American

▶ ● High-fat, low-fiber intake

▶ History of sexually transmitted infections (STIs)

▶ ● Taking opiates, decongestants, antihistamines, tricyclic anti-depressants (TCAs)

Signs and Symptoms

▶ Urinary hesitancy

▶ ● Bladder infection from decreased emptying

▶ ● Urinary urgency

  ▷ Backflow to kidneys

  ▷ May lead to death of kidney cells

▶ Weak or slow urinary stream

▶ Difficulty starting urination, maintaining stream, or both

▶ Straining, dripping, increased frequency

▶ Incomplete bladder emptying

▶ Nocturia

Diagnostic Tests

▶ Digital rectal exam (DRE)

  ▷ ● Healthy prostate tissue feels soft, rubbery, symmetrical, smooth, regular, and even.

    ▶ Consistency like tip of nose

  ▷ ● Anything firmer is suspicious for malignancy.

▶ Urinalysis

  ▷ ● No hematuria, glucosuria, infection

▶ ● Postvoid catheterization

  ▷ Identifies residual urine in bladder

▶ Blood urea nitrogen (BUN) and creatinine

  ▷ Renal function

  ▷ May be abnormal with upper urinary tract obstruction or retention

▶ ● Prostate-specific antigen (PSA)

  ▷ Increases as gland enlarges.

  ▷ Identifies prostate involvement.

    ▷ Normal <10 ng/mL.

    ▷ >10 ng/mL may be cancer.

    ▷ Increased 1–24 hours post DRE; avoid lab work-up during this period.

    ▷ Serum PSA testing is controversial; the US Preventive Services Task Force (USPSTF) recommends against screening for prostate cancer with PSA (2017).

► Urinary flowmetry studies

    ▷ Postvoid residual urine

► Other studies

    ▷ Urodynamic studies, transrectal ultrasound, intravenous pyelogram (IVP), abdominal ultrasound

Differential Diagnoses

► Diseases associated with increased urination

    ▷ Congestive heart failure (CHF)

► Bladder neck contracture or cancer

► Prostate cancer

► Infectious or inflammatory disease

    ▷ Prostatitis, cystitis, urethritis

► Neurological disease

► Urethral strictures

Management

► Increase fluids.

► Catheterize.

► Instruct patient to void with urge; don't wait.

► Transurethral resection of prostate.

► Transurethral laser prostatectomy.

► Determine American Urological Association (AUA) symptom index (SI) score, which is a validated, short, self-administered questionnaire used to assess the severity of three storage symptoms (frequency, nocturia, urgency) and four voiding symptoms (feeling of incomplete emptying, intermittency, straining, and a weak stream; McVary et al. 2010).

    ▷ If SI ≤ 8 (moderate), watchful waiting

    ▷ If SI ≥ 8 (moderate-to-severe and symptomatic), consider medications

► Alpha blockers relax muscles.

    ▷ Flomax (tamsulosin) 0.4 mg p.o. daily

    ▷ Hytrin (terazosin) 1–10 mg p.o. daily

    ▷ Cardura (doxazosin) 0.4–8 mg p.o. daily

    ▷ Rapaflo (silodosin) 8 mg p.o. daily

▶ • 5-Alpha reductase inhibitors shrink prostate.

   ▷ Proscar (finasteride) 5 mg p.o. daily

   ▷ Avodart (dutasteride) 0.5 mg p.o. daily

▶ Combination therapy (alpha blockers + 5-alpha reductase inhibitors) and anticholinergic therapy.

▶ • Anticholinergic agents are appropriate and effective treatment alternatives for management in men without an elevated postvoid residual and when urinary frequency symptoms are predominantly irritative (McVary et al. 2010).

   ▷ Prior to initiation of anticholinergic therapy, baseline postvoid residual (PVR) urine should be assessed.

   ▷ Anticholinergic agents should be used with caution in patients with a PVR greater than 250–300 mL.

Prevention

▶ None known

Prostatitis

▶ Prostate gland inflammation or infection

▶ • Bacterial infection from bladder infection, STI, or chemical reaction secondary to BPH

▶ Most common urologic disease in men

▶ • Residual urine in the urethra after urination backs up into the prostate and irritates prostate gland tissue

▶ 50–70 percent of cases in the United States from infection

▶ National Institutes of Health (NIH) categories of prostatitis (National Institute of Diabetes and Digestive and Kidney Diseases [NIDDK] 2014):

   I. Acute bacterial prostatitis

   II. Chronic bacterial prostatitis

   III. Chronic nonbacterial prostatitis or chronic pelvic pain syndrome (prostatodynia)

   IV. Asymptomatic inflammatory prostatitis

Risk Factors

▶ Iatrogenic

▶ • Recent medical urinary tract manipulation

▶ • Exposure to STI

▶ Abscess elsewhere in the body

▶ Age older than 50 years

▶ • Anal intercourse

▶ Urinary tract abnormalities

▶ • Recent or recurrent urinary tract infection (UTI) or BPH

Signs and Symptoms

- ▶ • Hematuria, dysuria
- ▶ • Burning, straining, urgency, frequency
- ▶ • Pain with bowel movements or ejaculation
- ▶ • Pain
  - ▷ Lower back, above pubic bone, between genitals and anus, tip of penis, or urethra

Diagnostic Tests

- ▶ • DRE
  - ▷ Most important in nonacute patients.
  - ▷ Exam needs to be done gently or withheld until after treatment has begun because of exquisite tenderness and risk of spreading infection into bloodstream.
- ▶ • Prostate massage
  - ▷ Expels fluids for analysis for microorganisms
- ▶ • Sequential urine test after prostate massage
  - ▷ Three samples:
    1. Measured amount of urine
    2. Sample after prostate massage
    3. Final urine sample
- ▶ • PSA
  - ▷ Elevated level indicates prostate problem
- ▶ • Blood cultures for acute prostatitis
- ▶ Complete blood count (CBC), BUN, and creatinine
- ▶ • Urine cytology in older adults
  - ▷ Bladder cancer screening
- ▶ • Penile discharge culture for STIs
- ▶ Urodynamic tests
  - ▷ Evaluate suspected prostatodynia
- ▶ • Needle biopsy
  - ▷ Rule out cancer
- ▶ • Imaging tests
  - ▷ Ultrasound, IVP, magnetic resonance imaging (MRI), computed tomography (CT) scan

Differential Diagnoses

I. Any of four types of prostatitis (NIDDK 2014)

II. Acute bacterial prostatitis

III.   Chronic bacterial prostatitis

IV.   Chronic prostatitis/chronic pelvic pain syndrome

V.   Asymptomatic inflammatory prostatitis

▶   BPH

▶   Urethral stricture

▶   Bladder or prostate cancer

▶   Renal calculi

▶   Other infections

▷   Epididymitis, cystitis, urethritis, abscess

Management

▶   Avoid irritants:

▷ ○ Alcohol, caffeine, over-the-counter (OTC) antihistamines and decongestants

▶ ○Sexual abstinence during first 2 weeks of acute illness.

▶ ○ Increase ejaculation frequency in nonacute states.

▶   Adequate hydration.

▶   Rest.

▶ ○ Sitz baths for 20 minutes, two to three times daily and p.r.n. for pain.

▶ ○Whirlpool baths, hot compresses.

▷   Not recommended for acute bacterial prostatitis

▶   Anxiety treatment.

▶   Meditation, biofeedback, yoga, and exercise.

▶ ○ Refer to urologist if:

▷   No improvement within 48 hours of treatment;

▷   Over age 50 years with symptoms, recurrent prostatitis, acute bacterial prostatitis; or

▷   BPH may be confounding the problem.

▶   Hospitalization with systemic involvement

▷   Intravenous (IV) antibiotics

▷   Treatment of suspected septicemia

▶ ○ Reevaluation

▷   Acute prostatitis

▶   In 48–72 hours, then 2–4 weeks

▷   Chronic prostatitis

▶   In 4–6 weeks

▶   Pharmacologic

▷   Acute or chronic bacterial prostatitis (see table 11–1 below)

TABLE 11–1.
PROSTATITIS PHARMACOLOGIC TREATMENT

PROSTATITIS	NONBACTERIAL PROSTATITIS
Antibiotics	Nonsteroidal anti-inflammatory drugs (NSAIDs)
Trimethoprim-sulfamethoxazole (Bactrim DS) 160/800 mg, 1 p.o. q12h × 4–6 weeks	Hyperthermia therapy
	5-Alpha reductase inhibitors
Ciprofloxacin 500 mg p.o. q12h × 4–6 weeks	Finasteride 5 mg p.o. daily
Levofloxacin 500 mg p.o. once daily × 4–6 weeks	Dutasteride (Avodart) 0.5 mg p.o. daily
Antispasmodics Baclofen 5 mg p.o. t.i.d. × 3 days then 10 mg p.o. t.i.d. × 3 days then 15 mg p.o. t.i.d. × 3 days then 20 mg p.o. t.i.d. × 3 days Maintenance dose: 40–80 mg p.o. daily	
Detrol LA (tolterodine tartrate extended release) 4 mg p.o. daily	

Prevention

▶ Good hygiene

▶ Good hydration

Testicular Torsion

▶ Spermatic cord twists, cutting blood supply to testicles and scrotal tissue and causing ischemia or infarction if untreated.

▶ May be due to anatomically abnormal, free-floating testicle not fixated in the scrotum that twists around its own blood supply.

▶ May be precipitated by trauma, sudden pulling movements on the cremasteric muscle (jumping into cold water, riding a bicycle), sexual activity, cold, or exercise.

▶ In some cases, there is no clear cause.

▶ Testicular torsion requires emergency surgery to prevent necrosis of testicle.

Risk Factors

▶ High risk at ages 15–35 years (most common between ages 12 and 18 years)

▶ Paraplegia

▶ Heavy exercise

▶ Sexual activity

▶ Cold

Signs and Symptoms

▶ Sudden onset of acute testicular or groin pain

▶ Rising of affected testicle

- Afebrile
- Patient is usually lying down and in acute distress.

Diagnostic Tests

- Physical exam.
- Patient usually lying down in acute distress
- Acute tenderness, edema, and erythema of testicle that extends to entire scrotum.
- Testicle is horizontal and elevated in scrotum.
- Negative cremasteric reflex.
- If only the testicle appendage is twisted, a "blue dot sign" is at superior aspect of testicle—small, palpable lump on superior pole of the epididymis.
- Doppler ultrasound will show no blood flow.

Differential Diagnoses

- Ischemia
- Trauma
- Infectious causes
- Inflammatory conditions (Henoch-Scholein purpura)
- Hernia
- Acute-on-chronic events (spermatocele, hydrocele, varicocele; Cohen, Gans, and Slaughenhoupt 2016)
- Testicular mass
  - Rule out cancer

Management

- Emergency referral to urologist
- Preoperative management
  - Elevate scrotum
  - Apply ice pack
  - Manual reduction prior to surgical intervention
- Surgical intervention to relieve torsion and orchiopexy (Cohen, Gans, and Slaughenhoupt)
  - The testis salvage rate approaches 100 percent in patients who undergo detorsion within 6 hours of the start of pain, 20 percent viability rate if detorsion occurs after more than 12 hours, and virtually no viability if detorsion is delayed more than 24 hours.

Prevention

- None known

Epididymitis

▶ An acute bacterial intrascrotal infection associated with painful enlargement of the epididymis.

▶ Most cases are infectious.

▶ • Sexually transmitted:
  ▷ Men younger than age 35 years
  ▷ Associated with urethritis
  ▷ Caused by *Chlamydia trachomatis* or *Neisseria gonorrhoeae*
  ▷ Heterosexual men <35 years old
    ▶ 70 percent caused by *C. trachomatis*
    ▶ *N. gonorrhoeae* in majority of remaining cases
    ▶ Some have combination of both

▶ • Nonsexually transmitted:
  ▷ Older men (over age 35)
  ▷ Associated with UTI and prostatitis
  ▷ Caused by gram-negative rods
  ▷ Route of infection probably urethra to ejaculatory duct to vas deferens to epididymis
  ▷ Urinary tract instrumentation surgery
  ▷ Systemic disease
  ▷ Immunosuppression

Risk Factors

▶ • Exposure to STIs
  ▷ Up to 30 days before symptom onset
▶ • Anatomical abnormalities
▶ • Instrumentation or surgery

Signs and Symptoms

▶ • Presents symmetrically.
▶ • Testicular pain and edema.
▶ • Edema may double testicle size in 3–4 hours.
▶ • Pain begins in scrotum, may radiate to spermatic cord or flank.
▶ • Commonly gradual onset.
▶ • May follow physical strain, trauma, sexual activity.
▶ Associated symptoms:
  ▷ • Urethritis
  ▷ • Pain at tip of penis and urethral discharge

▷ Cystitis

▷ Irritative voiding symptoms

► Epididymal tenderness and swelling.

► Fever, urethral discharge, voiding complaints in 50 percent

► If presentation is unilateral scrotal pain, *must* quickly rule out testicular torsion, testicular tumor, or chronic infection not responsive to appropriate antimicrobial therapy.

Diagnostic Tests

► Gram stain urethral exudate or intraurethral swab to diagnose gonococcal infection

► Culture same for gonorrhea and chlamydia

► Urinalysis, urine culture

▷ Diagnose concurrent UTI, especially in nonsexually transmitted types

► Syphilis serology

► CBC shows leukocytosis

► Human immunodeficiency virus (HIV) testing and counseling

► Ultrasound

▷ Differentiates testicular torsion from epididymitis

► CT and MRI scans

▷ Used occasionally to differentiate cysts, hydrocele, hernia, cancerous tissue

► Radionuclide scan, Doppler flow study, or surgical exploration

▷ For teens and young adults with acute unilateral testicular pain without urethritis

Differential Diagnoses

► Tumor

► Abscess, cyst

► Testicular torsion, infarction, cancer

► Mumps orchitis

► Hydrocele, varicocele

Management

► Bed rest

▷ Until fever and local inflammation subside

► Scrotal elevation and support

► Briefs underwear

► Avoid sexual and physical strain until resolved

► Antimicrobial therapy

▷ Age under 35 years

► Likely gonorrhea or chlamydia

▶ • Ceftriaxone (Rocephin) 250 mg intramuscularly (IM) single dose *and* doxycycline 100 mg p.o. b.i.d. × 10 days

▷ Age over 35 years

▶ High likelihood of enteric organisms

▶ • Levofloxacin 500 mg once a day × 10 days

▶ • Ofloxacin (Floxin) 300 mg p.o. b.i.d. × 10 days

▶ Analgesics for fever and inflammation

▷ NSAIDs, acetaminophen

Prevention

▶ Safe sexual practices

Prostate Cancer

▶ Malignant neoplasm of the prostate gland

▶ Most common malignancy in US men; third most common cause of cancer death in men older than 55 years

▶ Approximately 317,000 new US cases and more than 41,000 US deaths annually

▶ ◦ More common in African American men

▶ ◦ Asymptomatic in 80 percent of patients

Risk Factors

▶ ▪ Older than 60 years (rare before 50 years); risk increases with age

▶ Exposure to carcinogens

▶ • History of STIs

▶ Family history

▶ Higher prevalence in African American people

▶ • Possibly vasectomy, dietary fat

Signs and Symptoms

▶ Dysuria, difficulty voiding

▶ Increased urinary frequency

▶ Hematuria, urinary retention

▶ ◦ Back or hip pain

▶ Spinal cord compression from intradural metastases

▶ Deep vein thrombosis

▶ Pulmonary emboli

▶ • Myelophthisis anemia

▷ Replacement of hematopoietic tissue by abnormal tissue

Diagnostic Tests

- ▶ • DRE
  - ▷ Findings depend on stage of cancer
  - ▷ • Posterior surfaces of lateral lobes, where carcinoma begins, most frequently palpable
  - ▷ • Prostate is nodular, hard, irregular
  - ▷ Median sulcus obliterated
- ▶ • Local extraprostatic tumor extension into seminal vesicles
  - ▷ Often detected by DRE
- ▶ • Scrotal or lower extremity lymphedema
  - ▷ Extensive disease
- ▶ CBC, urinalysis, urine culture, and sensitivity workup for urinary symptoms
- ▶ • Serum alkaline phosphatase elevated in late-stage bone metastasis
- ▶ • PSA: Normal value < 4 ng/mL
  - ▷ PSA normal in 40 percent with cancer
  - ▷ PSA > 4 ng/mL
    - ▶ Possible cancer
  - ▷ Higher value on different tests or level >10 ng/mL
    - ▶ Recommend prostatic biopsy
- ▶ Imaging
  - ▷ • Transrectal prostatic biopsy with rapid-fire spring-loaded needle under sonography most accurate
- ▶ CT scan
- ▶ MRI
- ▶ Bone scan

Differential Diagnoses

- ▶ BPH
- ▶ Prostatitis
- ▶ Prostatic or bladder stones
- ▶ Bladder cancer

Management

- ▶ Watchful waiting option
  - ▷ • Asymptomatic patients with less than 10-year life expectancy
  - ▷ Low-grade tumors not necessarily treated
- ▶ Androgen deprivation or chemical castration
  - ▷ Flutamide (Eulexin) 250 mg p.o. t.i.d.

▷ Leuprolide (Lupron) 1 mg subcutaneously (SC) daily with flutamide (Eulexin) 75 mg IM monthly

▶ Radiation therapy

▶ Radium seeds

▶ Chemotherapy

▶ Surgical interventions

▷ Total prostatoseminovesiculectomy

▶ Oldest treatment

▶ Radical perineal prostatectomy and radical retropubic prostatectomy

Prevention

▶ Healthy lifestyle: Healthy diet, exercise, maintain optimal weight

Testicular Cancer

▶ Germinal or nongerminal carcinoma of the testicles

▶ Cause is unknown, but a strong link has been found with cryptorchid testis

▶ Second most common cancer of men ages 20–40 years, and number one cancer killer of 15- to 35-year-olds

▶ Greater than 95 percent cure rate if there is no metastasis, and 80 percent are curable in metastatic disease

Risk Factors

▶ Caucasian, higher social class, rural setting, unmarried

▶ Cryptorchidism or family history

▶ Klinefelter's syndrome

▶ Exposure to intrapartum estrogen (diethylstilbestrol [DES])

Signs and Symptoms

▶ Painless swelling, testicular mass

▶ Sense of heaviness or thickening in scrotum or testicle

▶ Tender testicle

▷ If tumor bleeding or epididymitis present

▶ If metastasized

▷ Gynecomastia, supraclavicular lymphadenopathy, abdominal or neck mass, pain in groin, flank, or back

Diagnostic Tests

▶ One or more firm, tender or nontender tumors on one or both testicles

▶ Inguinal lymphadenopathy may be present

▶ Transillumination

▷ Normal rosy glow absent

▶ Darkness of tumor visible

▶ ◄ Serum alpha fetoprotein

▶ Presence of seminomatous germ-cell tumors

▶ •Serum beta human chorionic gonadotropin

▷ Positive in 70–100 percent of seminomatous testicular carcinomas

▶ Ultrasound

▷ Distinguishes inguinal hernia, epididymitis or orchitis, hematomas, hydrocele, spermatocele

▶ Chest X-ray (CXR), CT scan, pedal lymphangiography

▷ Determines staging

Differential Diagnoses

▶ Inguinal hernia

▶ Epididymitis

▶ Orchitis

▶ Hematomas

▶ Hydrocele, spermatocele

Management

▶ Refer to oncologist

▶ Seminomas

▷ Orchiectomy or radiation

▶ Nonseminomas

▷ Surgery, radiation, combination chemotherapy

▶ Metastasis

▷ Radiation and chemotherapy

▶ • Sperm banking

▶ Self-examinations monthly if at high risk

Prevention

▶ Healthy lifestyle: Healthy diet, exercise, maintain optimal weight

▶ ◄ Testicular self-examination

WOMEN'S HEALTH

Menstruation

▶ In absence of fertilized ovum, ovarian corpus luteum undergoes regression within 9–11 days of ovulation.

▶ Estrogen and progesterone production decrease and menses ensues.

▶ Normal menstrual cycle is 23–39 days (average 29).

▶ Menstrual cycle shortens as menopause approaches.

▶ Menstrual period usually lasts 2–7 days, with the majority of blood loss in the first few days.

▶ Presence of clots or bleeding after more than 1 week is excessive blood loss.

▶ Abnormal bleeding may occur during normal ovulation or in its absence.

▶ Menorrhagia

  ▷ Bleeding normal in timing but excessive in amount and duration

▶ Mittelschmerz

  ▷ Normal ovulation accompanied by midcycle vaginal staining and pelvic pain (usually right side)

  ▷ Occurs in context of ovarian follicle rupture and release

Hormonal Contraception

▶ Estrogen or progesterone pills, patches, injections, or rings to prevent pregnancy, used to suppress follicle-stimulating hormone (FSH) and luteinizing hormone (LH), inhibit ovulation, alter endometrium, thicken cervical mucus, and alter ovum transport to prevent pregnancy.

▶ Use with caution in women with the following conditions or risk factors:

  ▷ Migraines triggered by oral contraceptives,

  ▷ Hypertension,

  ▷ Diabetes mellitus,

  ▷ Smoking

  ▷ Major surgery with immobilization planned in next 4 weeks,

  ▷ Undiagnosed uterine bleeding,

  ▷ Sickle cell disease,

  ▷ Lactation,

  ▷ Active cholecystitis,

  ▷ History of heart or renal disease,

  ▷ Family history of dyslipidemia or death from MI before 50 years of age, or

  ▷ Current impaired liver function including hepatic adenoma or liver cancer.

- Contraindications
  - ▷ Thrombophlebitis or thromboembolic disorder
  - ▷ Cerebrovascular accident (CVA), coronary artery disease (CAD), or ischemic heart disease (IHD)
  - ▷ Breast cancer: History of, known, or suspected
  - ▷ Estrogen-dependent neoplasia
  - ▷ Pregnancy
- Adverse effects
  - ▷ Menstrual changes
  - ▷ Bleeding, spotting, missed menses
  - ▷ Fluid retention, nausea, vomiting
  - ▷ Telangiectasia
  - ▷ Stomach cramps, bloating
  - ▷ Progestin effects
    - Breast tenderness, enlargement, discharge
    - Headaches
    - Hypertension
    - Androgenic effects
    - Increased appetite, weight gain
    - Depression
    - Higher low-density lipoprotein (LDL), lower high-density lipoprotein (HDL)
    - Carbohydrate intolerance
  - ▷ Breakthrough bleeding
    - Any bleeding that is not attributable to normal menstrual flow
    - Risk factors
      - ▷ First 4 months of use
      - ▷ Missed pills, pregnancy
      - ▷ Vomiting, diarrhea
      - ▷ Cervical inflammation, polyp
      - ▷ Pelvic infection or other gynecological pathology
    - Management
      - ▷ Address causes
      - ▷ If bleeding not because of causes
        - Higher progestin pill often effective for bleeding at any point in cycle
        - Higher estrogen pill only effective if bleeding is in first 2 weeks of cycle or no withdrawal bleeding

Abnormal Uterine Bleeding

▶ "Abnormal uterine bleeding (AUB) may be acute or chronic and is defined as bleeding from the uterine corpus that is abnormal in regularity, volume, frequency, or duration and occurs in the absence of pregnancy" (Committee on Gynecologic Practice 2013 p. 1).

▶ The etiologies of AUB are classified as

  ▷ Uterine structural abnormalities or

  ▷ Not related to uterine structural abnormalities.

▶ Categorized following the acronym PALM–COEIN (Committee on Gynecologic Practice 2013 p.5):

  ▷ Polyp

  ▷ Adenomyosis

  ▷ Leiomyoma

  ▷ Malignancy and hyperplasia

  ▷ Coagulopathy

  ▷ Ovulatory dysfunction

  ▷ Endometrial

  ▷ Iatrogenic

  ▷ Not otherwise classified

Diagnostic Tests

▶ CBC.

▶ Pregnancy test.

▶ Consider von Willebrand–ristocetin cofactor activity, von Willebrand factor antigen, factor VIII and antiphospholipid antibody syndrome.

▶ A workup for thyroid disorders, liver disorder, sepsis, or leukemia may be indicated.

▶ Endometrial tissue sampling

  ▷ If over 45 years old, as a first-line test

  ▷ If younger than 45 years old, test those with

    ▶ A history of unopposed estrogen exposure (such as seen in patients with obesity or polycystic ovary syndrome),

    ▶ Failed medical management, or

    ▶ Persistent AUB.

▶ Pelvic ultrasound examination (Committee on Gynecologic Practice 2013)

Differential Diagnoses

▶ Ovulatory bleeding

▶ Normal variant

▶ Mittelschmerz

- ▶ Uterine fibroids
- ▶ Cervical inflammation
- ▶ Polyps
- ▶ Endometrial cancer
- ▶ Pelvic inflammatory disease (PID)
- ▶ Intrauterine device (IUD)
- ▶ Anovulatory bleeding
- ▶ Hypothalamic dysfunction, hypothyroidism, polycystic ovary syndrome
- ▶ Puberty, perimenopause
- ▶ Stress, excessive exercise, weight loss
- ▶ Excessive androgen, prolactin, cortisol
- ▶ Oral contraceptives—low estrogen
- ▶ Postmenopausal bleeding
- ▶ Endometrial pathology
- ▶ Cancer
- ▶ Cervical pathology
- ▶ Erosion
- ▶ Vaginal pathology
- ▶ Atrophic vaginitis
- ▶ Pregnancy, ectopic pregnancy, failing pregnancy
- ▶ Postabortion (retained products of gestation)

Management

- ▶ Hormonal management
  - ▷ Combined oral contraceptives (OCs)
  - ▷ Oral progestins
- ▶ Treat underlying cause.
- ▶ Refer to gynecologist for treatment of underlying cause.

Prevention

- ▶ Maintain optimal weight.
- ▶ Take oral contraceptives as prescribed.

Amenorrhea

- ▶ Permanent or temporary absence of menstrual periods
- ▶ May result from disturbance in hypothalamus, pituitary, ovaries, or uterus

Risk Factors

▶   Varies according to underlying etiology

▶   ▪ Endocrine disorders

▷   Excess androgen, cortisol, or prolactin

▷   Hypothalamic dysfunction

▶   ▪ Serious emotional stress or psychopathology

▶   ▪ Dieting

▷   Anorexia nervosa with severe weight loss

▶   Serious concurrent illness

▶   ▪ Medications

▷   Phenothiazines, antidepressants, antihypertensives, chemotherapy and radiation complications, systemic steroids, gonadotropin-releasing hormone (GnRH) antagonists

▷   Oral contraceptives

▶   ▪ Increased exercise

▷   Competitive long-distance running

▶   Idiopathic

Signs and Symptoms

▶   Lack of menses

▶   Reflective of underlying causes

▷   Physiologic

▶   Occurs with pregnancy, lactation, and menopause

▷   ▪ Primary

▶   Menstrual periods have not begun by age 16 years.

▶   Approximately 30 percent with primary causes have associated genetic abnormalities.

▶   Constitutional delay in puberty.

▶   Congenital defects in steroid synthesis.

▶   Late-onset adrenal hyperplasia.

▷   ▪ Secondary

▶   Absence of menstrual periods for 3 consecutive cycles *or* for more than 6 months after previously menstruating

▷   ▪ Pregnancy is the most common cause, followed by polycystic ovary syndrome, hypothalamic amenorrhea, thyroid dysfunction, hyperprolactinemia, and ovarian failure.

▶   Medications

▷   ▪ Phenothiazines, antidepressants, antihypertensives, chemotherapy and radiation complications, systemic steroids, GnRH antagonists

▶ Surgery

▷ Oophorectomy, hysterectomy

▶ Outflow tract obstruction

▷ Severe cervical stenosis, severe endometrial scarring and obliteration of endometrium, vaginal scarring, labial fusion

Diagnostic Tests

▶ Rule out pregnancy

▶ Work-up depends on history and physical

▶ ● Primary

▷ Secondary sex characteristics absent or poorly defined

▶ Karyotype to rule out genetic etiology

▷ Breast tissue absent or poorly developed and uterus absent

▶ ● Test FSH

▷ Elevated: Ovarian failure

▷ If low , suggests pituitary or hypothalamic dysfunction

▶ Do karyotype to rule out ovarian dysgenesis

▷ Breast tissue present but uterus absent

▶ Test serum testosterone

▶ If at male level, do karyotype for testicular feminization

▷ Breast tissue and uterus present

▶ ● Test serum prolactin

▶ Elevated: Include pituitary tumor in differential

▶ ● Normal: Begin progesterone challenge test

▷ If work up negative, begin work up for secondary amenorrhea

▶ ● Secondary

▷ Serum prolactin, CBC, erythrocyte sedimentation rate (ESR), thyroid-stimulating hormone (TSH), bone age, DSH/ LH, liver function tests (LFTs), BUN and creatinine, urinalysis, urine human chorionic gonadotropin (HCG), karyotyping, dehydroepiandrostenedione sulfate (DHEAS) levels, androstenedione, testosterone, adrenal suppression test for 17-hydroxyprogesterone

▶ ● Progesterone challenge: Provera 10 mg p.o. daily × 5 days

▷ Positive test

▶ ● Withdrawal bleeding within 7 days of last Provera pill

▶ Suggests adequate endogenous estrogen present to prime endometrium

▶ Suggests anovulation

▶ Presence of intact outflow tract, functioning endometrium, ovary, pituitary, central nervous system (CNS)

▷ Negative test

▶ No withdrawal bleeding

▶ Suggests inadequate estrogen to prime uterus or absent endometrial cavity

▶ ○ If negative progesterone challenge, wait 2 weeks then prescribe conjugated estrogen 1.25 mg daily × 21 days, *or* 2 mg estradiol p.o. daily for 21 days with Provera 10 mg p.o. for last 5 days of estrogen, *or* combination oral contraceptives (monophasic) 1 tablet p.o. × 21 days

▷ If prolactin normal, and there is no galactorrhea, no further work-up needed

▷ ○ Positive test

▶ Withdrawal bleeding within 14 days

▷ ○ Negative test

▶ No withdrawal bleeding

▶ Suggests end-organ failure

▶ Probably due to congenital malformation or distortion of uterus, vagina

▶ ○ Repeat estrogen-Provera challenge to confirm

▷ If negative, obtain TSH or thyroid panel, FSH:LH, and LH:FSH ratios

▶ TSH elevated suggests hypothyroidism

▶ TSH low or undetectable suggests hyperthyroidism

▶ LH or LH:FSH ratio > 3, include polycystic ovary syndrome (PCOS) in differential

▶ If LH normal or low, include hypothalamic or pituitary regulation defect in differential

▶ Low LH and FSH suggests hypothalamic etiology

▶ High LH and FSH suggests ovarian failure or menopause secondary to radiation, chemotherapy, autoimmune disorder, chromosomal disorder

▷ If Cushing's is suspected:

▶ Check adrenocorticotrophic hormone (ACTH), DHEAS, urinary free cortisol

▶ ○ Pelvic ultrasound if abnormality found in exam or when PCOS suspected

▷ If galactorrhea or elevated prolactin

▶ MRI of sella turcica to assess for adenoma, necrosis, or ischemia (Sheehan syndrome)

▶ Coned-down X-ray of sella turcica also appropriate

Differential Diagnoses

▶ Pregnancy

▶ Chromosomal abnormality

▶ Menopause

Management

- ▶ ● Refer to endocrinologist for pituitary adenoma, PCOS.
    - ▷ Pituitary adenoma may need surgical intervention or bromocriptine (Pardoll) treatment
- ▶ Increase caloric intake if underweight.
- ▶ Encourage adequate calcium intake, reduce excessive exercise.
- ▶ Stress management, refer to eating disorder center if needed.
- ▶ Refer to gynecologist if no withdrawal bleeding, nonresponse to treatment, prolonged amenorrhea recurs, fertility, or for hormone replacement therapy (HRT) management.
- ▶ If positive Provera challenge
    - ▷ Give Provera monthly, 10 mg p.o. daily × 10 days minimum *or*
    - ▷ Progesterone 100–200 mg p.o. daily (days 14–16 until menses onset) for 3–6 cycles *or*
    - ▷ Combined OCs for minimum of 3–6 cycles
    - ▷ Start hormone therapy with OC or HRT regimen if no menses present for more than 6 months (or sooner if estradiol levels < 20 or FSH levels > 20)
    - ▷ Better not to use progestin-only contraception until regular cycles recur
    - ▷ If no withdrawal bleeding occurs, further evaluation is needed

Prevention

- ▶ Patient education to include
    - ▷ Maintain appropriate weight and
    - ▷ Avoid excessive exercise

Ectopic Pregnancy

- ▶ Implantation of embryo outside of the uterus, such as in fallopian tubes

Risk Factors

- ▶ ᵃ History of PID
- ▶ Prior ectopic pregnancy
- ▶ ● Tubal surgery to enhance fertility
- ▶ ● Use of intrauterine devices
- ▶ ● Ovulation-inducing drugs
    - ▷ Alter steroid hormone levels and affect tube motility

Signs and Symptoms

- ▶ ● Unilateral abdominal pain
- ▶ ● Menses delayed 1–2 weeks, followed by recurrent spotting
- ▶ ● Hypotension, hemorrhagic shock, and death with tubal rupture

Diagnostic Tests

- ▶ • Beta HCG
- ▶ • Pelvic and abdominal exams
- ▶ • Ultrasound

Differential Diagnoses

- ▶ Abortion complications
- ▶ Appendicitis
- ▶ Cervical cancer
- ▶ Dysmenorrhea
- ▶ Early loss of pregnancy
- ▶ Hemorrhagic or hypovolemic shock
- ▶ Placenta previa

Management

- ▶ Immediate surgical intervention (laparoscopic or laparotomy)

Prevention

- ▶ None known

Gynecological Pain

- ▶ The uterus, cervix, and adnexa share the same sympathetic nerve pathway as the gastrointestinal tract, rendering distinction of pain origin difficult
- ▶ Types of pain
  - ▷ • Acute pain
    - ▶ Pelvic inflammatory disease
    - ▶ Ectopic pregnancy
    - ▶ Torsion of fallopian tube, ovary, or ovarian cyst
    - ▶ Extrapelvic disease
    - ▶ Appendicitis
  - ▷ • Chronic pain
    - ▶ Benign neoplasms
    - ▶ Malignancy
    - ▶ Psychogenic pain
- ▶ Recurrent pain with menstruation
  - ▷ Dysmenorrhea
  - ▷ Primary dysmenorrhea
  - ▷ Pain just prior to or during menses

    ▷ Secondary dysmenorrhea

    ▷ Endometriosis

    ▷ Adenomyosis

    ▷ Chronic PID

    ▷ Intrauterine devices

    ▷ Mittelschmerz (midcycle pain)

    ▷ Leaking ovarian cysts

▶ Nongynecologic pathology

    ▷ Adhesions

    ▷ Irritable bowel syndrome

    ▷ Dysfunctional bowel

Risk Factors

▶ STIs

▶ History of PID

▶ History of sexual abuse

Signs and Symptoms

▶ Abdominal low midline pain, cramping

    ▷ May radiate to back or thighs, occurs in waves

    ▷ Lasts 1–2 days

    ▷ Headache, diarrhea, vasomotor flushing, nausea

▶ Associated symptoms indicate underlying problem

    ▷ Fever, unilateral pain, dizziness, unusual bleeding, dyspareunia

▶ Primary dysmenorrhea

    ▷ Fatigue, nervousness, irritability, dizziness, syncope, bloating, headache, mood changes, nausea or vomiting, constipation or diarrhea

Diagnostic Tests

▶ Ultrasound

▶ Urinalysis

▶ Pregnancy test

▶ CT scan

▶ Cultures

Differential Diagnoses

▶ Pregnancy, ectopic gestation

▶ Endometriosis, fibroids

▶ STIs, PID

- ▶ Leiomyoma
- ▶ Chronic pelvic pain syndromes
- ▶ IBS, urinary tract disorder
- ▶ Cancer

Management

- ▶ Treat causes of secondary dysmenorrhea
- ▶ Primary dysmenorrhea
  - ▷ Supportive
    - ▶ Patient education: Eat regularly, dry or moist heat to abdomen for pain relief
  - ▷ Transcutaneous electrical nerve stimulator (TENS)
  - ▷ NSAIDs
    - ▶ Most effective when taken before pain begins
  - ▷ Control menses with oral contraceptives
    - ▶ Contraceptive pills for 3 cycles without allowing withdrawal bleeding
    - ▶ Use first day start system
    - ▶ After 3 cycles, may respond and then take NSAIDs
- ▶ Follow up every 2–3 months to evaluate efficacy of treatment

Prevention

- ▶ Practice safe sex
- ▶ Maintain optimal weight
- ▶ Exercise

Polycystic Ovary Syndrome (PCOS)

- ▶ Most common hormonal disorder and cause of reproductive-age female infertility of unknown etiology
- ▶ Clinical presentation of hyperandrogenism (obesity, hirsutism, acne), menstrual irregularities, erratic fertility patterns or infertility, insulin resistance, and hyperinsulinemia

Risk Factors

- ▶ Android-pattern obesity

Signs and Symptoms

- ▶ Obesity
- ▶ Hirsutism
- ▶ Acne triad
- ▶ History of menstrual irregularities
- ▶ History of erratic fertility patterns

▶ Hyperinsulinemia, insulin resistance

▶ Complex hormonal irregularities

▶ Associated health conditions

▶ Diabetes

▶ Hypertension or hypercholesterolemia

Diagnostic Tests

▶ No single test for PCOS

▶ ₀ LH high normal

▶ ₀ FSH low normal

▶ ₀ Serum testosterone elevated

▶ ₀ DHEAS elevated

▶ ₀ Prolactin

▷ To rule out pituitary tumor

▶ ₀ Fasting blood sugar, lipid profile

▶ ₀ Overnight dexamethasone suppression test

▶ ₀ Vaginal ultrasound

▷ Identifies ovarian cysts, thickened endometrium

▷ Appearance of ovaries usually enlarged with numerous small cysts along outer edge of each ovary (appear polycystic)

▶ Consider endometrial biopsy for prolonged erratic bleeding to rule out endometrial cancer

Differential Diagnoses

▶ Adrenal

▷ Tumor, Cushing's syndrome, adult-onset adrenal hyperplasia

▶ HAIR-AN (hyperandrogenism, insulin resistance, and acanthosis nigricans) syndrome

▶ Ovarian

▷ Tumor, ovarian insensitivity syndrome

▶ Hepatic disease

▷ Alters estrogen clearance metabolism

▶ Thyroid disease

▷ May affect feedback loops

▶ Prolactinoma

Management

▶ Limit processed foods and refined carbs

▶ Increase dietary whole grains, fruits, vegetables, lean meats

- Exercise, weight control
  - ▷ Improve lipid profile
  - ▷ Reduce insulin resistance
  - ▷ Goal BMI < 27
    - ▶ Insulin resistance uncommon with low BMI
    - ▶ Improves fertility, menstrual cycles
    - ▶ Reduces hirsutism
- Monthly Provera 10 mg p.o. daily × 10–14 days at end of each month *or* oral contraceptives
- Bromocriptine (Parlodel) if high prolactin
- Spironolactone (Aldactone) reduces androgen
- Metformin (Glucophage)
  - ▷ Improves insulin sensitivity, lowers LH and androgen, and improves fertility

Prevention

- ▶ None known

Pelvic Prolapse

- ▶ Loss of normal pelvic support structures, allowing organ descent and herniation
- ▶ Symptoms depend on degree and location
- ▶ Presentation
  - ▷ Prolapsed uterus
  - ▷ Uterine or vaginal prolapse
    - ▶ Cystocele
  - ▷ Bladder bulges into vagina
    - ▶ Rectocele
  - ▷ Rectum bulges into vagina
    - ▶ Enterocele
  - ▷ Small intestines bulge into vagina
- ▶ Graded by severity
  - ▷ Mild
    - ▶ Descending halfway to vaginal introitus
  - ▷ Moderate
    - ▶ Descent to introitus
  - ▷ Severe
    - ▶ Prolapse beyond introitus

Risk Factors

► Vaginal deliveries

► Delivering large babies

► Aging

► Chronic cough

► Constipation or straining

► Fibroids or tumors

► Genetics

► Heavy lifting

► Menopause

► Obesity

► Pelvic surgery

► Spinal cord injuries

Signs and Symptoms

► Pelvic pressure, heaviness

► Protrusion or bulge into vagina

► Walking and exercise are irritants

► Incomplete rectal emptying

► Low back pain, pelvic ache

Diagnostic Tests

► Pelvic ultrasound

  ▷ Distinguishes prolapse from other pathology

► MRI

  ▷ Used for staging prolapse

Differential Diagnoses

► Cystitis

► Early loss of pregnancy

► Ectopic pregnancy

► Neoplasm

► Ovarian cysts

► Vaginitis

Management

► Mild to moderate

  ▷ Avoid stress to pelvic floor (heavy lifting, obesity, high-impact aerobics)

> ▷ Kegel exercises

> ▷ Weighted vaginal cones

► • Severe

> ▷ Intravaginal pessary

>> ► If surgery not wanted or not a consideration

► Referral to gynecologic surgeon for surgical repair

Prevention

► Regular Kegel exercises

► Avoid straining or heavy lifting

► Maintain optimal weight

Abnormal Cervical Cytology

Cervical Cancer

► • Dysplasia of cervical cells, which may appear normal or have small ulcerated lesions (cervical intraepithelial neoplasia [CIN]).

► 85 percent of cervical cancers are squamous cell carcinoma, which accounts for almost 20 percent of all gynecological cancers.

► Prognosis depends on stage and type of cervical cancer and tumor size.

Risk Factors

► • Early-age coitus

► • Multiple sex partners (three or more)

> ▷ Full-service sex workers have fourfold risk

► Male partner who has sex with multiple partners

► • Long-term OCs

► • Smoking

► • History of human papilloma virus (HPV)

► • DES exposure

► Low economic status

► • STIs

> ▷ More than 3

> ▷ HPV, herpes simplex virus (HSV)

Signs and Symptoms

► • Altered vaginal discharge

► • Unusual color or amount of vaginal bleeding

► • Post-douche or postcoital bleeding

▶ ◦ Postmenopausal bleeding

▶ ◦ Dyspareunia

▶ ◦ Pelvic pain

Diagnostic Tests

▶ Regular pelvic exams and Pap smears can detect precancerous cervical lesions.

▶ ◦ Pap smear

▷ Most accurate, specific for carcinoma or invasive cancer and high-grade lesions

▶ ◦ Cervical tissue biopsy.

▶ ◦ Colposcopy

▷ False negatives can occur from sampling or detection errors

▶ CXR, CT scan, MRI, and positron emission tomography (PET) scan

▷ Determine stage of cervical cancer

Differential Diagnoses

▶ Cervicitis

▶ Endometrial cancer

▶ PID

▶ Vaginitis

Management

▶ Refer all abnormal Pap smears to a gynecologist.

▷ ◦ Benign inflammation

▶ Follow up in 3 months

▷ Precancerous changes in cervix treated with cryosurgery, cauterization, or laser surgery.

▷ ◦ Cryotherapy

▶ For noninvasive small lesions without endocervical extension

▷ Laser surgery

▶ Appropriate for large lesions

▷ Loop electrosurgical excision procedure (LEEP)

▶ Appropriate when CIN is clearly visible

▷ Cone biopsy for higher-grade invasive lesions.

▷ Radiation therapy, chemotherapy, surgery not indicated unless invasion is suspected.

Prevention

▶ ◦ Gardasil and Cervarix vaccines can prevent HPV infection.

▶ Condom use.

Endometrial Cancer

▶ Endometrial cancer (also referred to as corpus uterine cancer or corpus cancer) is the most common gynecologic cancer in the developing world, with adenocarcinoma of the endometrium the most common type.

▶ Malignant transformation of glands and endometrial stroma; adenocarcinoma.

▶ 80–90 percent present with painless abnormal bleeding.

▶ Average age at onset 60.

▶ No simple and reliable ways to test for uterine cancer in women who do not have any signs or symptoms (Centers for Disease Control and Prevention [CDC] 2017).

▶ Stages

I. In uterus only

II. Into connective tissue

III. Into pelvis

IV. Beyond pelvis

Risk Factors

▶ Atypical endometrial hyperplasia

▶ Nulliparity, early menarche, late menopause

▶ Unopposed (i.e., without progesterone) estrogen therapy

▶ Obesity

▶ Diabetes

▶ Cigarette smoking

▶ Tamoxifen

▶ Age

▷ Approximately 75 percent are postmenopausal

▶ Lynch syndrome or hereditary nonpolyposis colorectal cancer (Cancer.net 2016)

Signs and Symptoms

▶ Pelvic pain and tenderness

▶ Uterine or adnexal enlargement

▶ Cervical lesions, hemorrhoids

▶ Painless abnormal bleeding

▶ Postmenopausal bleeding

Diagnostic Tests

▶ Pap smear

▷ All over age 40 years with abnormal Pap should be referred for endometrial biopsy.

▶ CBC

- ▶ Ultrasound
- ▶ Endometrial biopsy
  - ▷ ● Endometrial thickness
    - ▶ <5 mm: Atrophy
    - ▶ >15 mm: Hypertrophy

Differential Diagnoses

- ▶ Endometrial hyperplasia
- ▶ Cervical cancer
- ▶ Vaginal cancer
- ▶ Hemorrhoids
- ▶ Bleeding disorders
- ▶ Polyps

Management

- ▶ ● Surgery
  - ▷ Hysterectomy
- ▶ Radiation
- ▶ Chemotherapy
- ▶ Hormone therapy

Prevention

- ▶ No effective preventive measures

Ovarian Cancer

- ▶ Malignant transformation of glands and endometrial stroma; adenocarcinoma in ovaries, fallopian tube, or peritoneal lining (called primary peritoneal cancer)
- ▶ Fifth leading cause of cancer death among US women
- ▶ No effective screening available

Risk Factors

- ▶ ● Low parity, multiparity, or delayed childbearing
- ▶ ● Infertility
- ▶ ● Late menopause
- ▶ ● Anovulatory disorders
- ▶ ● BRCA mutation
- ▶ ● Lynch syndrome

Signs and Symptoms

- ▶ Few symptoms in early stages
- ▶ ● Abdominal fullness

▶ ▪ Pelvic pain

▶ ▫ Bloating, constipation

▶ ▫ Dysuria, difficulty urinating

▶ ▫ Weight loss, anorexia

   ▷ Weight loss and anorexia are poor prognostic signs

▶ ▫ Rule out cancer if ovary is palpable postmenopause

Diagnostic Tests

▶ ▪ Transvaginal ultrasound

   ▷ Imaging to identify masses and endometrial thickening

▶ ▫ CA-125

   ▷ CA-125 higher than 35 units suggests cancer

▶ ▫ Pelvic ultrasound

   ▷ Visualization of ovaries, fallopian tubes, uterus, and bladder

▶ CBC, complete metabolic panel

Differential Diagnosis

▶ Ovarian cyst

▶ Ovarian torsion

▶ Polycystic ovaries

▶ Endometriosis

▶ Gastrointestinal disorder

Management

▶ Surgery

▶ Chemotherapy

Prevention

▶ ▫ Known BRCA carriers may have ovaries removed after childbearing is complete.

Breast Cancer

▶ Malignancy of the breast.

▶ ▪ Most people diagnosed with breast cancer have no risk factors.

▶ Lifetime risk of breast cancer (to age 85 years) is 1:8, with increasing incidence after age 50 years.

▶ Most common cancer death in women older than 65 years.

   ▷ Invasive

      ▶ Tumor no longer contained within basement membrane.

      ▶ Originates from epithelial cells lining mammary ducts.

      ▶ Subtypes include medullary, papillary, tubular, and colloid.

      ▶ Invasive lobar carcinoma arises from mammary lobule.

▶ Screening

▷ See "Screening," chapter 4

Risk Factors

▶ Female

▶ Advanced age

▶ Early menarche

▶ Late menopause

▶ Use of combination estrogen-progesterone hormones after menopause

▶ Nulliparity

▶ Women who took the drug DES

▶ Alcohol consumption

▶ Family history or personal history of invasive breast cancer, ductal carcinoma in situ or lobular carcinoma in situ, or a history of breast biopsies that show benign proliferative

▶ Increased breast density

▶ Exposure to ionizing radiation, especially during puberty or young adulthood

▶ Inheritance of detrimental genetic mutations such as the BRCA mutation

Signs and Symptoms

▶ Nipple retraction, ulceration, eczema, tenderness, discharge

▶ Lump or thickening of breast or axilla

▷ Breast lump most common and has hard, indistinct borders

▶ Edema or erythema of breast skin

▶ Change in breast shape or skin texture

Diagnostic Tests

▶ Negative tests are not necessarily diagnostic in the presence of a palpable breast mass.

▷ Mammogram

▷ Ultrasound evaluation

▶ Determines solid or cystic lesion

▷ Fine-needle or core biopsy

▷ CBC, LFTs, chemistries, estrogen and progesterone receptor determination

▷ Chest X-ray, CT scan, ultrasound

▷ Assess lymph node involvement after biopsy

Differential Diagnoses

▶ Benign proliferative breast disease

▶ Benign lesions, lipoma, fibroadenoma

▶ Necrosis, infection, abscess

▶ Fibrocystic changes

▶ Intraductal papilloma

Management

▶ Surgical intervention

▶ Lumpectomy, mastectomy, sentinel node biopsy, axillary lymph node dissection

▶ Chemotherapy, hormonal or biological therapies

▶ Radiation

Prevention

▶ ◉ Patient education to include

▷ Avoid tobacco,

▷ Maintain optimal weight,

▷ Limit alcohol,

▷ Exercise, and

▷ Limit exposure to radiation.

REFERENCES

American College of Obstetricians and Gynecologists. 2012. "Abnormal Uterine Bleeding." FAQ 095: Gynecologic Problems. https://www.acog.org/-/media/For-Patients/faq095.pdf?dmc=1& ts=20161108T0048490959.

———. 2015. "ACOG Statement on Revised American Cancer Society Recommendations on Breast Cancer Screening." http://www.acog.org/About-ACOG/News-Room/Statements/2015/ ACOG-Statement-on-Recommendations-on-Breast-Cancer Screening.

Breastcancer.org. 2017. "What to Do if Your Genetic Test Results Are Positive." http://www. breastcancer.org/symptoms/testing/genetic/pos_results.

Cancer.Net. 2016. "Uterine Cancer: Risk Factors and Prevention." American Society of Clinical Oncology. http://www.cancer.net/cancer-types/uterine-cancer/risk-factors-and-prevention.

Centers for Disease Control and Prevention. 2015. "Gonococcal Infections." In "Sexually Transmitted Diseases Treatment Guidelines, 2015," supplement, *Morbidity and Mortality Weekly Report* 64 (3): 60–68. http://www.cdc.gov/std/tg2015/gonorrhea.htm.

———. 2017. "What Should I Know about Screening?" Gynecologic Cancers. https://www.cdc. gov/cancer/uterine/basic_info/screening.htm.

Cohen, S., W. Gans, and B. Slaughenoupt. 2016. "Medical Student Curriculum: Acute Scrotum." American Urological Association Educational Programs. https://www.auanet.org/education/ acute-scrotum.cfm.

Committee on Gynecologic Practice. 2013. "Management of Acute Abnormal Uterine Bleeding in Nonpregnant Reproductive-Aged Women." *American College of Obstetricians and Gynecologists Committee Opinion* no. 557, April. https://www.acog.org/-/media/Committee-Opinions/Committee-on-Gynecologic-Practice/co557.pdf?dmc=1&ts=20170807T1545067837.

Dunphy, L., J. Winland-Brown, B. Porter, and D. Thomas, eds. 2015. *Primary Care: The Art and Science of Advanced Practice Nursing.* 4th ed. Philadelphia: F. A. Davis.

McVary, K. T., C. G. Roehrborn, A. L. Avins, M. J. Barry, R. C. Bruskewitz, R. F. Donnell, H. E. Foster Jr., et al. 2010. *American Urological Association Guideline: Management of Benign Prostatic Hyperplasia.* Rev. ed. N.p.: American Urological Association Education and Research, Inc. https://www.auanet.org/education/guidelines/benign-prostatic-hyperplasia.cfm.

National Institute of Diabetes and Digestive and Kidney Diseases. 2014. *Prostatitis: Inflammation of the Prostate.* NIH Publication No. 14–4553. National Kidney and Urologic Diseases Information Clearinghouse. https://www.niddk.nih.gov/health-information/urologic-diseases/prostate-problems/prostatitis-inflammation-prostate.

Urology Care Foundation. 2017. "What Is Benign Prostatic Hyperplasia (BPH)?" http://www.urologyhealth.org/urologic-conditions/benign-prostatic-hyperplasia-(bph).

US Preventive Services Task Force. 2012. "Prostate Cancer: Screening." https://www.uspreventiveservicestaskforce.org/Page/Document/UpdateSummaryFinal/prostate-cancer-screening.

CHAPTER 12

GENITOURINARY, RENAL, AND SEXUALLY TRANSMITTED DISEASES

LEARNING OBJECTIVES

▶ Recognize common disorders of the genitourinary system and analyze processes for making differential diagnoses.

▷ Risk factors

▷ Signs and symptoms

▷ Diagnostic tests

▷ Differential diagnoses

▶ Describe treatment and management of genitourinary disorders.

▷ Management

▷ Prevention

RENAL AND UROLOGICAL CONSIDERATIONS FOR OLDER ADULTS

▶ Avoid nephrotoxic substances (such as IV contrast) when possible.

▶ Adjust medication dosing for decreased renal clearance and narrowed therapeutic index.

▶ Glomerular filtration rate (GFR) is the standard measure of renal function.

▶ Serum creatinine is *not* a reliable indicator of renal function in older persons.

▶ Renal function in older adults is best estimated by calculating creatinine clearance.

▶ Proteinuria indicates the kidney is leaking protein, usually from glomerular disease.

TABLE 12–1.
GENITOURINARY SYSTEM AGE-RELATED CHANGES

SYMPTOM	AGE-RELATED CHANGES
Drug toxicity	Decreases in renal blood flow, drugs are not excreted; contributed to by a decreased GFR and tubular resorption.
In men: Slower reaction time for erection with diminished ejaculation	Reduced testosterone production. Prostate hypertrophy. Penile arteries and veins sclerose.
Urinary frequency Urgency Nocturia	Bladder capacity drops to about 250 cc (from 500 cc). Ureters, bladder, and urethra lose muscle tone, elasticity. Sensory changes may delay voiding until bladder is full.
Stress incontinence Dribbling	Estrogen deficiency in women causes tissue changes and pelvic floor relaxation. Prostate enlargement in men. Atrophy of periurethral structures.
Retention	In men, enlarged prostate presses urethra closed. In women, cystocele can close it off.

Note: GFR = glomerular filtration rate

URINARY TRACT INFECTION (UTI)

► Lower UTI is an infection in one of the lower structures of the urinary tract; most often refers to inflammation in the bladder (cystitis).

► Uncomplicated UTI: Infection in an otherwise healthy patient with anatomically and functionally normal urinary tract.

► Complicated UTI: Infection associated with factors increasing colonization and decreasing efficacy of therapy:

▷ ● Anatomic or functional abnormality of urinary tract (enlarged prostate, stone disease, diverticulum, neurogenic bladder, etc.)

▷ ● Immunocompromised

▷ ● Multidrug-resistant bacteria

(Badalato and Kaufmann 2016)

► ● Most UTIs are caused by ascending infections from the urethra.

► UTI is the most common bacterial infection in women. The most common causative organisms are

▷ Gram-negative

► ● *E. coli* (80–90 percent)

► ● *Proteus mirabilis*

► ● *Klebsiella pneumoniae*

► ● *Enterobacter* species (sp.)

▷ Gram-positive *(Staphylococcus saprophyticus)* is commonly detected in sexually active women, but rarely in men.

▷ ● In symptomatic women with significant pyuria but no significant bacteriuria, suspect *Chlamydia trachomatis.*

▷ Viruses may be associated with hemorrhagic cystitis.

Risk Factors

▶ Female

▶ Sexual activity

▶ Pregnancy

▶ Diabetes

▶ Prior UTI

▶ Urinary stasis—retention

▶ Urinary tract structural abnormalities

▶ Urinary tract instrumentation

▶ Dysfunctional voiding patterns

▶ Impaired bladder innervation

▶ Immunocompromised state

▶ Aging

▷ Pelvic floor relaxation, benign prostatic hypertrophy (BPH), prostatitis, incontinence, cognitive impairment

Signs and Symptoms

▶ Dysuria

▶ Urgency, frequency

▶ Fever, chills

▶ Nausea

▶ Hematuria

▶ In older adults, altered mental status, agitation, anorexia, falls

▶ ● Urinalysis shows bacteria and white blood cells

▷ ● Pyuria (without infection) in 30 percent of asymptomatic older adults.

▷ ● Urine culture: >100,000 bacteria/mL indicates infection.

Diagnostic Tests

▶ Clean-catch or straight catheter urine collection

▶ Urinalysis and urine culture

▶ Blood urea nitrogen (BUN), creatinine, electrolytes, complete blood count (CBC)

▶ Blood cultures for severe cases

Differential Diagnoses

▶ Urethritis

▶ Diabetes

▶ Pyelonephritis

▶ Renal calculi

▶ Vaginitis

▶ Encopresis

▶ Female urethral syndrome

▶ Prostatitis

▶ Meatal stenosis

▶ Dysfunctional voiding

▶ Sexually transmitted infections (STIs)

▶ Balanitis

▶ Sexual abuse

▶ Foreign body

Management

▶ Antibiotic therapy

▶ Uncomplicated UTI (cystitis, some pyelonephritis)

   ▷ ● Nitrofurantoin 100 mg b.i.d. × 5 days or a 3-day course of oral trimethoprim/sulfamethoxazole (TMP/SMX) is 95 percent effective.

   ▷ ● If TMP/SMX resistance is >10–20 percent (US West coast, Europe), consider fluoroquinolones.

   ▷ Only use fluoroquinolones or beta-lactams if one of these recommended antibiotics cannot be used because of availability, allergy, or tolerance.

▶ Other uncomplicated UTI

   ▷ ● A full 7–10-day antibiotic course should be used in patients with diabetes, symptom duration before treatment of more than 7 days, pregnancy, age over 65 years, or past history of pyelonephritis or UTI with resistant organisms.

▶ Complicated UTI (acute pyelonephritis)

   ▷ Patients who are candidates for outpatient therapy may be treated with:

      ▶ ● Oral ciprofloxacin 500 mg b.i.d. × 7 days

      ▶ ● Once daily oral fluoroquinolone (ciprofloxacin 1000 mg ER × 7 days or levofloxacin 750 mg × 5 days)

- ▶ • Oral TMP/SMX double strength (DS) b.i.d. × 14 days (not for *Enterococcus* or *Pseudomonas*)
- ▶ Use of initial one-time IV agent (ceftriaxone 1 g, aminoglycoside, fluoroquinolone)
- ▶ Treat for 14 days
- ▷ For inpatient management (Kreshover, Ramasamy, and Singla 2016):
  - ▶ IV fluoroquinolone
  - ▶ Aminoglycoside with or without ampicillin
  - ▶ Third-generation cephalosporin
  - ▶ Extended-spectrum penicillin
  - ▶ Carbapenem
  - ▶ Switch from parenteral to oral therapy at 48 hours after clinically well
  - ▶ • Treat for 14 days

Prevention

- ▶ Hygiene measures
  - ▷ Women: Wipe from front to back
  - ▷ Men: Care of uncircumcised penis
- ▶ Complete voiding.
- ▶ Void after coitus.
- ▶ Do not "hold" voiding—prevent stasis.
- ▶ Hydration.

PYELONEPHRITIS

- ▶ Acute bacterial infection of soft tissue of renal parenchyma and pelvis, or other portion of upper urinary tract, typically producing signs and symptoms of systemic toxicity.
- ▶ • 75 percent of cases caused by *E. coli*; 10–15 percent by *Staphylococcus aureus* or *saprophyticus*; 10–15 percent by gram-negative species *P. mirabilis*, *K. pneumoniae*, or *Enterobacter* sp.
- ▶ • Most common route of infection is ascension from the bladder.

Risk Factors

- ▶ Urinary tract abnormalities or instrumentation
- ▶ Calculi
- ▶ Urinary catheterization
- ▶ Diabetes

▶ Immunocompromise

▶ Recent pyelonephritis

▶ BPH

▶ Pregnancy

▶ Fecal incontinence

▶ Recent lower UTI

Signs and Symptoms

▶ • Shaking, chills, malaise

▶ • Myalgia

▶ Abdominal or flank pain

▶ • Costovertebral angle tenderness

▶ • Fever >102°F

▶ • Hematuria, dysuria, frequency, urgency

▶ Nausea, vomiting

▶ • Urine dipstick may show casts, nitrates

▶ • Urinalysis shows bacteria and white blood cells (WBCs), possible proteinuria, leukocyte esterase, pyuria

▶ Urine culture and sensitivity identify pathogens and antibiotic sensitivity

Diagnostic Tests

▶ Urinalysis

▶ Urine culture

  ▷ • Gram stain before initiating antibiotic therapy to determine presence of gram-negative pathogens

▶ Voiding cystourethrogram, intravenous pyelogram (IVP), renal scan, cystoscopy

  ▷ Identify structural abnormality

▶ Abdominal and pelvic computed tomography (CT) scan

  ▷ Visualize renal abscess

Differential Diagnoses

▶ Calculi

▶ Prostatitis

▶ Kidney tuberculosis

▶ Acute lower back pain

▶ Tumors

Management

▶ Fluids.

▶ Recheck in 24 hours.

▶ ○ Repeat culture 2 weeks after therapy complete and again at 12 weeks.

▶ Antibiotic therapy.

▷ Treat for 14 days

▷ ○ Trimethoprim/sulfamethoxazole (TMP/SMZ) 160/800 mg or DS b.i.d.

▷ ○ Ciprofloxacin 500 mg q12h or 1 g extended release daily

▷ ○ Ofloxacin 200–300mg q12h

▶ For mild disease, a patient who is compliant and has no nausea, vomiting, dehydration, or septicemia, oral therapy is appropriate.

▷ Otherwise, initiate parenteral therapy, then switch to oral therapy for 14 days when afebrile for 24 hours (usually 72 hours after start of treatment).

▶ ○ Chronic pyelonephritis requires antibiotic therapy for 3–6 months.

▶ ○ Older adults should be hospitalized and started on an aminoglycoside with dosage adjusted for weight and renal function.

Prevention

▶ Hygiene measures:

▷ Women: Wipe from front to back

▷ Men: Care of uncircumcised penis

▶ Complete voiding.

▶ Void after coitus.

▶ Do not "hold" voiding—prevent stasis.

▶ Hydration.

HEMATURIA

▶ Presence of red blood cells (RBCs) in urine, microscopic (>3 RBC/high-power field [HPF]) or gross (visible to naked eye).

▶ May be due to infection, glomerulonephritis, stones, polycystic disease, hydronephrosis, renal vascular disease, tuberculosis, connective tissue disease, or medications; most commonly seen in prostatitis, cystitis, stones, and in older adults with neoplasms or BPH.

▶ Often no specific cause for hematuria is found.

Risk Factors

▶ UTI

▶ Renal calculi

▶ Environmental exposure to elements that cause bladder cancer

Signs and Symptoms

▶ ○ Painless hematuria

▶ ○ Urinary frequency

▶ ○ Dysuria

▶ ○ Flank pain

Diagnostic Tests

▶ Urinalysis

▶ ○ Three-tube test may identify source of bleeding

▷ Tube 1: Initial stream

▶ Urethral lesions

▷ Tube 2: Midstream

▶ Bladder

▷ Tube 3: End stream

▶ Bladder trigone

▷ Triangular region of internal bladder formed by two ureteral orifices and internal urethral orifice

▶ BUN and creatinine

▶ Renal ultrasound, cystourethrogram, CT scan, magnetic resonance imaging (MRI)

▷ Performed based on presentation

▶ STI cultures, Gram stain

▶ Midstream collection

▶ Ultrasound

▶ ○ Cystoscopy is recommended (Kreshover, Ramasamy, and Singla 2016)

▷ ○ For all patients at least 35 years of age with microhematuria,

▷ ○ For all patients who present with gross hematuria, and

▷ ○ At the discretion of the clinician based on the presence of risk factors for malignancy in patients younger than 35 years of age with microhematuria.

Differential Diagnoses

▶ Hemorrhagic cystitis

▶ Bladder cancer

▶ Ingestion of dyes and pigments

▶ Glomerulonephritis

▶ Pyelonephritis

▶ Renal calculi

▶ Pelvic inflammatory disease (PID)

Management

▶ Find and treat underlying cause.

▶ Often no treatment indicated.

▶ If protein and blood are present, rule out kidney disease.

▶ Patients with persistent hematuria after a negative initial evaluation, repeat evaluation at 48–72 months because 3 percent of this group will be subsequently diagnosed with a urologic malignancy (Kreshover, Ramasamy, and Singla 2016).

Prevention

▶ Patient education to include

▷ Maintain hydration and

▷ Prevent urinary tract infections.

ACUTE KIDNEY INJURY

▶ Defined as any of the following (Kidney Disease: Improving Global Outcomes [KDIGO] 2012 p. 8):

▷ Increase in serum creatinine (SCr) by >0.3 mg/dL within 48 hours

▷ Increase in SCr to >1.5 times baseline, which is known or presumed to have occurred within the prior 7 days

▷ Urine volume < 0.5 mL/kg/h for 6 hours

▶ Rapid loss of kidneys' ability to remove wastes, balance fluids and electrolytes; occurs over days to weeks.

▶ Associated with rapidly worsening azotemia (elevated BUN and creatinine).

▶ Many causes are reversible; many can also lead to death.

▶ Three stages of acute kidney injury (KDIGO 2012):

▷ Stage 1: 1.0- to 1.5-fold increase in serum creatinine or a decline in urinary output to 0.5 mL/ kg/h over 6–12 hours

▷ ◖ Stage 2: 2.0- to 2.9-fold increase in serum creatinine or decline in urinary output to 0.5 mL/ kg/h over 12 hours or longer

▷ ●Stage 3: 3-fold or greater increase in serum creatinine or decline in urinary output to less than 0.3 mL/ kg/h for 24 hours or longer or anuria for 12 hours or longer

TABLE 12–2.
ACUTE KIDNEY INJURY CLASSIFIED BY LOCATION OF PROBLEM

PRERENAL	INTRARENAL	POSTRENAL
Underlying kidney function may be normal, but intravascular volume depletion (vomiting or diarrhea) or decreased arterial pressure (heart failure or sepsis) reduces GFR Volume loss Cardiac and liver disease	Tubular: Ischemia or nephrotoxicity Glomerular: Interstitial blood vessels, glomeruli inflammation Vascular: Arterial catheter, anticoagulation, vascular surgery Nephrotoxic medications, recent exposure to radiographic contrast agents	Obstruction of urinary flow by prostatic hypertrophy

Risk Factors

▶   Obstruction

▶ ● Drug toxicity (angiotensin-converting enzyme inhibitor [ACEI])

▶   Rapidly progressive glomerulonephritis

▶ ◔ Rhabdomyolysis

▶   Chemotherapy

▶ ◦ Radiographic contrast agents

Signs and Symptoms

▶   Early stages may be asymptomatic

▶ ● Bruising, bleeding

▶ ◦ Anorexia, fatigue

▶ ◦ Mental status changes

     ▷   Seizures, confusion

▶ ● Uremic encephalopathy

     ▷   Mental status decline

     ▷ ● *Asterixis* (liver flap)

         ▶   Hand tremor when wrist extended, sometimes said to resemble a bird flapping its wings

▶ ◦ Flank pain

▶ ◦ Hypertension (HTN)

- ▶ Nausea and vomiting, anorexia
- ▶ Shortness of breath (SOB), edema, weight gain
- ▶ Polyuria
- ▶ Oliguria
  - ▷ Urine output less than 400 cc daily
- ▶ Anuria
  - ▷ Urine output less than 100 cc daily
- ▶ Elevated BUN and creatinine ratio
- ▶ Anemia
  - ▷ Caused by uremic platelet dysfunction

Diagnostic Tests

- ▶ Urinalysis
  - ▷ Most important noninvasive measure
  - ▷ Guides differential diagnosis and work-up
- ▶ Urine electrolytes
  - ▷ Helpful in distinguishing prerenal from intrinsic renal causes of acute kidney injury
- ▶ Medication review
- ▶ CBC, BUN, and creatinine
- ▶ 24-hour urine
- ▶ Renal ultrasound

Differential Diagnoses

- ▶ Abdominal aneurysm
- ▶ Alcohol toxicity
- ▶ Chronic renal failure
- ▶ Diabetic ketoacidosis
- ▶ Gastrointestinal (GI) bleeding
- ▶ Heart failure
- ▶ Renal calculi
- ▶ Sickle cell anemia
- ▶ Metabolic acidosis
- ▶ Obstructive uropathy
- ▶ Urinary obstruction
- ▶ Urinary tract infection

▶ Dehydration

▶ Protein overloading

▶ Steroid use

Management

▶ ● Immediately refer to urologist or nephrologist.

▶ Identify and reverse cause.

▶ Rule out obstruction from benign prostatic hypertrophy.

▶ ● Renal dialysis for aggressive treatment (hyperkalemia, acidosis, volume overload).

▶ ● Avoid urinary catheters when possible because they greatly increase the risk of infection.

Prevention

▶ Maintain hydration.

▶ Avoid nephrotoxic agents.

▶ Optimal blood glucose control.

▶ Optimal blood pressure control.

ACUTE GLOMERULONEPHRITIS

▶ Glomerular inflammation or injury resulting from an immune response following an immunologic injury (deposition of antigen-antibody complexes from the bloodstream in glomeruli).

▶ ● Diffuse inflammatory changes and abrupt hematuria with RBC casts and mild proteinuria, 1–2 weeks after strep infection.

▶ Latent period 7–21 days from onset of infection to nephritis.

Risk Factors

▶ ● Strep infection

▶ ● Systemic lupus erythematosus

▶ ● Goodpasture syndrome: Rare autoimmune disease in which antibodies attack the kidneys and lungs

▶ ● Amyloidosis: Abnormal protein build-up in the organs and tissues

▶ ● Wegener's granulomatosis: Rare disease that causes inflammation of the blood vessels

▶ ● Polyarteritis nodosa: Disease in which cells attack arteries

Signs and Symptoms

- ▶ • Recent strep infection (within 2–3 weeks)
- ▶ • Edema (90 percent of cases)
- ▶ • Especially face, hands, feet
- ▶ • HTN (75 percent of cases)
- ▶ Fever
- ▶ Abdominal or flank pain
- ▶ • Azotemia
- ▶ Malaise, fatigue
- ▶ • Abrupt hematuria, oliguria, anuria
- ▶ • Proteinuria
- ▶ • Antistreptolysin O (ASO) increased in 60–80 percent of cases
- ▶ • Total serum complement decreased

Diagnostic Tests

- ▶ • Urinalysis
- ▶ • Throat and skin cultures for strep
- ▶ • ASO
- ▶ • Total serum complement
  - ▷ Monitors proteins in immune system
  - ▷ Decreased in septicemia, shock, infections
- ▶ • Renal biopsy confirms diagnosis

Differential Diagnoses

- ▶ Systemic lupus erythematosus
- ▶ Anaphylactoid purpura
- ▶ Subacute bacterial endocarditis
- ▶ Congestive heart failure

Management

- ▶ • Inpatient treatment until edema and HTN controlled
- ▶ • Fluid restrictions
- ▶ • Protein restriction if azotemia and metabolic acidosis present
- ▶ • Avoidance of potassium-rich foods
- ▶ • Low sodium

▶ Possible dialysis

▶ Strep infection

　▷ • Penicillin 400,000 U intramuscularly (IM) or 250 mg p.o. q6h or 500 mg p.o. q12h × 10 days

　▷ • Erythromycin 400 mg q12h × 10 days

▶ Acidosis

　▷ • Sodium bicarbonate 1.2–2.4 g daily if symptomatic or bicarbonate < 15

▶ HTN

　▷ • Diuretics

　▷ • Furosemide 0.5–1 mg/kg IV or 2 mg/kg p.o. b.i.d. or t.i.d.

▶ Vasodilators

　▷ • Apresoline 0.25–1 mg/kg q.i.d. *or* nifedipine 0.25 mg/kg p.o. p.r.n. or q.i.d.

▶ • Usually spontaneous diuresis occurs within 7–10 days after onset

Prevention

▶ Treat strep infections.

▶ Optimal blood pressure control.

▶ Optimal blood glucose control.

CHRONIC KIDNEY DISEASE (CKD)

▶ Decreased glomerular filtration rate with progressive, irreversible kidney damage.

▶ • 70–75 percent of end-stage renal disease is due to HTN and diabetes mellitus (DM).

▶ • Stages (National Kidney Foundation 2002):

　▷ Stage 1: Normal or high GFR (GFR > 90 mL/min)

　▷ Stage 2: Mild CKD (GFR = 60–89 mL/min)

　▷ Stage 3A: Moderate CKD (GFR = 45–59 mL/min)

　▷ Stage 3B: Moderate CKD (GFR = 30–44 mL/min)

　▷ Stage 4: Severe CKD (GFR = 15–29 mL/min)

　▷ Stage 5: End stage CKD (GFR < 15 mL/min); dialysis indicated

Risk Factors

▶ Diabetes

▶ Hypertension

▶ Family history of kidney failure

▶ Increasing age

▶   African, Hispanic, Asian, Pacific Island, or Native American descent

▶ ◢ Multiple myeloma, BPH, HTN, DM

Signs and Symptoms

▶   Fatigue, insomnia

▶   Poor appetite

▶   Muscle cramping at night

▶   Facial, ankle, pedal edema

▶   Urticaria

▶   Nocturia

Diagnostic Tests

▶ ◢ Urinalysis or microalbumin

　▷   Shows protein

▶ ◢ 24-hour urine

　▷   Shows protein excretion and decreased creatinine clearance

▶ ◢ CBC, complete metabolic panel, electrolytes, BUN

　▷   Creatinine not a reliable indicator of renal function in older adults

▶ ◢ Renal ultrasound, biopsy.

▶ ◢ GFR

　▷   Calculated using Cockroft-Gault formula; older adults with low GFR should be assessed for other markers of CKD such as HTN and proteinuria.

　▷   Cockroft-Gault formula:

　　▶ $C_{Cr} = (140 - age) \times weight\ (kg) \div (S_{Cr} \times 72)$ ($\times\ 0.85$ if female to account for less muscle mass)

Differential Diagnoses

▶   Systemic lupus erythematosus

▶   Renal artery stenosis

▶   Urinary obstruction

▶   Wegener's granulomatosis

▶   Acute kidney injury

▶   Polycystic kidney disease

▶   Glomerulonephritis

▶   Diabetic nephropathy

▶   Goodpasture syndrome

▶ Multiple myeloma

▶ Nephrolithiasis or nephrosclerosis

Management

▶ Discontinue offending medications, if possible.

▶ Evaluate hydration status.

▶ Monitor daily weights, edema.

▶ Correct volume depletion or overload.

▶ Monitor intake and output

▶ Treat comorbidities.

▶ Monitor CBC for anemia of chronic disease.

▶ Maintain low-protein diet.

▶ Control glucose.

▶ Manage lipids.

▶ Avoid contrast dyes, nephrotoxic drugs (NSAIDs).

▶ ACEIs or angiotensin receptor blockers (ARBs) for blood pressure control (nephroprotective).

Prevention

▶ Maintain hydration.

▶ Avoid nephrotoxic agents.

▶ Optimal blood glucose control.

▶ Optimal blood pressure control.

END-STAGE RENAL DISEASE (ESRD)

▶ End-stage kidney disease is the last stage of chronic kidney disease, in which kidney function is failing and unable to sustain life.

Risk Factors

▶ Chronic kidney disease (CKD)

▶ Diabetes

▶ Injury or trauma to the kidneys

▶ Major blood loss

Signs and Symptoms

▶ Oliguria, anuria

▶ General malaise, fatigue

- ▶ Drowsiness, confusion
- ▶ Pruritis, muscle cramping
- ▶ Weight loss, anorexia
- ▶ Nausea and vomiting, excessive thirst, hiccups
- ▶ Edema
- ▶ Paresthesia in hands and feet
- ▶ Bruising, nosebleeds, bloody stool
- ▶ Sleep problems

Diagnostic Tests

- ▶ Kidney function tests
- ▶ GFR
- ▶ CBC, complete metabolic panel, renal panel, magnesium
- ▶ Erythropoietin
- ▶ Parathyroid hormone
- ▶ Bone density test

Differential Diagnoses

- ▶ Acute kidney injury
- ▶ Alport syndrome
- ▶ Genetic condition with progressive kidney decline, hearing loss, and eye abnormalities
- ▶ Diabetic nephropathy
- ▶ Glomerulonephritis
- ▶ Goodpasture syndrome
  - ▷ Autoimmune disease in which the body produces antibodies against collagen in the lungs and kidneys
- ▶ Multiple myeloma
- ▶ Nephrolithiasis or nephrosclerosis
- ▶ Polycystic kidney disease

Management

- ▶ Dialysis
- ▶ Transplantation
- ▶ Antihypertensives
- ▶ Diabetes control

► ⸱ Anemia treatment
  ▷ Dietary iron or supplements
  ▷ Erythropoietin
  ▷ Blood transfusions
► ⁕ Low-protein, low-salt diet
► Limit foods high in potassium, phosphorous
► Calcium and vitamin D supplements
► ⁕ Phosphate binders to keep phosphate levels down
  ▷ � Calcium salts
    ► Carbonate, lactate, or acetate
  ▷ � Aluminum hydroxide (Alu-Caps)
► � Fluid restrictions
  ▷ For patients on dialysis, 700–1,000 mL/day, plus urine output
► Palliation

Prevention

► Maintain hydration.
► Avoid nephrotoxic agents.
► Optimal blood glucose control.
► Optimal blood pressure control.

URINARY INCONTINENCE

► Involuntary loss of urine from weakened or overactive bladder sphincter and detrusor muscles.
► Approximately 20 million women and 6 million men in the United States have urinary incontinence or have experienced it at some time in their lives.
► See table 12–3 for the types of urinary incontinence.
► ⦁ Reversible causes: DRIP
  ▷ **D**elirium
  ▷ **R**estricted mobility from illness, injury, restraints
  ▷ **I**nfection, Inflammation, Impaction
  ▷ **P**olyuria from diabetes, caffeine intake, volume overload or
  ▷ **P**harmaceuticals (diuretics, anticholinergic agents, psychotropics)
► DRIP management
  ▷ Identify and treat reversible causes

TABLE 12–3.
INCONTINENCE TYPES

TYPE	CAUSE	SIGNS AND SYMPTOMS
Stress	Increased intra-abdominal pressure Weak pelvic floor or sphincter muscle at bladder neck	Leakage with sneezing, coughing, bearing down
Urge	Overactive bladder Bladder muscles contract and override urethral sphincter muscles	Leakage after abrupt urge to void
Mixed	Combined urge and stress	Combined urge and stress
Overflow	Weak bladder muscles Nerve damage Urine flow blockage (tumors; enlarged prostate) Constipation Medications	Constant dribbling because of incomplete emptying
Functional	Neuro-urologic and lower urinary tract dysfunction (delirium, psychiatric disorders, urinary infection, impaired mobility)	Inability to get to toilet because of pain and other limitations

Risk Factors

▶ • Women

▷ Weakened and stretched pelvic muscles after childbirth

▷ Hysterectomy

▷ Postmenopausal vaginal or urethral thinning and drying

▶ • Men

▷ BPH

▷ Prostate surgery

▶ Advanced age

▶ Weakened pelvic floor muscles

▶ High-impact exercise

▶ Smoking

▶ Medicines

▷ Alpha-adrenergic blockers

▶ Relax muscles

▷ Terazosin

▷ Alpha-adrenergic agonists (e.g., pseudoephedrine)

▶ Tighten muscles

▶ Cause overflow incontinence

- ▷ Diuretics
- ▷ Colchicine
  - ▶ Urge incontinence
- ▷ Caffeine, sedatives, antidepressants, antipsychotics, antihistamines
- ▶ Constipation
- ▶ Obesity
- ▶ Urinary tract infections
- ▶ Vascular disease
- ▶ Neurological disorders
- ▶ Diabetes
- ▶ Multiple sclerosis
- ▶ Alzheimer's disease

History

- ▶ Onset and course
- ▶ Precipitating factors
- ▶ Timing, frequency, and volume of incontinence
- ▶ Diet: Fluids, alcohol, caffeine intake
- ▶ Lower urinary tract symptoms
- ▶ Bowel habits
- ▶ Sexual function
- ▶ Medications
- ▶ Voiding diary
- ▶ Patient goals

Physical Exam

- ▶ Neurological, physical (including pelvic, rectal, and prostate exams), and psychological exams
- ▶ Evidence of fluid retention
- ▶ Observation of leakage
- ▶ Mobility and mental status
- ▶ Odor

Diagnostic Tests

- ▶ Urinalysis, culture and sensitivity
  - ▷ Identifies UTI

▶ ⁖Serum BUN, creatinine

▶ ⁖ Glucose

▶ ⁘ Urodynamic studies (postvoiding residual [PVR] < 100 = normal)

Differential Diagnoses

▶ Cystitis

▶ Multiple sclerosis

▶ Prostatitis

▶ Urinary obstruction

▶ Uterine prolapse

▶ Vaginitis

▶ Urinary tract infection

▶ Spinal cord neoplasms, trauma, disease, epidural abscess

Management

▶ Antibiotics for UTI

▶ ⁖ Behavior therapy

▷   Timed or prompted voiding; no caffeine or alcohol

▶ ⁖ Weight loss

▶ ⁖ Increase fluid

▷   Stop 2–3 hours before bedtime

▶ ⁖ Pelvic floor exercises

▷   Kegel exercises strengthen pelvic floor muscles that support the uterus, bladder, small intestine, and rectum.

▶ ⁖ Pessary insertion

▷   Firm ring that presses against vaginal and urethral walls to decrease urine leakage

▷   Fitted into vagina to support uterus, bladder, and rectum

▶ ⁖ Medications

▷   Acetylcholine antagonists

▶   Side effects: Tachycardia, hyperthermia, mydriasis, dry skin, dry mucus membranes, decreased bowel sounds, urinary retention, hallucinations, psychosis, seizures, coma

▶   Side effects worse in frail older adults

▶ Intermittent catheterization

▶ Condom catheter for men

- ▶ Surgery

  - ▷ Urethral bulking: Injections to build urethral thickness to prevent leakage.

  - ▷ Suburethral slings: Slings placed under urethra to help prevent urinary leaks.

  - ▷ Sacral nerve modulation or stimulation: Implanted device sends electrical pulses to sacral nerves to reduce incontinence.

  - ▷ Botox therapy: Botox injections block contractions of overactive bladder, while surrounding muscles still function.

Prevention

- ▶ Kegel exercises
- ▶ Avoid constipation
- ▶ Exercise
- ▶ Maintain optimal weight
- ▶ Bladder training

SEXUAL DYSFUNCTION

- ▶ Disorders of sexual desire, arousal, and orgasm, and sexual pain disorders
- ▶ Sexual function influenced by ethnicity, culture, emotional state, previous sexual experiences, age, disease, and drug use
- ▶ Can occur at any age but erectile dysfunction and premature or delayed ejaculation more common in men older than 70 years

Risk Factors

- ▶ Age-related changes

  - ▷ Women

    - ▶ Vaginal wall dryness and thinning and uterine contractions cause dyspareunia, tearing of vaginal wall, slowed sexual response.

  - ▷ Men

    - ▶ Loss of penile firmness, slowed sexual response, erectile dysfunction, longer time to ejaculate, longer interval between erections

- ▶ Prostatectomy
- ▶ Loss of partner
- ▶ Estrogen deficiency
- ▶ History of sexual abuse
- ▶ Medications or drug abuse
- ▶ Depression or stress

▶ Medical conditions

▶ • Coronary artery disease (CAD), HTN, sleep apnea, diabetes, arthritis

Signs and Symptoms •

▶ Premature or delayed ejaculation

▶ Erectile dysfunction or dyspareunia

▶ Loss of libido

▶ Lower urinary tract symptoms

▶ Difficulty reaching orgasm

▶ Vaginal dryness

Diagnostic Tests

▶ Sexual history

▷ Living situation, sexual activity

▷ Partners: Men, women, both?

▷ Married, girlfriend, or boyfriend?

▷ Ever treated for STI?

▷ Experimented with drugs or alcohol?

▷ Ask gender-neutral questions to build trust: Avoid gender stereotypes. Avoid making assumptions about the gender of patient's partner(s).

▷ Topics that cover sexual behaviors or feelings that need discussion:

▶ Concerns about sexual identity

▶ Sexual behavior that increases risk of disease

▶ Harassment of or by others

▶ Worry about masturbating or touching body

Differential Diagnoses

▶ Vulvodynia

▶ Vaginismus

▶ Dyspareunia

▶ Sexual aversion

▶ Cancer

▶ Epispadias

▶ Widow or widower syndrome

▶ Performance anxiety

▶ Malnutrition

▶ Medications

▷ Antidepressants, antipsychotics, antihypertensives, antiulcer drugs, hyperlipidemia medications

Management

▶ ⁹ Antidepressants

▶ Psychological behavior therapies for sexual disorders

▶ ⁰ Alternative medicine herbals

▷ Ginseng, gingko, yohimbe

▶ Men

▷ ⁰ Erectile dysfunction

▶ Phosphodiesterase type 5 inhibitors

▶ Sildenafil (Viagra), tadalafil (Cialis), vardenafil (Levitra)

▶ Vasodilators injected into penis

▶ Papaverine, phentolamine, or alprostadil and combinations (Caverject, Edex, Trimix)

▶ Penile vacuum devices

▶ Vascular or penile implant surgery

▶ Women

▷ ⁹ Postmenopausal vaginal dryness

▶ Over-the-counter (OTC) creams and preparations for vaginal dryness.

▶ Estrogen therapy—patch or cream.

▶ Testosterone may increase sexual drive.

Prevention

▶ None known

SEXUALLY TRANSMITTED INFECTIONS (STIS)

▶ Infections caused by bacteria, parasites, and viruses contracted by having sex with an infected person

▶ Most common: Chlamydia, genital herpes, gonorrhea, syphilis, human papilloma virus (HPV), trichomoniasis, human immunodeficiency virus (HIV), or acquired immune deficiency syndrome (AIDS)

Risk Factors (all STIs)

▶ Women more susceptible than men

▶ Sexual activity at young age

- ▶ Multiple sex partners

- ▶ Unprotected vaginal, anal, or oral sex

- ▶ Sexual contact with high-risk or infected partner

- ▶ Immunocompromised

- ▶ Substance abuse

Chlamydia

- ▶ *Chlamydia trachomatis* is the most common sexually transmitted bacterium in the United States, with over 4 million infections annually.

- ▶ Incubation period can range from days to months, averaging 1–3 weeks to months.

- ▶ If untreated:

  - ▷ Women

    - ▶ ●Can lead to PID, fallopian tube damage and infertility, increased risk of ectopic pregnancy, premature birth; can be passed from mother to child during childbirth

  - ▷ Men

    - ▶ ● Can cause nongonococcal urethritis (NGU), epididymitis, proctitis

Signs and Symptoms

- ▶ Often asymptomatic

- ▶ Vary by gender; see table 12–4

Diagnostic Tests

- ▶ ● Culture

  - ▷ Most definitive, but takes 3–9 days

- ▶ ● Enzyme immunoassay (EIA) for screening

  - ▷ Results in 30–120 minutes

TABLE 12–4.
CHLAMYDIA SIGNS AND SYMPTOMS BY GENDER ●

FEMALE	MALE
Vaginal discharge, itching, burning	Thick, cloudy, penile discharge
Dysuria, dysmenorrhea	Itching or burning at penal orifice
Intramenstrual spotting	Testicular pain and swelling
Postcoital bleeding	Dysuria
Abdominal or pelvic pain	
Dyspareunia	
Fever	

Differential Diagnoses

▶ Candidiasis

▶ Conjunctivitis

▶ Ectopic pregnancy

▶ Endometriosis

▶ Gonorrhea

▶ Herpes simplex

▶ Trichomoniasis

▶ Orchitis

▶ Pelvic inflammatory disease

▶ Reactive arthritis

▶ UTI

Management

▶ Antibiotics

▶ Oral antibiotic therapy for 7–10 days

▶ • Azithromycin 1 g orally in a single dose

▶ • Erythromycin base 500 mg orally four times a day for 7 days

▶ Erythromycin ethylsuccinate 800 mg orally four times a day for 7 days

▶ Levofloxacin 500 mg orally once daily for 7 days

▶ Ofloxacin 300 mg orally twice a day for 7 days

▶ If patient is pregnant

▷ Azithromycin 1 g orally in a single dose

▷ Amoxicillin 500 mg orally three times a day for 7 days

▷ Erythromycin base 500 mg orally four times a day for 7 days

▷ Erythromycin base 250 mg orally four times a day for 14 days

▷ Erythromycin ethylsuccinate 800 mg orally four times a day for 7 days

▷ Erythromycin ethylsuccinate 400 mg orally four times a day for 14 days (CDC 2015b)

Prevention

▶ Education for prevention

▷ Safe sex practices

▷ Trace and treat contacts

Genital Herpes

▶ See also "Herpes Simplex" in chapter 6.

▶ Herpes simplex virus (HSV) II is a sexually transmitted virus; HSV I can also be transmitted sexually, usually involving the sacral nerve root ganglia (S2–S5) in genital HSV infections.

▶ HSV II reactivates more frequently in the genital region and is transmitted sexually.

▶ Incubation period is 1–20 days.

Signs and Symptoms

▶ Single or multiple clusters of small, painful vesicles on red base or open sores that sequence as follows:

1. Prodrome tingling, burning, itching sensation in legs, buttocks, or genitals
2. Erythematous papules
3. Tiny vesicles become pustular and ulcerate
4. Dry to yellow crust within 5–7 days

▶ Spontaneously disappears in few weeks.

▶ Herpes virus remains in the body and may reoccur.

Diagnostic Tests

▶ Polymerase chain reaction (PCR) blood test

▷ Most common test (very accurate)

▷ Identifies genital herpes when no symptoms

▷ Identifies viral DNA

▶ Cell culture

▷ Scraping lesion identifies presence of herpes

▶ Type-specific HSV serologic assays are based on the HSV-specific glycoprotein G2 (HSV-2) and glycoprotein G1 (HSV-1)

▷ Differentiates HSV I and HSV II

▶ When possible, test for other STIs (syphilis, gonorrhea, chlamydia, HIV)

Differential Diagnoses

▶ Syphilis

Management

▶ Initial treatment (choose one)

▷ Acyclovir 400 mg p.o. t.i.d. for 7–10 days

▷ Acyclovir 200 mg p.o. five times a day for 7–10 days

▷ Valacyclovir 1 g p.o. b.i.d. for 7–10 days

▷ Famciclovir 250 mg p.o. t.i.d. for 7–10 days

▶ Suppressive therapy (choose one)

  ▷ Acyclovir 400 mg p.o. b.i.d.

  ▷ Valacyclovir 500 mg p.o. once a day

  ▷ Valacyclovir 1 g p.o. once a day

  ▷ Famciclovir 250 mg p.o. b.i.d.

▶ Episodic therapy (choose one)

  ▷ Acyclovir 400 mg p.o. t.i.d. for 5 days

  ▷ Acyclovir 800 mg p.o. b.i.d. for 5 days

  ▷ Acyclovir 800 mg p.o. t.i.d. for 2 days

  ▷ Valacyclovir 500 mg p.o. b.i.d. for 3 days

  ▷ Valacyclovir 1 g p.o. t.i.d. for 5 days

  ▷ Famciclovir 125 mg p.o. b.i.d. for 5 days

  ▷ Famciclovir 1 g p.o. b.i.d. for 1 day

  ▷ Famciclovir 500 mg p.o. once, followed by 250 mg p.o. b.i.d. for 2 days

Prevention

▶ Education for prevention

  ▷ Safe sex practices

  ▷ Trace and treat contacts

Gonorrhea

▶ *Neisseria gonorrhoeae* is a gram-negative diplococcal sexually transmitted bacterial infection present in human exudate and mucus.

▶ Incubation is 2–10 days.

▶ Greatest incidence is in sexually active 15- to 29-year-olds.

▶ Symptoms in infected men occur early so treatment is started before complications arise but symptoms in many infected women are delayed until complications develop.

▶ Incidence of gonorrhea infections among men who have sex with men is 10 times greater.

▶ Can cause ophthalmic gonorrhea and can be disseminated.

Signs and Symptoms

▶ White, yellow, or green purulent penile or vaginal discharge

▶ Burning urination

▶ Dyspareunia

▶ Vaginal bleeding or discharge

Diagnostic Tests

▶ Annual screening recommended for all sexually active women younger than 25 years and for older women at increased risk for infection (e.g., those who have a new sex partner, more than one sex partner, a sex partner with concurrent partners, or a sex partner who has an STI)

▶ Cervical or urethral culture using modified Thayer Martin media

▶ Nucleic acid amplification on first void in males

▶ DNA probe

Differential Diagnoses

▶ PID

▶ Nongonococcal cervicitis or pharyngitis

▶ Urethritis

▶ Proctitis

▶ Vaginitis

▶ Chlamydia

▶ Arthritis

Management

▶ Uncomplicated gonococcal infections of the cervix, urethra, and rectum

▷ Ceftriaxone 250 mg IM in a single dose *plus*

▷ Azithromycin 1g p.o. in a single dose *or*

▷ If ceftriaxone is not available:

▶ Cefixime 400 mg p.o. in a single dose *plus*

▶ Azithromycin 1 g p.o. in a single dose

▶ Uncomplicated gonococcal infections of the pharynx

▷ Ceftriaxone 250 mg IM in a single dose *plus*

▷ Azithromycin 1 g p.o. in a single dose

▶ Disseminated gonococcal infection

▷ Ceftriaxone 1 g IM or IV q24h *plus*

▷ Azithromycin 1 g p.o. in a single dose

▷ Alternative regimens

▶ Cefotaxime 1 g IV q8h *or*

▶ Ceftizoxime 1 g IV q8h *plus*

▶ Azithromycin 1 g p.o. in a single dose

▶ Coexistent chlamydial infections are common

▷ Tetracycline or macrolide antibiotic concurrently

▷ Doxycyline 100 mg p.o. b.i.d. × 7 days

▷ Azithromycin 1 g p.o.

Prevention

▶ Safe sex practices.

▶ Abstain from sexual activity for 7 days after treatment and until all sex partners are adequately treated.

▶ Recent sex partners (i.e., persons having sexual contact with the infected patient within the 60 days preceding onset of symptoms or gonorrhea diagnosis) should be referred for evaluation, testing, and presumptive dual treatment.

Chancroid

▶ Gram-negative bacillus *Haemophilus ducreyi* is a sexually transmitted bacterium that causes genital ulcerations.

▶ Transmission occurs from direct contact with infected lesions.

▶ Predominant in Africa and Southwest Asia; most diagnosed cases in the United States are among people who travel to where infection is common.

▶ Incubation period from 3–5 days to 2 weeks.

Risk Factors

▶ ● Residing in endemic areas

▶ ● Uncircumcised male

Signs and Symptoms

▶ ● Painful unilateral inguinal lymphadenopathy in 50 percent

▷ Occurs in 1–2 weeks

▶ ● Painful, small lump 1/8–2 inches in diameter with sharply defined borders

▷ Vesicopustule with necrotic base

▷ Erythema with undermined edges

▷ Multiple lesions and inguinal adenitis common

▶ Women

▷ Multiple lesions

▷ Ulcers on labia majora

▷ ● "Kissing ulcers" on opposite surfaces of labia

▶ Men

▷ ● Single lesion

▷ Ulcer on foreskin, groove behind penile head or shaft, penal orifice, scrotum

Diagnostic Tests

▶ A probable diagnosis of chancroid can be made if *all* of the following criteria are met:

▷ Patient has one or more painful genital ulcers.

▷ Clinical presentation, appearance of genital ulcers and, if present, regional lymphadenopathy are typical for chancroid.

▷ Patient has no evidence of *T. pallidum* infection by darkfield examination of ulcer exudate or by a serologic test for syphilis performed at least 7 days after onset of ulcers.

▷ HSV PCR test or HSV culture performed on the ulcer exudate is negative.

Differential Diagnoses

▶ Syphilis

▶ Herpes

Management

▶ Antibiotics

▷ Azithromycin 1 g p.o. in a single dose *or*

▷ Ceftriaxone 250 mg IM in a single dose *or*

▷ Ciprofloxacin 500 mg p.o. b.i.d for 3 days *or*

▷ Erythromycin base 500 mg p.o. t.i.d. for 7 days

▶ Patients should be reexamined 3–7 days after initiation of therapy.

▶ ● Sex partners of patients who have chancroid should be examined and treated if they had sexual contact with the patient during the 10 days preceding the patient's onset of symptoms.

Prevention

▶ Education for prevention:

▷ Safe sex practices

▶ Treat sexual partners as needed.

Syphilis

▶ Sexually transmitted *Treponema pallidum* spirochete bacterium causes syphilis.

▶ Incubation period is 3 weeks to 3 months.

TABLE 12–5.
SIGNS AND SYMPTOMS OF SYPHILIS

PRIMARY	SECONDARY	TERTIARY
Small, painless chancre on genitals, mouth, skin, or rectum	Palm and sole rash	Paralysis, blindness, dementia, deafness, impotence, death when untreated
Heals in 3–6 weeks	Mucous patches in mouth, vagina, or penis	
Chancre area lymphadenopathy	Condylomata lata on genitals, skin folds	
	Fever, malaise, muscle aches, joint pain, appetite loss, vision changes, hair loss, lymphadenopathy	

Diagnostic Tests

▶ ◦ VDRL (Venereal Disease Research Laboratory)

▷ 78–86 percent sensitivity for primary syphilis

▷ 100 percent sensitivity for secondary syphilis

▷ 95–98 percent sensitivity for tertiary syphilis

▶ ◦ RPR (rapid plasma reagin)

▶ Fluorescent treponemal antibody absorbed (FTA-ABS)

Differential Diagnoses

▶ Candidiasis

▶ Chancroid

▶ Condyloma acuminata

▶ Cystitis in females

▶ Herpes

▶ Drug eruptions

▶ HIV

▶ Lymphogranuloma venereum

▶ Urethritis

▶ Urinary tract infection

▶ Varicella zoster

▶ Yaws

Management

▶ Primary or secondary syphilis

▷ Benzathine penicillin G 2.4 million units IM in a single dose

▷ Penicillin allergy

▶ Any person with penicillin allergy should be treated in consultation with infectious disease specialist.

▷ Doxycycline 100 mg p.o. b.i.d. for 14 days

▷ Tetracycline 500 mg p.o.. q.i.d. for 14 days

▶ Tertiary (gummas and cardiac syphilis, but not neurosyphilis)

▷ Benzathine penicillin G 7.2 million units total, administered as three doses of 2.4 million units IM each at 1-week intervals (Centers for Disease Control and Prevention [CDC] 2016c)

Prevention

▶ Education for prevention:

▷ Safe sex practices

▶ Treat sexual partners as needed.

Human Papillomavirus (HPV) and Genital Warts

▶ Human papillomavirus is a sexually transmitted virus that causes genital warts, and is the most common sexually transmitted infection (STI).

▶ Over 40 types of HPV exist.

▶ Approximately 20 million Americans are currently infected; 6 million are newly infected annually.

▶ Incubation period is 2 weeks to 8 months.

▶ HPV affects 50 percent of sexually active men and women at some point.

▶ Most who are infected do not even know it.

▶ ● Ninety percent of cases of HPV are cleared by the immune system within 2 years.

▶ HPV can infect the mouth, throat, genitals, and anus, but rarely causes warts in the throat.

▶ The majority of genital warts appear 2–3 months after HPV infection.

▶ ● Infected persons may have recurrent respiratory papillomatosis.

▶ Some warts cause cancer of cervix, vulva, vagina, penis, anus, or oropharynx.

▶ The types that cause genital warts do not cause cancer.

▶ There is no way to detect who among the infected will develop cancer or other health problems; few with genital warts develop symptoms or health issues.

Signs and Symptoms

▶ ● Various sizes and shapes of flesh-colored macular or papular bumps or clusters on genitals or mouth

Diagnostic Tests

▶ ● Diagnosis of anogenital warts is usually made by visual inspection.

▷ Can be confirmed by biopsy, which is indicated if lesions are atypical (e.g., pigmented, indurated, affixed to underlying tissue, bleeding, or ulcerated lesions).

▷ Biopsy might also be indicated in the following circumstances, particularly if the patient is immunocompromised (including those infected with HIV; CDC 2015a):

▶ The diagnosis is uncertain;

▶ The lesions do not respond to standard therapy; or

▶ The disease worsens during therapy.

▶ ● HPV testing is not recommended for anogenital wart diagnosis, because test results are not confirmatory and do not guide genital wart management (CDC 2015a).

▶ Test for concomitant STDs: HIV, gonorrhea, syphilis, chlamydia.

Differential Diagnoses

▶ Herpes simplex

▶ Syphilis

Management

▶ • Most HPV infections clear spontaneously, so antivirals are not recommended.

▶ Recommended regimens for external anogenital warts (i.e., penis, groin, scrotum, vulva, perineum, external anus, and perianus):

   ▷ Patient-applied

      ▶ Imiquimod 3.75 percent or 5 percent cream *or*

      ▶ Podofilox 0.5 percent solution or gel *or*

      ▶ Sinecatechins 15 percent ointment

   ▷ Provider-administered

      ▶ • Cryotherapy with liquid nitrogen or cryoprobe *or*

      ▶ • Surgical removal by tangential scissor excision, tangential shave excision, curettage, laser, or electrosurgery *or*

      ▶ • Trichloroacetic acid (TCA) or bichloroacetic acid (BCA) 80–90 percent solution

▶ • Pap smear

   ▷ Cervical cancer screening: Start at age 21 years and continue through age 65 years to prevent invasive cervical cancer.

   ▷ Pap testing is recommended every 3 years from ages 21–29.

   ▷ During ages 30–65 years, women should either receive a Pap test every 3 years or a Pap test plus HPV co-test every 5 years; co-testing can be done by either collecting one swab for the Pap test and another for the HPV test or by using the remaining liquid cytology material for the HPV test.

   ▷ • Because of the high negative predictive value of two tests, women who test negative for both HPV and Pap test should not be screened again for 5 years.

   ▷ Cervical screening programs should screen women who have received HPV vaccination in the same manner as unvaccinated women (CDC 2016b).

   ▷ • Anal Pap smears for men who receive anal sex.

Prevention

▶ Vaccination (see table 12–6):

   ▷ Protects against cancers caused by HPV when given at recommended ages

   ▷ • Vaccinate at age 11–12 years

   ▷ • If not previously vaccinated, vaccinate up to age 26

▶ • Routine screening for cervical cancer in women aged 21 to 65 years old can prevent cervical cancer.

▶ Education for prevention:

   ▷ Latex condoms lower chance of HPV infection of genitals, mouth, throat, tongue, and anus.

   ▷ Monogamy reduces risk.

Trichomoniasis

▶ Sexually transmitted protozoan flagellate causes trichomoniasis.

▶ Trichomoniasis is the most prevalent nonviral sexually transmitted infection in the United States.

▶ Most common curable STI in the United States, with 3.7 million people infected.

▶ 30 percent never develop symptoms.

▶ Older women are more likely to be infected than younger women.

▶ ● Associated with adverse pregnancy outcomes, infertility, postoperative infections, and cervical neoplasia.

▶ Incubation period is 5–28 days.

Signs and Symptoms

▶ ● Men

▷ Itching, irritation inside penis, burning after urination, ejaculation, penile discharge

▶ ● Women

▷ Itching, burning, redness or soreness, discomfort with urination, malodorous thin or frothy yellow-green vaginal discharge.

▷ ● Vaginal pH > 4.5.

▷ Pap smear may show trichomonads.

▷ ● Positive whiff test

▶ ● Fishy odor when potassium hydroxide (KOH) applied to discharge ●

Diagnostic Tests

▶ ● NAAT (nucleic acid amplification test) is highly sensitive and more sensitive than wet-mount microscopy.

▶ ● Pap smear

▷ May show trichomonads

▶ ● KOH wet mount

▷ To rule out candidiasis

▷ Whiff test

Differential Diagnoses

▶ Bacterial vaginosis

▶ Vulvovaginal candidiasis

▶ Gonorrhea

▶ PID

▶ *Chlamydia trachomatis*

TABLE 12–6.
HPV VACCINATION REGIMEN

POPULATION	RECOMMENDED NUMBER OF HPV VACCINE DOSES	RECOMMENDED INTERVAL BETWEEN DOSES
Persons initiating HPV vaccination at ages 9 through 14 years,* except immunocompromised persons†	2	0, 6–12 months§
Persons initiating HPV vaccination at ages 15 through 26 years¶ and immunocompromised persons† initiating HPV vaccination at ages 9 through 26 years	3	0, 1–2, 6 months**

*ACIP recommends routine HPV vaccination for adolescents at age 11 or 12 years; vaccination may be given starting at age 9 years.

† Persons with primary or secondary immunocompromising conditions that might reduce cell-mediated or humoral immunity (see also: Medical conditions)

§ In a 2-dose schedule of HPV vaccine, the minimum interval between the first and second doses is 5 months.

¶ For persons who were not adequately vaccinated previously, ACIP recommends vaccination for females through age 26 years and for males through age 21 years; males ages 22 through 26 years may be vaccinated. Vaccination is recommended for some persons aged 22 through 26 years; see Medical conditions and Special populations.

** In a 3-dose schedule of HPV vaccine, the minimum intervals are 4 weeks between the first and second doses, 12 weeks between the second and third doses, and 5 months between the first and third doses.

Source: Meites, Kempe, and Markowitz 2016

Management

▶ Without treatment, lasts months or years

▶ Antibiotic therapy

▷ Anaerobe antibiotic

▷ Metronidazole 2 g single p.o. dose *or*

▷ Tinidazole 2 g p.o. single p.o. dose *or*

▷ Metronidazole 500 mg p.o. b.i.d. × 7 days

Prevention

▶ Education for prevention:

▷ Safe sex practices

▶ Treat sexual partners as needed.

Pelvic Inflammatory Disease (PID)

▶ Mixed microbial infection from vagina or cervix into uterus, lymphatics into parametria, fallopian tubes, ovaries, or pelvis weeks to months after exposure; commonly occurs as result of STI.

▶ Frequently caused by *streptococci, Chlamydia trachomatis, Escherichia coli, Neisseria gonorrhoeae, Mycoplasma* sp., anaerobic organisms (Bacteroides); most common causes are chlamydia and gonorrhea.

▶ One million women diagnosed with PID each year.

▶ About one in eight sexually active young women have PID before age 20 years.

▶ PID can cause scarring and result in infertility, ectopic pregnancy, or tubo-ovarian abscesses.

Risk Factors

▶ Multiple sex partners

▶ Infected partner

▶ History of PID or STI

▶ Intrauterine device (IUD)

▶ Surgical instrumentation

▷ Dilation and curettage (D&C) or induced abortion

Signs and Symptoms

▶ Little pain at first

▶ Lower abdominal pain

▶ Fever

▷ Only one third have fever > 101°F

▶ Malodorous vaginal discharge

▶ Dyspareunia

▶ Bleeding with intercourse

▶ Burning on urination

▶ Bleeding between periods

▶ Cervicitis

▷ Blood, ulcerations, nodules

▶ Classic triad

▷ Abdominal pain

▶ Tenderness with or without rebound

▷ Adnexal tenderness

▶ Unilateral or bilateral

▶ Adnexal masses may be palpable

▷ Cervical motion tenderness

▶ Chandelier sign: Cervical pain acute and startling

Diagnostic Tests

▶ Primarily based on history and physical

▶ Pelvic exam

   ▷ Cervical motion, uterine or adnexal tenderness

▶ WBC, C-reactive protein (CRP), erythrocyte sedimentation rate (ESR), HCG

▶ Gonorrhea, chlamydia testing

▶ Consider HIV testing

▶ Vaginal wet preps

   ▷ 10 WBC/HPF

   ▷ Look for trichomonads (could alter findings)

▶ Pelvic ultrasound or CT scan

   ▷ Rule out pregnancy

   ▷ Identify tubal masses

▶ Endometrial biopsy

▶ Laparoscopy

Differential Diagnoses

▶ Appendicitis

▶ Ectopic pregnancy

▶ Endometriosis

▶ Ruptured ovarian cyst

▶ Leiomyoma

▶ Acute enteritis

▶ Severe UTI or pyelonephritis

▶ Colitis

▶ Renal calculi

Management

▶ Antibiotic therapy (one of the following)

   ▷ Cefotetan 2 g IV q12h *plus* doxycycline 100 mg p.o. or IV q12h

   ▷ Cefoxitin 2 g IV q6h *plus* doxycycline 100 mg p.o. or IV q12h

   ▷ Clindamycin 900 mg IV q8h *plus* gentamicin loading dose IV or IM (2 mg/kg), followed by a maintenance dose (1.5 mg/kg) q8h

▶ Also treat partner(s)

▶ Surgical excision of abscesses

Prevention

▶ Education

  ▷ Condom use; abstinence; monogamy

  ▷ Have partners tested for STIs before engaging in sexual relationship

HIV and AIDS

▶ Human immunodeficiency virus (HIV) is a sexually transmitted viral infection that causes acquired immune deficiency syndrome (AIDS).

▶ While new HIV infections are highest in younger adults (ages 25–34 years), both new and long-term infections are also seen among older adults.

▶ More than a million people in the United States live with HIV and one in five is unaware of infection.

▶ The number of newly infected persons exceeds the number of deaths among HIV-infected persons, which results in a net increase of about 30,000 persons with HIV each year.

▶ Gay and bisexual men and men who have sex with men are most commonly, but not exclusively, affected.

▶ In the earliest stages of transmission in the United States, HIV in older adults was initially seen from blood transfusions but increasingly, it is being seen in older adults from sexual activity.

▶ Currently, 20 percent of HIV cases are older adults, and 11 percent of new cases of AIDS are in people older than 50 years old.

▶ The incubation period from HIV infection to AIDS ranges from months to 10 years.

▶ In the absence of treatment, the average disease progression from seroconversion to death in younger persons is 10–12 years. Older adults experience a more rapid downhill course, perhaps because of impaired T-cell replacement.

▶ Stages of infection

  ▷ Viral transmission

  ▷ Primary HIV infection

  ▷ Also called acute HIV infection

  ▷ Occurs in 80–90 percent of HIV-infected persons

  ▷ Seroconversion

  ▷ Asymptomatic chronic infection

  ▷ Symptomatic HIV infection

▶ AIDS: People with AIDS are defined by the CDC as HIV-positive persons with opportunistic infection (OI) such as esophageal candidiasis, tuberculosis, *Cryptococcus* meningitis, or *Pneumocystis carinii*; or HIV-positive person with CD4 cell count < 200 per mL or CD4 percent < 14.

▶ Advanced HIV infection

TABLE 12–7.
OPPORTUNISTIC INFECTIONS AND RELATED COMPLICATIONS

Bacterial and Mycobacterial	*Mycobacterium avium* complex, salmonellosis, syphilis and neurosyphillis, tuberculosis
Fungal	Aspergillosis, candidiasis, coccidioidomycosis, cryptococcal meningitis, histoplasmosis
Malignancies	Kaposi's sarcoma, non-Hodgkin lymphoma, primary central nervous system, lymphoma
Protozoal	Cryptosporidiosis, isosporiasis, microsporidiosis, *Pneumocystis carinii* pneumonia, toxoplasmosis
Viral	Cytomegalovirus, hepatitis, herpes simplex, herpes zoster, human papillomavirus, *Molluscum contagiosum*
Oral	Hairy leukoplakia, progressive multifocal leukoencephalopathy
Complications	**Neurological** AIDS dementia complex, peripheral neuropathy **Other Conditions** Aphthous ulcers, malabsorption, depression, diarrhea, thrombocytopenia, wasting syndrome, idiopathic thrombocytopenic purpura (ITP)

Signs and Symptoms

▶ • Fever, adenopathy, pharyngitis, rash, diarrhea, myalgias or arthralgias, headache, nausea and vomiting, hepatosplenomegaly, thrush.

▶ ◂ Asymptomatic infection

▷ Clinically asymptomatic

▷ Usually no physical findings

▷ Some with persistent generalized lymphadenopathy

▶ ◦ Early symptomatic HIV infection

▷ Stage B (formerly called AIDS-related complex [ARC])

▷ Thrush, oral hairy leukoplakia, peripheral neuropathy

▷ Cervical dysplasia, fever, night sweats, recurrent herpes zoster

▷ ITP, listeriosis

▶ Clinical conditions are more common and severe when HIV is present, but are not AIDS indicators.

Diagnostic Tests

▶ The USPSTF recommends that clinicians screen for HIV infection in adolescents and adults ages 15–65 years (US Preventive Services Task Force [USPSTF] 2013).

▶ HIV tests

▷ Antibody tests

▶ ◦ Enzyme-linked immunosorbent assays (ELISAs) that detect antibody to HIV are used as an initial test to screen for HIV infection.

▷ Laboratory-based

▷ Rapid tests

- ▶ Combination tests (antibody and antigen tests).
    - ▷ Fourth-generation HIV tests, detect both HIV antibody and antigens
- ▷ Nucleic acid tests (NATs)
    - ▶ Detect HIV the fastest by looking for HIV in the blood. It can take 7–28 days for NATs to detect HIV and they are very expensive.
- ▷ Confirmatory tests
    - ▶ HIV-1/HIV-2 differentiation immunoassay
    - ▶ Western blot (CDC 2016a; Bartlett and Sax 2016)
- ▶ See also CDC and Association of Public Health Laboratories (2014) poster for updated CDC testing recommendations.

Differential Diagnoses

- ▶ Influenza
- ▶ Malignancy
- ▶ Other viral infection

Management

- ▶ The most recent guideline from the Department of Health and Human Services (DHHS) Panel on Antiretroviral Guidelines for Adults and Adolescents (the Panel; 2016) recommends that all HIV-infected persons begin antiretroviral therapy (ART), regardless of CD4 T-cell count, to prevent HIV transmission and morbidity and mortality associated with HIV infection.
- ▶ Considerations for initiating antiretroviral medications:
    - ▷ HIV infection
    - ▷ History of AIDS-defining illness *or*
    - ▷ CD4 T-cell count < 350 *or*
    - ▷ CD4 T-cell count < 200 and history of AIDS
    - ▷ HIV-associated neuropathy
    - ▷ Coinfection with HPV when treatment for hepatitis B (HBV) is indicated
    - ▷ May consider for patients with CD4 T-cell counts > 350
    - ▷ Rapidly declining CD4 T-cell count
    - ▷ Viral load
    - ▷ Viral resistance testing
    - ▷ Patient adherence and barriers to adherence
    - ▷ Use drug cocktails (combination therapy)
- ▶ Antiretroviral medication classes:
    - ▷ Antiretroviral drugs (ARVs) approved by the Food and Drug Administration (FDA):
        - ▶ Nucleoside reverse transcriptase inhibitors: 12
        - ▶ Nonnucleoside reverse transcriptase inhibitors: 6
        - ▶ Protease inhibitors: 10

▶ Entry infusion inhibitors: 1

▶ Integrase inhibitors: 2

▶ Fixed-dose combination: 3

▶ Review current recommendations for initial antiretroviral therapy.

▷ The Panel's recommendations for antiretroviral-naïve patients (2016, p. F-1):

▶ Integrase strand transfer inhibitor-based regimens:

▷ Dolutegravir/abacavir/lamivudine—*only* for patients who are HLA-B*5701–negative (AI)

▷ Dolutegravir *plus* tenofovir disoproxil fumarate/emtricitabine *or* tenofovir alafenamide/emtricitabine (AII)

▷ Elvitegravir/cobicistat/tenofovir alafenamide/emtricitabine (AI)

▷ Elvitegravir/cobicistat/tenofovir disoproxil fumarate/emtricitabine (AI)

▷ Raltegravir *plus* tenofovir disoproxil fumarate/emtricitabine *or* tenofovir alafenamide/emtricitabine (AII)

▶ Protease inhibitor-based regimens:

▷ Darunavir/ritonavir *plus* tenofovir disoproxil fumarate/emtricitabine (AI) or tenofovir alafenamide/emtricitabine (AII)

▶ Medication management principles

▷ Educate on benefits and issues regarding ART.

▷ Counsel on strategies to optimize adherence.

▷ Must take each dose of antiretroviral prescription.

▷ Dose should be same time each day.

▷ Cannot substitute one medication for another.

▷ Attempt to initiate once-daily or b.i.d. dosing

▷ Observe patient for signs and symptoms of drug therapy.

▷ Monitor lab values.

▷ Treat abnormal lab values or a change in patient condition.

▶ Refer to an infectious disease specialist for evaluation and management of opportunistic infections (see table 12–7).

Prevention

▶ Safe sexual practices

▶ Preexposure prophylaxis (PrEP)

▷ To help prevent HIV infection in people at very high risk.

▷ A combination of two HIV medicines (tenofovir and emtricitabine).

▷ If taken daily, can significantly reduce risk of HIV infection from

▶ Sex by more than 90 percent, and

▶ Injection drug use by more than 70 percent (CDC 2017).

► Postexposure prophylaxis (PEP)

▷ Should be used only in emergency situations and must be started within 72 hours after possible exposure to HIV.

▷ For information on occupational exposure, see page 87 in chapter 5.

Additional Resources

AIDS.gov: https://www.hiv.gov/

FDA (antiretroviral drugs used in the treatment of HIV): http://www.fda.gov/ForPatients/Illness/HIVAIDS/Treatment/ucm118915.htm

CDC: https://www.cdc.gov/hiv/library/factsheets/index.html

University of California, San Francisco (HIV InSite): http://hivinsite.ucsf.edu/

International AIDS Society: http://www.iasociety.org/

The Body: http://www.thebody.com/

National Institutes of Health: "What to Start: Initial Combination Regimens for the Antiretroviral-Naïve Patient," https://aidsinfo.nih.gov/guidelines/html/1/adult-and-adolescent-arv-guidelines/11/what-to-start

REFERENCES

Badalato, G., and M. Kaufmann. 2016. "Adult UTI." American Urological Association Educational Programs. https://www.auanet.org/education/adult-uti.cfm.

Bartlett, J. G., and P. E. Sax. 2017. "Screening and Diagnostic Testing for HIV Infection." https://www.uptodate.com/contents/screening-and-diagnostic-testing-for-hiv-infection?source=machineLearning.

Centers for Disease Control and Prevention. N.d. "Interpretation of Hepatitis B Serologic Test Results." http://www.cdc.gov/hepatitis/HBV/PDFs/SerologicChartv8.pdf.

———. 2010. "Sexually Transmitted Diseases Treatment Guidelines, 2010," supplement, *Morbidity and Mortality Weekly Report* 59 (RR-12).

———. 2013. "Incidence, Prevalence, and Cost of Sexually Transmitted Infections in the United States." CDC Fact Sheet. http://www.cdc.gov/std/stats/sti-estimates-fact-sheet-feb-2013.pdf.

———. 2015a. "Anogenital Warts." In "Sexually Transmitted Diseases Treatment Guidelines, 2015," supplement, *Morbidity and Mortality Weekly* 64 (3): 86–90. http://www.cdc.gov/std/tg2015/warts.htm.

———. 2015b. "Chlamydial Infections." In "Sexually Transmitted Diseases Treatment Guidelines, 2015," supplement, *Morbidity and Mortality Weekly Report* 64 (3): 55–60. https://www.cdc.gov/std/tg2015/chlamydia.htm.

———. 2015c. "Diseases Characterized by Genital, Anal, or Perianal Ulcers." In "Sexually Transmitted Diseases Treatment Guidelines, 2015," supplement, *Morbidity and Mortality Weekly Report* 64 (3): 25–34. http://www.cdc.gov/std/tg2015/genital-ulcers.htm.

———. 2016a. "HIV testing." HIV/AIDS. http://www.cdc.gov/hiv/testing/index.html.

———. 2016b. "HPV-Associated Cancers and Precancers." In "Sexually Transmitted Diseases Treatment Guidelines, 2015," supplement, *Morbidity and Mortality Weekly Report* 64 (3): 90–100. http://www.cdc.gov/std/tg2015/hpv-cancer.htm.

———. 2016c. "Syphilis." In "Sexually Transmitted Diseases Treatment Guidelines, 2015," supplement, *Morbidity and Mortality Weekly Report* 64 (3): 34–49. http://www.cdc.gov/std/tg2015/syphilis.htm.

———. 2017. "PrEP." HIV Basics. https://www.cdc.gov/hiv/basics/prep.html.

Centers for Disease Control and Prevention and Association of Public Health Laboratories. 2014. "Quick Reference Guide—Laboratory Testing for the Diagnosis of HIV Infection: Updated Recommendations." Poster. https://stacks.cdc.gov/view/cdc/23446.

Kidney Disease: Improving Global Outcomes. 2012. *KDIGO Clinical Practice Guideline for Acute Kidney Injury, Kidney International Supplements* 2 (Suppl. 1): 1–138. http://www.kdigo.org/clinical_practice_guidelines/pdf/KDIGO AKI Guideline.pdf.

Kreshover, J., R. Ramasamy, and N. Singla. 2016. "Medical Student Curriculum: Hematuria." American Urological Association Educational Programs. https://www.auanet.org/education/hematuria.cfm.

Meites, E., A. Kempe, L. E. Markowitz. 2016. "Use of a 2-Dose Schedule for Human Papillomavirus Vaccination—Updated Recommendations of the Advisory Committee on Immunization Practices." *Morbidity and Mortality Weekly Report* 65 (49): 1405–8. http://dx.doi.org/10.15585/mmwr.mm6549a5.

National Kidney Foundation, Inc. 2002. "Part 4. Definition and Classification of Stages of Chronic Kidney Disease." In *KDOQI Clinical Practice Guidelines for Chronic Kidney Disease: Evaluation, Classification, and Stratification.* http://www2.kidney.org/professionals/KDOQI/guidelines_ckd/p4_class_g1.htm.

Panel on Antiretroviral Guidelines for Adults and Adolescents. 2016. *Guidelines for the Use of Antiretroviral Agents in HIV-1-Infected Adults and Adolescents.* N.p.: Department of Health and Human Services. https://aidsinfo.nih.gov/guidelines/html/1/adult-and-adolescent-arv-guidelines/11/what-to-start.

US Preventive Services Task Force. 2013. "Human Immunodeficiency Virus (HIV) Infection: Screening." https://www.uspreventiveservicestaskforce.org/Page/Document/UpdateSummaryFinal/human-immunodeficiency-virus-hiv-infection-screening.

CHAPTER 13

MUSCULOSKELETAL DISORDERS

LEARNING OBJECTIVES

▶ Recognize common musculoskeletal disorders and injuries and analyze processes used to make differential diagnoses.

▷ Risk factors

▷ Signs and symptoms

▷ Diagnostic tests

▷ Differential diagnoses

▶ Describe treatment and management of musculoskeletal disorders.

▷ Management

▷ Prevention

SYSTEMIC LUPUS ERYTHEMATOSUS (SLE)

▶ A chronic autoimmune, inflammatory disease that can affect joints, skin, kidneys, blood cells, brain, heart, and lungs.

▶ Lupus may be triggered by infections, medications, or sunlight.

▶ Lupus cannot be cured, but symptoms can be controlled.

▶ American College of Rheumatology's (ACR) eleven diagnostic criteria for SLE (must have four of eleven; Starkebaum 2016):

1. Malar rash

2. Discoid rash

3. Photosensitivity

4. Oral ulcers

5. Nonerosive arthritis

6. Pleuritic or pericarditis

7. Renal disorder

8. Neurologic disorder

9. Hematologic disorder

10. Immunologic disorder

11. Positive antinuclear antibody

Risk Factors

▶ Gender (more common in women)

▶ Age (most diagnosed between 15 and 40 years old)

▶ Race (more common in people of African, Hispanic, and Asian descent)

Signs and Symptoms

▶ Depend on systems affected

▶ Fatigue

▶ Fever

▶ Joint pain, stiffness, and swelling

▶ Butterfly-shaped rash on cheeks and bridge of the nose

▶ Skin lesions that appear or worsen with sun exposure (photosensitivity)

▶ Blanching of fingers or toes when exposed to cold or stressed (Raynaud's phenomenon)

▶ Shortness of breath or chest pain

▶ Dry eyes

▶ Headaches, confusion, and memory loss

Diagnostic Tests

▶ Antinuclear antibody (ANA) panel

▶ Complete blood count (CBC) with differential

▶ Chest X-ray

▶ Serum creatinine

▶ Urinalysis

▶ Complement components (C3 and C4)

▶ Coombs test—direct

▶ Cryoglobulins

▶ Erythrocyte sedimentation rate (ESR)

▶ C-reactive protein (CRP)

▶ Kidney function tests

▶ Liver function tests (LFTs)

▶ ✔ Rheumatoid factor

▶ ●Antiphospholipid antibodies and lupus anticoagulant test

▶ Kidney biopsy

(Starkebaum 2016)

Differential Diagnoses

▶ Acute pericarditis

▶ Antiphospholipid syndrome

▶ B-cell lymphoma

▶ Connective-tissue disease

▶ Fibromyalgia

▶ Hepatitis C

▶ Infectious mononucleosis

▶ Infective endocarditis

▶ Lyme disease

▶ Polymyositis

▶ Rheumatoid arthritis

▶ Scleroderma

▶ Sjögren's syndrome

Management

▶ ●Mild symptoms

▷ Bed rest, midafternoon naps, avoid fatigue

▷ Sun protection

▷ Topical glucocorticoids for isolated skin lesions

▷ NSAIDs

▷ Hydroxychloroquine

▶ ●Severe symptoms

▷ Glucocorticoids for life-threatening manifestations

▷ Pulse therapy in rapidly progressive renal failure, central nervous system (CNS) disease, and severe thrombocytopenia

▷ Immunosuppressant drugs (cyclophosphamide, chlorambucil, azathioprine) for steroid-resistant cases

▷ Coumadin to international normalized ratio (INR) > 3 with antiphospholipid antibodies and arterial or venous clotting

Prevention

▶ None known

GIANT-CELL ARTERITIS (GCA; TEMPORAL ARTERITIS)

▶ Giant-cell arteritis is a chronic systemic inflammatory vasculitis of unknown etiology that affects medium and large arteries and is the most common form of systemic vasculitis in adults.

▶ Giant-cell arteritis can cause systemic, neurologic, and ophthalmologic complications.

▶ Superficial temporal arteries are usually affected, but ophthalmic, occipital, vertebral, posterior ciliary, and proximal vertebral arteries may also be affected.

Risk Factors

▶ Over 50 years old (mean age 72 years)
▶ More common in women
▶ Genetics
▶ Infection

Signs and Symptoms

▶ Headache, scalp tenderness
▶ Visual symptoms
   ▷ Visual loss most significant cause of morbidity
▶ Jaw claudication, throat pain
▶ Nodular, enlarged, tender, or pulseless temporal artery
   ▷ May palpate specific area of pain
▶ Nonclassic presentation
   ▷ Respiratory involvement
   ▷ Fever to 104°F
   ▷ Rigors and chills

Diagnostic Tests

▶ Elevated ESR
▶ Elevated CRP
▶ CBC
   ▷ Normal WBC
   ▷ Mild anemia

▷ •Slightly elevated platelets

    ▶ If normal, probably not GCA

▶ •LFTs sometimes slightly elevated

▶ ◦Ultrasound

    ▷ May not be visualized in early stage

▶ ◢Temporal artery biopsy

    ▷ Vasculitis and multinucleated oversized cells

Differential Diagnoses

▶ Acute-angle glaucoma

▶ Iritis, uveitis

▶ Migraine

▶ Idiopathic facial pain

▶ Polymyalgia rheumatica

▶ Postherpetic neuralgia

▶ Retinal artery or vein occlusion

▶ Rheumatoid arthritis

▶ Transient ischemic attack (TIA)

Management

▶ ◦Prednisone 60–80 mg p.o. daily × 1–2 months, then taper.

    ▷ Follow-up in 72 hours after initiation of therapy

    ▷ ◢ESR when tapering steroids

▶ ◦Methylprednisolone 250–1,000 mg IV daily × 3 days (for acute visual changes)

▶ Monitor for steroid-related side effects and complications (diabetes, hypertension, edema, weight gain, cataracts).

▶ ◦Long-term steroid therapy.

    ▷ Usually 1–2 years on steroids

▶ ◦Thoracic aortic disease can occur years after initial diagnosis.

    ▷ Educate on symptoms of aortic disease.

        ▶ Claudication of arms or legs, bruits over affected arteries, stroke symptoms

Prevention

▶ None known

ARTHRITIS

▶ Arthritis is musculoskeletal disease manifested by inflammation of one or more joints.

▶ More than one hundred types of arthritis exist (see table 13–1).

▶ ❧ Primary symptoms are joint pain and stiffness that worsen with time.

TABLE 13–1.
CHARACTERISTICS OF OSTEO- AND RHEUMATOID ARTHRITIS

CHARACTERISTICS	OSTEOARTHRITIS	RHEUMATOID ARTHRITIS
X-ray findings	Joint space narrowing, osteophytes, subchondral sclerosis, cysts	Osteoporosis with or without subchondral bone destruction; joint deformities
Morning stiffness	Lasts <30 minutes	Lasts >1 hour
Joints involved	Spine, hips, knees, or distal fingers Asymmetric	Multiple small joints; symmetric joints (especially of hands); rare in spine
Lab findings	ESR < 20–40 Serum RF negative	Serum RF usually elevated; ESR usually elevated
Clinical findings	Joint pain, tenderness, hypertrophy and crepitus; may have some deformity; occasional fluid in joint	Joint deformity, muscle atrophy, and extra-articular soft tissue nodules; acute, red, warm, swollen, and tender

Note: RF = rheumatoid factor

Rheumatoid Arthritis (RA)

▶ RA is a chronic, systemic inflammatory disease of unknown cause that symmetrically affects synovial joints, and is the most common autoimmune arthritis.

▶ ❧ Small joint destruction and extra-articular symptoms predominate.

▶ Female:male ratio for developing RA is 3:1.

▶ ❧ Peak age of onset is between ages 20 and 40 years.

▶ Susceptibility is genetically determined and highly variable.

Risk Factors

▶ Family history of autoimmune disorders

▶ Onset usually in forties, though 5 percent of cases seen in children

Signs and Symptoms

▶ Prodromal symptoms

▶ ❧ Malaise and weight loss; physical or emotional stress are infrequent triggers

▶ ❧ Symmetrically affects joints

▶ ❧ Swelling, stiffness, warmth, tenderness, and pain

▶ ◦ Stiffness prominent in morning and subsides during day

▶ ◦ Duration of stiffness indicator of disease activity

▶ ◦ May develop permanent deformity

▶ ◦ Splenomegaly and lymph node enlargement in some

▶ ◦ May have vasculitis and other systemic inflammation

Diagnostic Tests

▶ ◦ RF

   ▷ Positive in 80 percent

▶ ◦ ANA

   ▷ Elevated in 20 percent

▶ ◦ ESR

   ▷ Elevated

   ▷ Correlates with degree of synovial inflammation

▶ ◦ CBC

   ▷ Hypochromic, normocytic anemia common

▶ ◦ Joint fluid aspiration

   ▷ Inflammatory changes: >3.5 cc translucent or opaque, yellow or opalescent fluid

   ▷ 3,000–50,000 WBC with >50 percent polymorphonuclear neutrophils (PMN)

   ▷ Negative culture

   ▷ Glucose present but lower than in serum

▶ X-ray

   ▷ Soft-tissue swelling, juxta-articular demineralization, lateral joint space narrowing and erosion

Differential Diagnoses

▶ Lupus

▶ Seronegative spondyloarthropathy

▶ Psoriatic, septic, osteoarthritis

▶ Gout

▶ Lyme disease

Management

▶ ◦ Goals of treatment (National Institute of Arthritis and Musculoskeletal and Skin Diseases 2017):

   ▷ Relieve pain

   ▷ Reduce inflammation

   ▷ Slow down or stop joint damage

▷ Improve a person's sense of wellbeing and ability to function

▷ Nonpharmacologic therapies:

▶ • Rest, splinting, physical and occupation therapy

▶ • Assistive devices

▷ Corrective surgery for joint deformities

▷ Follow-up at 3- to 6-month intervals

▶ Medications

▷ Aspirin (acetylsalicylic acid [ASA]) and NSAIDS.

▷ COX-2 inhibitors (Celebrex), but be cautious with sulfa allergy (Ogbru 2016).

▷ Disease-modifying antirheumatic drugs (DMARDs) should be started early.

▶ Methotrexate 10–15 mg p.o. once weekly and titrate up to maximum dose (25 mg/week) as tolerated

▶ Leflunomide (Arava) 100 mg p.o. daily ×3 days

▶ Sulfasalazine 500 mg daily and titrate to 500–1,000 mg p.o. q.i.d. with food

▷ Antimalarials

▶ Hydroxychloroquine (Plaquenil) 400–600 mg p.o. daily

▷ Proinflammatory cytokine TNF-alpha (tumor necrosis factor) inhibitors

▶ Etanercept (Enbrel) 50 mg subcutaneously (SC) weekly or 25 mg twice weekly

▶ Infliximab (Remicade) 3 mg/kg intravenously (IV) at 0, 2, and 6 weeks, then q8 weeks

▷ Gold sodium thiomalate

▶ 50 mg intramuscularly (IM) per week ×20 weeks

▶ Titrate to 50 mg per month if not tolerating methotrexate

▷ Corticosteroids

▶ Methylprednisolone 60–80 mg IM during acute flare

▶ Prednisone 2.5–7.5 mg p.o. daily

▶ Short-term relief: No more than 10 mg/day

▶ Report signs or symptoms of infection

▶ Good response in 60 percent

▷ Leflunomide (Arava), infliximab (Remicade), and etanercept (Enbrel) are expensive; insurance may not cover

▶ Monitor eye symptoms, neuropathy, myopathy

Prevention

▶ None known

Osteoarthritis (OA)

▶   OA is a joint disease with degeneration of cartilage and hypertrophy of articular margins in moveable joints, bone hypertrophy, formation of osteophytes and subchondral cysts, and sclerosis in synovial joints and vertebrae.

▶ • It is the most common musculoskeletal disorder in older adults, and can lead to serious functional decline.

▷   By age 75 years, 80 percent have signs of OA.

Risk Factors

▶   Advancing age

▶   Female sex

▶ • Athletic overuse or repetitive joint use

▶   Joint trauma from disease or injury

▶   Obesity

▶   Heredity

▶   Musculoskeletal disorders

▶ ● Metabolic or endocrine disorders

▷   Gout or hyperparathyroidism

Signs and Symptoms

▶ ● No systemic manifestations

▶ ● Joints asymmetrically affected

▶ ● Bony hypertrophy of joint

▶ ● Crepitus with movement

▷   Joint swelling may be present

▶   Common in terminal interphalangeal joints, cervical and lumbar spine, and weight-bearing joints

▷ • Usually affects knees, hips, cervical and lumbar spine, hands

▶   Joint pain, tenderness, and stiffness

▷ • Worsens with activity and is relieved by rest

▶   Joint instability in later stages

▷   Especially in knees

▶ ● Heberden's nodes

▷   Distal interphalangeal (DIP) joint swelling

▶ ● Bouchard's nodes

▷   Proximal interphalangeal (PIP) joint swelling

▶   Stiffness

▷ • Common in morning and after inactivity

▷ ● Usually lasts less than 30 minutes

Diagnostic Tests

▶ • Physical exam indicated by history of symptoms to rule out other types of arthritis

▶ • Functional status, mobility, muscle strength, deep-tendon reflexes (DTRs) assessments

▶ • Posture (kyphosis, lordosis, scoliosis)

▶ No specific lab tests

▶ X-rays as needed

     ▷ • Unequal, narrowed joint space; subchondral sclerosis; sharp articular margins; cysts and osteophytes

▶ CBC with differential if infection suspected

▶ ESR to rule out inflammatory condition

▶ Bone density (dual-energy X-ray absorptiometry [DXA] scan), ultrasound, computed tomography (CT) scan

Differential Diagnoses

▶ Rheumatoid arthritis

▶ Gout

▶ Septic arthritis

▶ Polymyalgia rheumatic

▶ Tendinitis

▶ Arthritis
(Heidari 2011)

Management

▶ • Physical activity is cornerstone of treatment

▶ • Physical therapy

▶ • Heat or cold to affected joints

▶ Weight loss

▶ Biofeedback

▶ Splinting, bracing, or assistive devices

▶ Acupuncture, massage

▶ Surgical intervention: Debridement, joint replacement

▶ Pain control to prevent functional decline and morbidity

     ▷ • First-line pharmacologic treatment is acetaminophen; second-line is NSAIDs, then intra-articular injections.

     ▷ Acetaminophen 2.6–4 g per day is effective and less toxic than NSAIDs.

     ▷ Salicylates or NSAIDs if acetaminophen fails.

     ▷ Short-term use of COX-2 inhibitor if no cardiovascular risk factors.

▷ Topical analgesic creams:

  ▶ Over-the-counter (OTC)

   ▷ Heat, BenGay, Capsaicin

  ▶ Prescription

   ▷ Diclofenac (Voltaren,) Lidocaine

▷ Narcotic pain relievers:

  ▶ Tramadol, opioids

▷ Glucosamine and chondroitin (controversial); may interfere with warfarin.

▷ Intra-articular joint injections:

  ▶ Corticosteroid for joint effusion and inflammation

  ▶ Hyalgan (sodium hyaluronate) or Synvisc (hylan G-F 20) knee injections

   ▷ Intra-articular triamcinolone 20–30 mg

   ▷ Should not be repeated more than three times per year

Prevention

▶ Maintain optimal weight, avoid obesity

▶ Avoid joint injuries

▶ Exercise

Gouty Arthritis (Gout)

▶ A group of metabolic diseases that causes inflammatory arthritis in peripheral joints by depositing uric acid or monosodium urate crystals in extracellular fluid.

▶ Primary gout is hereditary (defective purine metabolism or uric acid excretion).

▶ Secondary gout is caused by urate overproduction or uric acid underexcretion, resulting in hyperuricemia and crystal deposits.

▶ Classically affects proximal phalanx of great toe.

Risk Factors

▶ Obesity

▶ Hereditary

▶ Purine-rich diet

▶ Dehydration

▶ Starvation

▶ Alcohol

▶ Use of thiazide diuretics

Signs and Symptoms

▶ Classic presentation

  ▷ Sudden red, hot, swollen, exquisitely tender joint

▶ ● Acute attack

▷ Joint red, hot, swollen, exquisitely painful; fever, chills, malaise may accompany

▶ ● Chronic

▷ Chronic pain in more than one joint

▶ ● Late chronic stage

▷ Joint swelling, restricted motion

▶ ● Skin desquamation and pruritis during acute attack resolution

▶ ● Tophi: Sodium urate crystal deposits in soft tissue

▷ Seen in chronic tophaceous gout

▷ Usually occurs 2–10 years from onset of acute intermittent attacks

▶ ● Hyperuricemia

Diagnostic Tests

▶ ● Serum uric acid > 6.0 mg/dL, but serum uric acid level does not confirm or rule out diagnosis

▶ ● Elevated ESR

▶ ● Elevated leukocytes

▶ X-ray

▷ ● Normal in early disease

▷ ● Soft-tissue tophi may be visible if 5 mm in diameter

▷ ● Punched-out lesions in subchondral bone

▶ Usually first seen in metatarsophalangeal joint

▶ ● Joint aspiration

▷ Needle-shaped crystals present

Differential Diagnoses

▶ Septic joint

▶ Cellulitis

▶ Fracture

▶ Rheumatoid or pyogenic arthritis or pseudogout

▶ Acute rheumatic fever

Management

▶ Dietary modifications: Avoid

▷ ● Alcohol and

▷ ● Purines (organ meats, shellfish, peas, lentils, beans).

▶ Avoid causative medications.

▷ ● Salicylates, diuretics, pyrazinamide, ethambutol, nicotinic acid

▶ • Increase fluid intake to >3 liters daily.

▶ Weight loss

▶ Acute attack management

  ▷ The choice of pharmacologic agent should be based upon severity of pain and the number of joints involved.

  ▷ For attacks of mild/moderate gout severity (6 of 10 on a Visual Analogue Scale [VAS] of 0–10 pain), particularly those involving one or a few small joints or one or two large joints, initiate monotherapy.

  ▷ Combination therapy is appropriate to consider when the acute gout attack is characterized by severe pain, particularly in an acute polyarticular gout attack or an attack involving one or two large joints.

    ▶ NSAIDs

      ▷ If renal function is normal:

        ▶ • Naproxen 500 mg p.o. t.i.d. × 2–3 days or until symptoms subside

        ▶ • Indomethacin 50mg p.o. t.i.d. × 2–3 days and then 25 mg p.o. t.i.d. 4–10 days

        ▶ Then taper over 10–14 days

    ▶ Corticosteroids

      ▷ • Intra-articular methylprednisolone 20–40 mg single dose

        ▶ • Prednisone: Starting dosage of at least 0.5 mg/kg per day for 5–10 days, followed by discontinuation

  ▷ Colchicine

    ▶ • Loading dose of 1.2 mg, followed by 0.6 mg 1 hour later, followed by 0.6 mg once or twice daily until attack resolves

▶ Severe/refractory gout

  ▷ • Pegloticase is appropriate for patients with severe gout disease burden and refractoriness to, or intolerance of, conventional and appropriately dosed ULT.

  ▷ • Lesinurad (Zurampic; Khanna et al. 2012a, 2012b; Moses 2017)

    ▶ 100 mg/day (titrated every few weeks up to max 800 mg/day).

    ▶ First selective uric acid reabsorption inhibitor (SURI) approved by the FDA.

    ▶ Must be coadministered with an XOI.

    ▶ Monotherapy or higher than recommended doses are associated with an increased serum creatinine. Renal function should be assessed before initiating therapy and periodically thereafter. More frequent monitoring is required for an estimated CrCl < 60 mL/min. Do not initiate therapy if CrCl is <45 mL/min and discontinue if CrCl decreases persistently to <45 mL/min.

    ▶ May be used to treat high levels of uric acid.

Prevention

▶ Limit alcohol intake.

▶ Avoid purine-rich foods.

▶ Maintain optimal weight. Prevention of acute attacks

   ▷ Xanthine oxidase inhibitor (XOI): First-line pharmacologic urate-lowering therapy (ULT) approach in gout

      ▶ Allopurinol: Starting dosage of allopurinol should be no greater than 100 mg/day (and less than that in moderate-to-severe chronic kidney disease [CKD]), followed by gradual upward titration of the maintenance dose of 300 mg a day.

   ▷ Febuxostat (Uloric)

      ▶ Dose: 40 mg daily (up to 80 mg/day if uric acid is still >6 mg/dl after 2 weeks of therapy)

   ▷ Probenacid (if XOI not tolerated or contraindicated)

      ▶ Dose: 250 mg orally twice daily, gradually increased to up to 2 grams daily

Osteoporosis

▶ Metabolic disease of low bone mass and microarchitectural deterioration of bone tissue, leading to bone fragility and increased fracture risk.

▶ Bone resorption by osteoclasts is faster than new bone matrix formation by osteoblasts, resulting in bone demineralization. Trabecular bone turnover is faster than cortical bone turnover.

▶ Often not identified until pain caused by unrecognized fracture.

▶ World Health Organization (WHO) criteria for osteoporosis and osteopenia:

   ▷ Bone density in relation to young adult means

      ▶ Normal: T score within 1 standard deviation (SD)

      ▶ Osteopenia: −1 to −2.4 SD

      ▶ Osteoporosis: −2.5 SD and below

      ▶ Severe osteoporosis: −2.5 SD and below with history of fracture

▶ Z score (compared to age-matched individuals) not preferred because bone mass begins to decline near age 40.

Risk Factors

▶ Female, postmenopausal

▶ Inadequate calcium intake or vitamin D deficiency

▶ Petite frame, low weight (<127 pounds)

▶ Advanced age

▶ Genetic predisposition

▶ Caucasian or Asian

▶ Sedentary lifestyle

▶ Smoking

▶ Excess alcohol, protein, or caffeine

▶ • Chronic hyperthyroidism, hyperparathyroidism, Cushing's disease, or rheumatoid arthritis

▶ • Renal insufficiency

▶ • Medications: Corticosteroids, phenytoin, lithium, heparin

Signs and Symptoms

▶ • Gradual loss of height

▶ • Stooped posture

▶ • History of bone fracture after age 40 years

▷ Spine, hip, wrist

▶ • Back pain

▷ Vertebral fracture

▶ • Kyphosis in older adults

Diagnostic Tests

▶ Height and weight

▶ • Bone densitometry (DXA scan)

▷ Bone density at least 2.5 SD below peak density biochemical markers indicates osteoporosis.

▶ • X-ray

▷ Evident when >30 percent of bone is lost

▶ Bone scan or magnetic resonance imaging (MRI) to assess fracture

▶ CBC, ESR, renal and liver function, thyroid-stimulating hormone

▶ • Serum 25 (OH) vitamin D level

Differential Diagnoses

▶ Osteo- or rheumatoid arthritis

▶ Endocrine disorders

▶ Malnutrition and malabsorption syndromes

▶ Osteomalacia

▶ Metastatic bone disease

▶ Connective tissue disorder, Paget's disease

Management

▶ No cure for osteoporosis

▶ • Weight-bearing exercise

▶ • Calcium and vitamin D supplements (see table 13–2)

▶ • Bisphosphonates

▷ • Contraindicated with creatinine clearance (CrCl) < 35.

▷ • Take on empty stomach with 8 oz. water (preferably after 12-hour fast).

> ▹ • Sit upright for at least ½ hour.
> ▹ • No food or drink (except water) for ½ hour.
> ▹ • Weekly and monthly dosing preparations:
>> ▶ Alendronate (Fosamax); risedronate (Actonel); ibandronate (Boniva)
> ▹ Reclast annual infusion
>> ▶ • Report new onset or worsening heartburn.
>> ▶ • Encourage calcium and vitamin D supplementation.
▶ • Calcitonin (Miacalcin) daily SC injection
▶ Selective estrogen receptor modulators (SERMs) in women only
> ▹ • Raloxifene (Evista) 60 mg p.o. daily
▶ • Teriparatide (Forteo) daily SC injection for 18 months
> ▹ Only therapy that builds new bone
▶ • Monoclonal antibody
> ▹ Denosumab 60 mg every 6 months SC injection in the upper arm, upper thigh, or abdomen
▶ • Parathyroid (PTH) analog
> ▹ Teriparatide 20 mcg/day

Prevention

▶ Selective estrogen receptor modulators
▶ Patient education:
> ▹ Smoking avoidance
> ▹ Exercise
> ▹ Limited alcohol use
> ▹ Balanced diet with sufficient calcium and vitamin D consumption

FRACTURES

▶ Bone fractures can occur at any age.
▶ • In older adults, lower bone mineral density (BMD) can increase the risk of fractures.
▶ Artificial elevations in BMD in the spine related to OA and spurring means that BMD of the hip is often more reflective of fracture risk.
▶ Most common bone fractures among older adults:
> ▹ • Hip fractures can occur spontaneously because of osteoporosis or with falls.
> ▹ • Vertebral fractures can occur with sudden moves such as sneezing.
> ▹ • Colles's fracture of the distal radius occurs with fall and outstretched arm.

TABLE 13–2.
RECOMMENDED DAILY CALCIUM AND VITAMIN D INTAKE

CALCIUM		VITAMIN D	
WOMEN			
Age 50 and younger	1,000 mg daily (from food and supplements)	Under age 50	400–800 international units (IU) daily
Age 51 and older	1,200 mg daily (from food and supplements)	Age 50 and older	800–1,000 IU daily
MEN			
Age 70 and younger	1,000 mg daily (from food and supplements)	Under age 50	400–800 international units (IU) daily
Age 71 and older	1,200 mg daily (from food and supplements)	Age 50 and older	800–1,000 IU daily

Source: National Osteoporosis Foundation 2017

- ▶ Hip fracture most frequent in older adults
  - ▷ • Affected leg shortened and externally rotated; patient will not bear weight.
  - ▷ • 20 percent of hip fractures have 1-year mortality rate, especially in nursing home settings (Schnell et al. 2010).
  - ▷ • Leads to functional decline.
  - ▷ • 50 percent of hip fracture patients are admitted to nursing home.
  - ▷ • <30 percent regain prefracture physical function level.

- ▶ • Wrist fracture is second most frequent
  - ▷ Colles's fracture exquisitely tender to touch

- ▶ • Vertebral fracture
  - ▷ Back pain, kyphosis

Risk Factors

- ▶ • Extreme physical activity or sports
- ▶ Trauma
- ▶ • Falls
- ▶ • Osteoporosis or osteopenia
- ▶ Age
- ▶ Smoking
- ▶ Alcohol abuse
- ▶ • History of fractures
- ▶ • Calcium or vitamin D deficiency

Signs and Symptoms

- ▶ ○ Pain worse with movement
- ▶ ● Point tenderness over bone or referred pain
- ▶ ○ Muscle weakness
- ▶ ○ Rapid swelling, bruising, variable degree of deformity

Diagnostic Tests

- ▶ X-ray
- ▶ CT scan
- ▶ MRI
- ▶ Bone scan

Differential Diagnoses

- ▶ Depends on fracture site
- ▶ Soft tissue injury
- ▶ Vascular injury
- ▶ Bursitis or tendinitis
- ▶ Sprain, strain, or dislocation

Management

- ▶ Repair fractures
- ▶ Pain management
- ▶ ○ Rehabilitation

Prevention

- ▶ Wear protective and other safety gear.
- ▶ Avoid clutter to prevent trips and falls.
- ▶ ● Weight-bearing exercises to maintain bone density.
- ▶ ○ Diet rich in calcium and vitamin D.

CARPAL TUNNEL SYNDROME

- ▶ ● Compression or entrapment of median nerve of wrist, resulting in pain and paresthesia in fingers of affected extremity
- ▶ ● Mnemonic for causes: **PRAGMATIC**
    - ▷ **P**regnancy
    - ▷ **R**heumatoid **a**rthritis

▷   **G**rowth hormone

▷   **M**etabolic disorders

▷   **A**lcoholism

▷   **T**umors

▷   **I**diopathic

▷   **C**onnective tissue disorders

Risk Factors

▶ • Repetitive wrist flexion and extension movements

▶ • Collagen vascular disease

▶ • History of Colles's fracture

Signs and Symptoms

▶ • Hand, forearm, wrist numbness or pain that wakens patient at night

▶ • Tingling, numbness (pins and needles), or pain that worsens when using hand or wrist

▶ • Aching pain in mid-forearm

Differential Diagnoses

▶   Cervical radiculopathy in C6 or C7

▶   Brachial plexus syndrome

▶   Carpal navicular fracture

Diagnostic Tests

▶ • Tinel's sign

▷   Strike median nerve where it passes through carpal tunnel with index finger or middle finger.

▷   Positive if tingling radiates from wrist to hand along median nerve.

▶ • Phalen's sign

▷   With elbows on hard surface, force hands to flex for 1–2 minutes.

▷   Positive with paresthesia, numbness, and tingling of median nerve.

▶ • Carpal compression test

▷   Positive with numbness and tingling with direct pressure over carpal tunnel.

▶   X-rays

▷   May rule out fracture if history of trauma

▶ ◦ Electromyogram (EMG) or nerve conduction velocity (NCV) confirmatory.

▷ Symptoms must be present 6 months to ensure nerve conduction velocities and electromyography are accurate.

Management

▶ • Splinting at night

▶ Modification of work or hobby

▶ ◦ Vitamin B6 50–100 mg p.o. b.i.d.

▶ ◦ Acetaminophen up 4 g p.o. daily in divided doses

▶ ◦ NSAIDs with caution

▶ ◦ Corticosteroid

▷ Injection into carpal tunnel

▶ ◦ Surgical release

▷ If conservative methods fail

Prevention

▶ • Avoid repetitive wrist movement

▶ ◦ Wear wrist splints

▶ ◦ Take frequent breaks if occupation requires prolonged or repetitive flexing of the wrist

SHOULDER INJURIES

Rotator Cuff Injuries

▶ The rotator cuff is formed by four scapular-humeral muscles that function in counter-traction to abduction by deltoid muscles and connect to bone with ligaments that can tear.

▶ ◦ Tendinitis and tears are common in this area. Injury occurs with wear and tear, poor movement patterns, slouching, calcium deposits, or bone spurs caused by arthritis that can irritate or pinch the rotator cuff.

Risk Factors

▶ ◦ Repetitive overhead activity

▶ • Rheumatoid or osteoarthritis

▶ ◦ Previous shoulder injury

Signs and Symptoms

▶ ◦ Pain in shoulder girdle may radiate to deltoid

▶ ◦ May have felt "something give way" in shoulder

▶ • Inability to raise arm overhead

▶ • Weakness or inability to externally rotate arm

▶ • Unable to sleep on affected side

Diagnostic Tests

▶   X-ray

▶   MRI

▶   Ultrasound

Differential Diagnoses

▶   Tendinitis

▶   Cervical neck injury

▶   Frozen shoulder

▶   Bursitis

Management

▶ • Physical therapy

▶ • Passive range of motion (ROM) exercise

▶ • Ice or heat

▶ • NSAIDs used with caution

▶ • Pain medications

▶ • Local corticosteroid injection

▶ • Surgical intervention for complete cuff tear

Prevention

▶ • Strengthen rotator cuff muscles.

▶ • Avoid lifting heavy objects.

▶ • Avoid prolonged overhead movements.

Adhesive Capsulitis (Frozen Shoulder)

▶ • Result of shoulder immobility from pain of trauma or neuropathy (can occur in weeks)

Risk Factors

▶ • Repetitive overhead activity

▶ • Rheumatoid or osteoarthritis

▶   Previous shoulder injury

Signs and Symptoms

▶   May or may not have history of trauma

▶ • Progressive loss of motion

- ▶ Minimal to severe pain
- ▶ Three stages
    1. • Freezing: Slowly increasing pain until shoulder loses range of motion. Lasts 6 weeks to 9 months.
    2. • Frozen: Pain improves, stiffness remains. Lasts 4–6 months.
    3. • Thawing: Motion slowly improves. Return to normal in 6 months to 2 years.

Differential Diagnoses

- ▶ Rotator cuff injury
- ▶ OA
- ▶ Bursitis

Management

- ▶ • Physical therapy
- ▶ • NSAIDs
- ▶ • Pain medications
- ▶ • Local corticosteroid injection
- ▶ • Surgical intervention

Prevention

- ▶ • Shoulder stretching and strengthening exercises

KNEE INJURIES

- ▶ Common primary care symptoms attributable to osteoarthritis, trauma, overuse, meniscus or ligament tears

Risk Factors

- ▶ • Contact or running sports
- ▶ • Poor conditioning
- ▶ • Osteoarthritis
- ▶ • Poorly fitted footwear

Signs and Symptoms

- ▶ Vary according to location
    - ▷ • Lateral collateral ligament tear
        - ▶ Joint laxity
    - ▷ • Posterior cruciate ligament
        - ▶ Joint instability, knee giving way

▷ •Anterior cruciate tear

▶ Joint insufficiency or instability

▷ • Meniscal tear or loose bodies

▶ "Locking" joint

Diagnostic Tests

▶ Radiographs are of limited utility.

▶ MRI only if results will change treatment.

▶ Maneuvers specific to involved ligament or meniscus.

▶ **Medial collateral ligament (MCL) tear**

▷ Sudden valgus stress with medial knee pain and tenderness when palpated

▷ May report "pop" sensation

▷ Localized swelling over 1–4 hours

▷ Tenderness on palpation

▷• Positive anterior drawer

▶ Patient supine with hip flexed 45°, knee flexed 90°, foot in neutral position. Examiner sits on foot with both hands behind proximal tibia, and thumbs on tibial joint line while applying anterior force to proximal tibia.

▷ Increased anterior tibial displacement compared to the other leg is a positive test.

▷• Positive Lachman's test

▶ Patient supine, knee flexed 20°–30° and externally rotated. Examiner's one hand behind tibia, other on thigh with thumb on tibial tuberosity, pulls anteriorly on tibia.

▷ Anterior translation with a soft, mushy endpoint is a positive test.

▶ **Lateral collateral ligament (LCL) tear**

▷ Direct blow to knee's medial aspect

▷ Tenderness over LCL

▷ Varying degree of joint laxity

▷ Small or absent effusion

▷ • Positive varus test

▶ Examiner places hand on end of femur at medial side of knee, other hand on lateral side of tibia while pushing knee with both hands as patient rotates hip.

▷ If a soft spot is felt, test is positive.

▶ **Posterior cruciate ligament (PCL) tear**

▷ Forced hyperextension from direct blow to anterior or proximal knee while flexed and foot planted

▷   Mild to moderate effusion

▷   Positive posterior drawer and Godfrey's test

▷ ● Positive posterior drawer test

    ▶   Patient is supine, knee flexed 90°. Examiner sits on toes to stabilize foot and grasps proximal lower leg at tibial joint line, and translates lower leg posteriorly.

        ▷   Lack of end feel or excessive posterior translation is positive.

▷ ● Positive Godfrey's test

    ▶   Patient supine with hip and knee flexed 90°, while examiner stabilizes hip and knee along tibia longitudinal axis.

        ▷   Tibia resting more inferiorly than contralateral side is positive

▶ **Anterior cruciate ligament (ACL) tear**

▷   Posterolateral joint pain, tenderness, edema immediately after sudden deceleration, jumping

▷ ● Weight-bearing difficult; sense of knee instability

▷ ● Effusion or hemarthrosis

▷ ● Positive anterior drawer test

    ▶   Patient supine with hip flexed 45°, knee flexed 90°, foot in neutral position. Examiner sits on foot with both hands behind proximal tibia, and thumbs on tibial joint line while applying anterior force to proximal tibia.

        ▷   Increased anterior tibial displacement compared to other leg is positive.

▷ ● Positive Lachman's test

    ▶   Patient supine, knee flexed 20°–30° and externally rotated. Examiner's one hand behind tibia, other on thigh with thumb on tibial tuberosity. Pull anteriorly on tibia.

        ▷   Anterior translation with a soft or a mushy endpoint indicates a positive test.

▶ **Meniscal tear**

▷   Pain with twisting of knee (e.g., getting in or out of automobile)

▷ ● More difficult going down stairs than up

▷ ● Sense of knee "locking," "giving way"

▷ ● Edema, tenderness over medial or lateral tibial joint

▷ ● Positive McMurray's test

    ▶   Apply valgus stress to the knee with one hand while the other hand extends and rotates the leg externally.

        ▷   Pain or audible click is positive.

Differential Diagnoses

- ▶ OA
- ▶ Ligament injuries
- ▶ Cartilage injuries
- ▶ Baker's cyst
- ▶ Effusion

Management

- ▶ Conservative therapy
- ▶ Rest, ice, immobilization
- ▶ Reduce weight-bearing
- ▶ Range of motion to prevent stiffness
- ▶ Refer to orthopedic department

Prevention

- ▶ Exercise to maintain strength and flexibility through hip and leg.
- ▶ Avoid overuse or overtraining.
- ▶ Proper footwear.

POLYMYALGIA RHEUMATICA (PMR)

- ▶ PMR is a syndrome characterized by aching and morning stiffness in proximal joints (shoulder and pelvic girdles).
- ▶ The shoulder girdle is first affected, and may start unilaterally, but then becomes bilateral.
- ▶ The pelvic girdle is often affected. Persons with PMR have difficulty standing up without pushing up with their arms.
- ▶ The exact cause of PMR is not known.
- ▶ It is more common among northern Europeans.
- ▶ Temporal arteritis (TA) frequently occurs with PMR.

Risk Factors

- ▶ Genetics
  - ▷ 50 years or older
- ▶ Giant-cell arteritis

Signs and Symptoms

▶ • Malaise, night sweats, weight loss

▶ • Proximal joint weakness

▶ • Painful or difficult joint movement

▶ Possible low-grade fever

Diagnostic Tests

▶ • ESR

▷ Essential to diagnose

▷ • Must be at least 40–50 mm/h

▶ Rheumatoid factor negative

▶ Temporal artery biopsy if symptoms consistent with temporal arteritis

Differential Diagnoses

▶ Amyloidosis

▶ Depression

▶ Fibromyalgia

▶ Giant-cell arteritis

▶ Hypothyroidism

▶ Multiple myeloma

▶ Rheumatoid or osteoarthritis

▶ Polymyositis

Management

▶ • Corticosteroids

▷ Start prednisone between 12.5 and 25 mg p.o. daily and taper to 10 mg per day within 4 to 8 weeks. For relapse therapy, oral prednisone should be increased to the dose the patient was taking before relapse and then decreased gradually over 4 to 8 weeks to the dose at which the relapse occurred. Once remission is achieved, daily oral prednisone can be tapered by 1 mg every 4 weeks or by 1.25 mg using an alternate day schedule until the prednisone is discontinued.

▶ If signs and symptoms consistent with temporal arteritis, immediately start high-dose prednisone

Prevention

▶ None known

ADDITIONAL JOINT INJURIES

TABLE 13–3.
OTHER JOINT INJURIES

CONDITION	DESCRIPTION	JOINTS COMMONLY AFFECTED	DIAGNOSES
Bursitis	Synovial fluid–filled bursal sac that cushions and reduces friction in joints becomes inflamed	Shoulder, elbow, hip, knee, ankle	Subacromial, olecranon, trochanteric, prepatellar, or retrocalcaneal bursitis
Tendinitis	Overuse syndrome of collagen fibrils, sheathed in connective tissue, that provide elasticity and strength to muscle and bone	Shoulder, wrist, elbow, knee, ankle	Patellar, de Quervain's, Achilles, or rotator cuff tendinitis. Medial or lateral epicondylitis
Muscle strain	Tearing of muscle fibers causing pain, swelling, decreased function	Shoulder, wrist	Deltoid muscle strain. Radiocarpal muscle strain
Ligament sprain	Stretching and tearing of ligaments	Knee, ankle	Collateral ligament sprain. Ankle ligament sprain

LOW BACK PAIN

▶ Low back pain is primarily due to mechanical causes, and is associated with spondylosis from normal wear and tear in spinal joints, discs, and bones.

Risk Factors

▶ Mechanical or metabolic disorder

▶ Autoimmune connective tissue disorders

▶ Tumors

▶ Infections

▶ Arteriovenous malformation

Signs and Symptoms

▶ Quality of the pain

▷ ● Herniated disk or radiculopathy associated with paresthesia or sciatic-type pain

▶ Burning pain in buttock or leg

▷ ● Bladder or bowel incontinence with large central disk herniation

▷ ● Stiffness usually associated with muscle injury

Diagnostic Tests

- ▶ ● Straight leg raising (SLR) indicates nerve root irritation.
  - ▷ ● Positive if symptoms recur with leg elevated 30°–60°.
  - ▷ Pain at >60° is nonspecific.
- ▶ ● Passive leg raises
  - ▷ Pain with <60° elevation
- ▶ Neurological exam of lower extremities detects small deficits of disk disease.
- ▶ ● Schober's test
  - ▷ Shows ankylosing spondylitis.
  - ▷ Make a mark 10 cm above and 5 cm below S1.
  - ▷ Patient bends forward as far as possible.
  - ▷ Distance should increase by at least 5 cm.
- ▶ X-ray
  - ▷ Helps identify degenerative changes, vertebral alignment, fracture, bone tumors, disk space height
- ▶ Serum studies usually are not needed.
- ▶ ESR or CRP elevated in infection.
- ▶ ● HLA-B27 (human lymphocyte antigen) elevated in ankylosing spondylitis.

Differential Diagnoses

- ▶ ● If saddle anesthesia or incontinence, rule out cauda equina
  - ▷ Medical emergency
  - ▷ Severe compression of spinal nerve roots
  - ▷ Urgent treatment to prevent permanent incontinence and leg paralysis
  - ▷ Leg pain, numbness, weakness
  - ▷ Severe or worsening paresthesia in buttocks (saddle anesthesia) and lower extremities
  - ▷ Incontinence
- ▶ ● Lumbar radiculopathy
  - ▷ Pain radiates down one or both buttocks or legs
  - ▷ Can be caused by herniated disk
  - ▷ Sciatica form of radiculopathy compressing sciatic nerve causes shock-like or burning low back pain
- ▶ ● Spondylolisthesis
  - ▷ Vertebra of lower spine slips out of place, pinching nerves exiting the spinal column

- ▶ • Spinal stenosis
  - ▷ Narrowing of spinal column puts pressure on spinal cord and nerves
  - ▷ Pain or numbness with walking
  - ▷ Over time, weakness and sensory loss in affected leg
- ▶ • Herniated disc
  - ▷ Due to spinal degenerative joint disease
  - ▷ Ruptured nucleus pulposus through annulus fibrosis of intervertebral disk
  - ▷ Compresses spinal cord or irritates nerve root
  - ▷ Usually unilateral; can cause central herniation
  - ▷ Unusual for older adults to have acute disc herniation

Management

- ▶ • Immediate referral for worsening neurological deficits
- ▶ Most resolve with conservative treatment in 4–6 weeks
- ▶ Refer when no response to conservative treatment
- ▶ • OTC acetaminophen or aspirin (ASA)
- ▶ • NSAIDs
  - ▷ Ibuprofen, ketoprofen, naproxen, COX-2 inhibitors
- ▶ • Analgesics: Topical and oral
- ▶ • Antidepressants
  - ▷ Tricyclics, serotonin and norepinephrine reuptake inhibitors (SNRIs) for low back pain
- ▶ • Muscle relaxants
- ▶ • Anticonvulsants
  - ▷ Effective in radiculopathy and radicular pain
- ▶ • Topical analgesics
  - ▷ Creams and sprays to reduce inflammation, stimulate blood supply
- ▶ • Corticosteroid injections
- ▶ • No activity restriction
- ▶ Surgical intervention

Prevention

- ▶ Proper body mechanics with lifting.
- ▶ Lower back and core strengthening exercises.
- ▶ Proper posture when sitting.
- ▶ Avoid sitting for prolonged periods.

NECK PAIN

- ▶ Neck injury or damage causing pain in neck, trapezius, rhomboid, or parascapular muscles; occipital headache
- ▶ May be acute or chronic

Risk Factors

- ▶ Precipitating event or trauma
- ▶ Poor posture
- ▶ Muscle strain
- ▶ Tumors
- ▶ Degenerative diseases

Signs and Symptoms

- ▶ Pain on movement
- ▶ • Restricted neck movement
- ▶ • Neurologic symptoms
- ▶ • Paresthesia
- ▶ • Dizziness or vertigo
- ▶ • Drop attacks

Diagnostic Studies

- ▶ X-rays
- ▶ MRI
- ▶ Myelogram
- ▶ CT scan
- ▶ EMG (confirms radiculopathy)

Differential Diagnoses

- ▶ Tumor or metastatic disease
- ▶ Meningitis
- ▶ Rheumatoid or PMR
- ▶ Compression fracture
- ▶ Torticollis
- ▶ Ankylosing spondylitis
- ▶ Cervical herniated disk

Management

▶ . Heat

▶ ◦ Soft cervical collar

▶ ◦ Analgesics

    ▷ OTC acetaminophen or ASA, or prescription opioids

▶ ◦ NSAIDs

    ▷ Ibuprofen, ketoprofen, naproxen

▶ ◦ Topical analgesics

    ▷ Creams and sprays to reduce inflammation, stimulate blood flow

▶ ◦ Neck exercises to strengthen as tolerated

▶ Surgery for decompression if indicated

Prevention

▶ Proper posture

▶ Proper work ergonomics

▶ Proper sleep positions

▶ Strengthening and stretching exercises

GAIT DISORDERS

▶ Deviation from normal gait from disease, injury, or aging.

▶ ◦ May be the result of aging changes in which sway while standing increases and postural support responses are slowed.

▶ ◦ Stride is shorter and broad-based, speed declines, and arm swing decreases.

Risk Factors

▶ Sensory deficits

▶ ◦ Neurologic disorders

    ▷ Dementia, Parkinson's disease, normal pressure hydrocephalus (NPH)

    ▷ Cerebellar disease, peripheral neuropathy, stroke with hemiparesis

▶ ◦ Frontal lobe apraxia of gait

▶ Medications

▶ Substance abuse

Signs and Symptoms

▶ ◦ Propulsive gait

    ▷ Stooped, stiff posture with head and neck bent forward

- ▶ ' Scissors gait
    - ▷ Legs flexed slightly at hips and knees, like crouching
    - ▷ Knees and thighs hitting or crossing in scissors-like movement
- ▶ ' Spastic gait
    - ▷ Stiff, foot-dragging walk from long muscle contraction
- ▶ ' Steppage gait
    - ▷ Foot drop causing toes to scrape ground while walking, so leg has to be lifted higher than normal
- ▶ ' Waddling gait
    - ▷ Duck-like walk
- ▶ ' Poor balance
- ▶ ' Frequent falls clinically significant

Diagnostic Tests

- ▶ ' History
    - ▷ Time course of problem
    - ▷ Additional symptoms
    - ▷ Medication
    - ▷ Frequent falls
    - ▷ Interference with function
    - ▷ Drug or alcohol use
    - ▷ Urinary or fecal incontinence
- ▶ ' Neurologic examination
    - ▷ Assess whether gait has a widened stance with lateral instability of the trunk.
    - ▷ ' Sensory ataxia destabilized by eye closure:
        - ▶ If <12 seconds of eye closure destabilizes, high risk for falling
    - ▷ ' Get-up-and-go test:
        - ▶ Assesses mobility and fall risk
        - ▶ Timed walk from getting up from seated position to a point 10 feet away
    - ▷ ' Tandem gait test:
        - ▶ Walk a straight line while touching heel of one foot to toe of other with each step
- ▶ Eye examination
    - ▷ Check vision difficulties
- ▶ Balance evaluation, toxic or metabolic causes
- ▶ Assess environmental safety
    - ▷ Footwear, home inspection for fall hazards

- ▶ Labs based on history and physical
    - ▷ • Blood chemistries, B12
- ▶ Cervical spine X-ray
- ▶ CT or MRI
    - ▷ For motor function deficits
    - ▷ Rule out mass lesion, subdural hematoma (SDH), NPH, cerebrovascular accident (CVA)

Differential Diagnoses

- ▶ Malignancy
- ▶ Cerebellar disorder
- ▶ CNS disorders
- ▶ Inner ear disorder

Management

- ▶ Specific to cause
- ▶ Properly fitted footwear
- ▶ Physical therapy
- ▶ Balance training
- ▶ Assistive devices
- ▶ Exercise

Prevention

- ▶ Fall prevention
    - ▷ Install adequate lighting, handrails on stairs, and grab bars by toilets and tubs.
    - ▷ Eliminate clutter and other tripping hazards in hallways and walkways.
    - ▷ Professional home fall assessment.

OSTEOMYELITIS

- ▶ Local infection of bone and surrounding tissue that is usually caused by bacteria.
- ▶ Considered an orthopedic emergency.
    - ▷ Delayed or inadequate treatment can lead to chronic infection.
- ▶ 75 percent report a recent trauma.

Risk Factors

- ▶ • Debilitating diseases
  - ▷   Cancer, diabetes, sickle cell anemia, salmonella, dialysis
- ▶ • Puncture wound
  - ▷   *Pseudomonas aeruginosa*
- ▶ • IV drug use
- ▶ • Poor blood supply
- ▶ • Recent injury

Signs and Symptoms

- ▶ • Pain, swelling, redness, heat at infection site
- ▶ • Sudden onset fever and chills, refusal to bear weight

Diagnostic Tests

- ▶   Elevated CBC, CRP, ESR
- ▶ • Positive blood cultures
- ▶   X-ray, bone scan, MRI
- ▶ • Needle aspiration at site
- ▶ • Bone biopsy positive for infection

Differential Diagnoses

- ▶   Septic or rheumatoid arthritis
- ▶   Toxic synovitis
- ▶   Cellulitis or myositis
- ▶   Sickle cell anemia
- ▶   Slipped capital femoral epiphysis
- ▶   Malignancy

Management

- ▶ • Acute infection
  - ▷   Antibiotic therapy for 4–6 weeks
- ▶ • Chronic infection
  - ▷   Oral antibiotics for 6–8 weeks
- ▶   Antibiotics, based on culture and sensitivity; must be able to penetrate bone

▷ Methicillin-sensitive *Staphylococcus aureus* (MSSA)

  ▶ Nafcillin or oxacillin 2 g IVPB q4h *or*

  ▶ Cephalosporin (cefazolin) 2 g IV q8h

▶ Methicillin-resistant *Staphylococcus aureus* (MRSA)

  ▶ Vancomycin 1g IV q12h *or*

  ▶ Linezolid 600 mg p.o. or IV q12h

  ▷ Gram-negative rods suspected

  ▶ Ceftriaxone 2g IV or cefotaxime 2 g IV q6–8h *or*

  ▶ Ceftazidime 2g IV q8h or cefepime 2 g IV q12h *plus*

  ▶ Fluoroquinolone (ciprofloxacin) IV 400 mg q12h or p.o. 750 mg q12h

  ▷ Anaerobes

  ▶ Clindamycin 600 mg IV q6h

▶ Surgical debridement

  ▷ Necrotic tissue, foreign materials, or skin closure of chronic wounds

▶ Amputation

  ▷ For resistant infection

Prevention

▶ Prevent skin wounds.

▶ Monitor skin wounds for signs of infection and treat early.

▶ Proper hand hygiene.

REFERENCES

CenterWatch. 2015. "Zurampic (Lesinurad)." http://www.centerwatch.com/drug-information/fda-approved-drugs/drug/100127/zurampic-lesinurad.

Goldberg, C. 2011. "Musculo-Skeletal Examination." A Practical Guide to Clinical Medicine. https://meded.ucsd.edu/clinicalmed/joints2.htm.

Heidari, B. 2011. "Knee Osteoarthritis Diagnosis, Treatment and Associated Factors of Progression: Part II." *Caspian Journal of Internal Medicine* 2 (3): 249–55.

Khanna, D., P. Khanna, J. Fitzgerald, M. Singh, S. Bae, T. Neogi, M. Pillinger, et al. 2012a. "2012 American College of Rheumatology Guidelines for Management of Gout. Part 1: Systematic Nonpharmacologic and Pharmacologic Therapeutic Approaches to Hyperuricemia." *Arthritis Care and Research* 64 (10): 1431–46. http://dx.doi.org/10.1002/acr.21772.

———. 2012b. "2012 American College of Rheumatology Guidelines for Management of Gout. Part 2: Therapy and Antiinflammatory Prophylaxis of Acute Gouty Arthritis." *Arthritis Care and Research* 64 (10): 1447–61. http://dx.doi.org/10.1002/acr.21773.

Moses, S. 2017. "Gouty Arthritis." In *Rheumatology Family Practice Notebook*. http://www.fpnotebook.com/Rheum/joint/GtyArthrts.htm#fpnContent-panel-id_12.

National Institute of Arthritis and Musculoskeletal and Skin Diseases. 2017. "Handout on Health: Rheumatoid Arthritis." http://www.niams.nih.gov/health%5Finfo/rheumatic%5Fdisease/#ra_2.

National Osteoporosis Foundation. 2017. "Calcium/Vitamin D." http://www.niams.nih.gov/health%5Finfo/rheumatic%5Fdisease/#ra_2.

Ogbru, O. 2016. "Cox-2 Inhibitors." MedicineNet. http://www.medicinenet.com/cox-2_inhibitors/article.htm.

Schnell, S., S. M. Friedman, D. A. Mendelson, K. W. Bingham, and S. L. Kates. 2010. "The 1-Year Mortality of Patients Treated in a Hip Fracture Program for Elders." *Geriatric Orthopaedic Surgery and Rehabilitation* 1 (1): 6–14. http://doi.org/10.1177/2151458510378105.

Starkebaum, G. A. 2016. "Systemic Lupus Erythematosus." Medical Encyclopedia. https://medlineplus.gov/ency/article/000435.htm.

CHAPTER 14

NEUROLOGIC SYSTEM DISORDERS

LEARNING OBJECTIVES

▶ Recognize common neurologic disorders.

   ▷ Risk factors

   ▷ Signs and symptoms

▶ Analyze processes useful to providing differential diagnosis for neurologic disorders.

   ▷ Diagnostic tests

   ▷ Differential diagnoses

▶ Describe treatment and management of neurologic disorders.

   ▷ Management

   ▷ Prevention

HEADACHE

▶ Various types (see table 14–1).

▶ Chronology is the most important history item.

▶ Evaluate location, duration, and quality.

▶ Associated activity (exertion, sleep, tension, relaxation)

▶ Timing of menstrual cycle.

▶ Presence of associated symptoms.

▶ Presence of "triggers."

TABLE 14–1.
HEADACHES BY TYPE

	TENSION	MIGRAINE	CLUSTER
Subtypes		**Classic migraine** with aura **Common migraine** without aura **Variant migraine** (see description following table 14–1)	
Risk Factors	Increased stress or fatigue Depression Anxiety	Fatigue Family history	Predominantly affects middle-aged men Often no family history of headache or migraine
Causes	Unknown Possibly head or neck muscle contractions related to various foods, activities, stressors	Related to dilation and excessive pulsation of external carotid artery branches	Not known May be precipitated by alcohol ingestion Possibly sudden histamine or serotonin release Hypothalamus may be involved Stress, glare, or ingestion of certain foods
Signs and Symptoms	Vague, nonspecific symptoms Poor concentration Daily vise-like or tight headaches Usually generalized, bilateral Most intense in neck or back of head Neurological symptoms Usually last several hours Gradual onset	Episodic unilateral, lateralized dull or throbbing headache Builds gradually, last several hours May be accompanied or preceded by focal neurologic disturbances (classic migraine) Nausea and vomiting Physical exam often normal Possible neurological deficits Visual disturbances: Field defects, luminous visual hallucinations (e.g., stars, sparks, or zigzag of lights) Aphasia, numbness, tingling, clumsiness, weakness Photophobia and phonophobia Careful exam for focal deficits or findings supportive of tumor Appears ill	Severe, unilateral, periorbital pain daily for several weeks Intense pain may initially imitate migraine, but cluster headaches are distinct Usually last <2 hours Pain-free months or weeks between attacks Usually nighttime, waking from sleep Ipsilateral rhinorrhea, nasal congestion, and eye redness may occur

	TENSION	MIGRAINE	CLUSTER
Diagnostic Tests	None specific Depends on intensity	Rule out organic causes Basic metabolic panel, complete blood count, VDRL, erythrocyte sedimentation rate Brain CT scan	History and physical exam MRI
Management	Over-the-counter analgesics Relaxation techniques When simple measures fail, a trial of antimigraine agents may be helpful	Avoid triggers Headache diary Relaxation and stress management Eliminate MSG, nitrates, and nitrites Stabilize or wean caffeine Trial of no alcohol **Acute migraine** • Rest in a dark, quiet room • Simple analgesic (such as aspirin) right away may provide some relief • Cafergot 1–2 tabs at onset and 1 tablet every 30 minutes up to 6 per attack, 10 per week • Imitrex (sumatriptan) 25 mg p.o. at onset then 100 mg q2h to max 300 mg/day • Imitrex 6 mg SC at onset, may repeat in 1 hour, to total of three times per day o Contraindicated in coronary artery disease, uncontrolled hypertension (HTN), Prinzmetal's angina	Imitrex Ergotamine aerosol Steroids 100 percent oxygen Sumatriptan (Imitrex) 6 mg subcutaneously (SC) or 20 mg nasal spray; may repeat in 24 hours Dihydroergotamine (DHE) 0.5 mg intranasal bilaterally Lidocaine 10 percent 1 mL intranasal bilaterally via swab ×5 min Capsaicin ipsilateral nostril via swab b.i.d. × 7 days

(continued)

	TENSION	MIGRAINE	CLUSTER
Prevention	Explore causes of chronic anxiety	Prophylactic therapy for >2–3 attacks per month • Aspirin or NSAIDs in chronic, low doses daily. • Propanolol 80–240 mg daily. • Amitriptyline 10–150 mg daily. • Imipramine 10–150 mg daily. • Clonidine 0.2–0.6 mg daily • Verapamil 80–160 mg daily. • Various ergotamines, MAO inhibitors, and antiserotonin drugs are also used for prophylaxis. • Botox for injection is indicated for the prophylaxis of headaches in adult patients with chronic migraine (≥15 days per month with headache lasting 4 hours a day or longer). Recommended total dose 155 units, as 0.1 mL (5 units) injections per each site divided across 7 head/neck muscles.	Ergotamine tartrate p.o., SC, or rectum • 2 mg p.o. daily • 0.5–1.0 mg p.o. at h.s. • 0.25 mg SC t.i.d. • 5 days weekly Tapering prednisone • Begin with 40 mg daily Methysergide 4–6 mg daily Verapamil 240–480 mg daily Lithium 300–600 mg daily

Note: VDRL = Venereal Disease Research Laboratory; MSG = monosodium glutamate; CT computed tomography; NSAIDS = nonsteroidal anti-inflammatory drugs; MAO = monoamine oxidase; MRI = magnetic resonance imaging; SC = subcutaneous

Source: American Migraine Foundation (AMF) 2016

Variant Migraine Syndromes

▶ • Hemiplegic migraine

▷ • Presents with hemiplegia, aphasia, speech disturbances followed by headache and associated symptoms

▷ Headache contralateral to hemiplegia

▷ Headache less symptomatic than hemiplegia

▶ • Abdominal migraine

▷ Episodic abdominal pain with nausea, vomiting, followed or accompanied by headache

▶ • Confusional migraine

▷ More common in younger children.

▷ Period of confusion and disorientation followed by vomiting and deep sleep, waking feeling well.

▷ Headache may not be described.

▶ • Basilar migraine

▷ Dizziness, vertigo, syncope, dysarthria preceding variable headaches and vomiting

MENINGITIS

▶ Central nervous system (CNS) infection of the pia, arachnoid meninges, and cerebral spinal fluid (CSF) of brain and spinal cord caused by viruses, bacteria, mycobacteria, spirochetes, fungi, protozoa, parasites, or chemical agents.

▶ United States has 20,000–25,000 new cases each year; higher prevalence is seen in fall and winter months when respiratory infections are common.

▶ Median age for infection is 25 years.

▶ Incidence is 15/100,000 and prevalence is 5/100,000.

▶ Mortality is 10–15 percent.

▶ Types:

▷ Bacterial

▶ Most commonly caused by *Neisseria meningitidis*, *Haemophilus influenzae* type B, and *Streptococcus pneumoniae*

▷ Chronic

▶ Most commonly caused by fungus, mycobacteria, spirochete, HIV, and neoplasms

▷ Aseptic

▶ No bacteria found in CSF; usually associated with a virus or with noninfectious causes such as a brain tumor or CVA

▶ Most common viral cause is enteroviruses (Dunphy et al. 2015)

Risk Factors

▶ • Poverty

▶ • Crowded living conditions

▷ Dormitories, barracks, nursing homes

▶ Immunodeficiency

▶ ˀ Recent respiratory or ear infection

▶ ˏ Endocarditis

▶ Penetrating head trauma

▶ Syphilis

▶ Lyme disease

Signs and Symptoms

▶ ˀ Rapid onset (24–48 hours).

▶ ˌ Most common subjective findings are headache, photophobia, and neck pain and stiffness (Dunphy et al. 2015).

▶ Most common objective findings are fever, chills, tachycardia, tachypnea, and signs of meningeal irritation, which include

▷ • Brudzinski's sign (hip and knee flexion when the neck is flexed) and

▷ • Kerning's sign (inability to fully extend legs).

▶ Progressive headache, neck or back pain, fever, nausea and vomiting, rash.

▶ ˸ Decreased level of consciousness.

▶ ˀ Cranial nerve III, IV, VII, VIII deficits.

▶ ˷ Focal motor deficits, seizure.

▶ ˶ Nuchal rigidity.

▶ Fever, chills, malaise

▶ Bacterial

▷ Headache, positive Kernig's sign, nuchal rigidity, hyperactive reflexes, fever, chills, malaise, nausea and vomiting, tachycardia, petechial or puerperal rash

▶ Viral

▷ Milder symptoms, fever, nausea and vomiting, neck, back pain, headache, irritability, photophobia

Diagnostic Tests

▶ ˙ Lumbar puncture

▶ Gold standard diagnosis

▷ Viral

▶ Some lymphocytes, normal glucose, moderately high protein, normal or slightly elevated opening pressure

▷ Bacterial

▶ Increased lymphocytes, decreased glucose, high protein, markedly elevated opening pressure

- ▶ Complete blood count (CBC), platelets, prothrombin time (PT), partial thromboplastin time (PTT), electrolytes, blood urea nitrogen (BUN), creatinine, glucose, arterial blood gasses as indicated
- ▶ Blood cultures
- ▶ ● Chest or sinus X-ray if exam indicates source of infection
- ▶ ● CT scan prior to spinal tap if space-occupying lesion is suspected
  - ▷ Brain abscess, subdural empyema or hematoma, tumor

Differential Diagnoses

- ▶ Aseptic meningitis
- ▶ Encephalitis
- ▶ Brain abscess
- ▶ Meningeal irritation
  - ▷ Sarcoidosis, lupus, cancer, medications, chemical irritants
- ▶ Endocarditis, bacteremia
  (Ferri 2016)

Management

- ▶ ● Immediate hospitalization for IV antibiotics for bacterial meningitis and supportive care.
- ▶ Maintain airway, breathing, circulation.
- ▶ ● Inform family and contacts of postexposure prophylaxis.
- ▶ Educate about disease, treatment, prognosis.
- ▶ ● Intravenous antimicrobials, usually 10–14 days, for bacterial meningitis.
  - ▷ Cefotaxime or ceftriaxone 2 g q4h
  - ▷ Vancomycin 1 g q12h
  - ▷ Acyclovir 10 mg/kg q8h for 10 days
- ▶ ● Corticosteroids.
- ▶ ● Osmotic diuretics for cerebral edema.
- ▶ Universal precautions for certain bacterial strains.

Prevention

- ▶ Meningococcal vaccination
- ▶ Pneumococcal vaccination
- ▶ Flu vaccination

AMYOTROPHIC LATERAL SCLEROSIS (ALS) OR LOU GEHRIG'S DISEASE

▶ ● Progressive, degenerative disease involving destruction of both anterior horn cells, corticospinal tracts of the brainstem (especially the cranial motor nerves), and spinal cord, resulting in progressive muscle weakness

▶ Most common degenerative disease of the motor neuron system

▶ Occurs slightly more in Caucasians

▶ ● Fatal within 5–10 years, secondary to muscle weakness at phrenic nerve

Risk Factors

▶ Heredity

▶ ● Occurs between 40 and 70 years of age

▶ ● More common in men

▶ ● Smokers twice as likely to develop ALS

▶ ● Exposure to lead

Signs and Symptoms

▶ ● Muscle weakness, atrophy, and cramping

▶ ● Wasting in hand muscles

▶ ● Tripping, stumbling

▶ ● Dysphagia, dysarthria, dysphonia

▶ ● Fasciculations

   ▷ Muscle fiber contractions causing flickering movement under the skin

Differential Diagnoses

▶ Brainstem gliomas

▶ Central cord syndrome

▶ Lyme disease

▶ Multiple sclerosis

▶ Neurosarcoidosis

▶ Polymyositis

▶ Primary lateral sclerosis

▶ Spinal muscular atrophy

Management

▶ Supportive care

  ▷ Eventually nasogastric or percutaneous endoscopic gastrostomy (PEG) feeding tube, or ventilator

▶ • Rilutek 50 mg p.o. q12h on an empty stomach

  ▷ Slows progression of ALS

Prevention

▶ None known

MYASTHENIA GRAVIS (MG)

▶ • Chronic autoimmune neuromuscular disease characterized by varying degrees of weakness of the skeletal (voluntary) muscles as a result of antibodies that block acetylcholine receptors at neuromuscular junctions and prevent muscle contraction

▶ Occurs in approximately 10–15 people per 100,000

Risk Factors

▶ Age

  ▷ Early onset: 20–30 years

  ▷ Late onset: After age 50 years

▶ • Women are more likely to be affected than men

▶ Heredity

  ▷ Increased chance of MG if family member has it

Signs and Symptoms

▶ • Bulbar symptoms common

  ▷ Ptosis, diplopia, dysarthria, dysphagia

▶ • Fluctuating muscle weakness that is more severe in the evening and after exertion

  ▷ • Weakness worse in proximal muscles, diaphragm, neck

  ▷ • Ocular and facial muscles almost always affected

Diagnostic Tests

▶ • Tensilon test

  ▷ Acetylcholine is a neurotransmitter released by nerves to stimulate muscles.

  ▷ Tensilon (edrophonium) prevents breakdown of acetylcholine.

  ▷ Injection of Tensilon that results in increased muscle strength indicates MG.

▶ ○ Acetylcholine receptor antibody

▷ Found in 85 percent with MG

▶ ○ Anti-MuSK (muscle-specific Kinase) antibodies

▷ Present in 40 percent with seronegative myasthenia gravis test

▶ Rheumatoid factor (RF) and antinuclear antibody (ANA)

▷ Rule out lupus and rheumatoid arthritis.

▶ Thyroid function tests

▷ Rule out Graves's disease or hyperthyroidism.

▶ X-ray

▷ Rule out thymoma or other mass.

▶ CT scan

▷ Rule out thymoma or other mass, especially in older adults.

▶ ● Electromyography

▷ Repetitive nerve stimulation checks for characteristic MG patterns

Differential Diagnoses

▶ ALS

▶ Basilar artery thrombosis

▶ Botulism

▶ Brainstem gliomas

▶ Chronic myelogenous leukemia

▶ Lambert-Eaton MG syndrome

▶ Multiple sclerosis

▶ Myocardial infarction

▶ Neurosarcoidosis

▶ Polymyositis

▶ Pulmonary embolism

Management

▶ Comfort, rest, positioning, assess swallowing prior to giving medications and meals

▶ Education

▷ ● Avoidance of medication triggers

▶ Aminoglycosides and quinolone antibiotics, class I and II antiarrhythmics

▷ Class I antiarrhythmics

> ► Quinidine, procainamide, disopyramide, lidocaine, Dilantin, mexiletine, flecainide, propafenone, moricizine

> ▷ Class II antiarrhythmics

> ► Propranolol, esmolol, timolol, metoprolol, atenolol

▷ ⦿ Prednisone 15–20 mg p.o. daily

▷ ⦿ Titrate in 5 mg increments until maximal response or 1 mg/kg daily

► Anticholinesterase inhibitors

> ▷ Pyridostigmine bromide (Mestinon) 30–60 mg p.o. q4–6h

> ▷ Neostigmine bromide (Prostigmine) 15–375 mg p.o. daily in divided doses

> > ► Average dose 150 mg daily

> > ► Maximum response in 2–3 months

► Immunosuppressants to reduce autoimmune response

> ▷ Azathioprine (Imuran) 50 mg p.o. daily

> > ► Titrate 2–3mg/kg daily

> > ► Maximum response in 6–12 months

> ▷ Mycophenolate mofetil (CellCept)

> > ► Dosage not established. One gram PO twice daily has been used with adjunctive corticosteroids or other nonsteroidal immunosuppressive medications (Providers' Digital Reference 2017).

> > ► Titrate to 2–3 mg daily.

> > ► Effects within 2–8 weeks.

> ▷ Cyclosporine (Sandimmune, Neoral) 5 mg/kg p.o. daily

> > ► Effects within 1–2 months

► ⦿ Plasmapheresis

> ▷ Removes antibodies that block neuromuscular receptor sites

► ⦿ Intravenous immunoglobulin (IVIg)

> ▷ Infuses normal antibodies to alter immune response

► ⦿ Thymectomy

> ▷ Removal of thymus gland

> > ► Stops production of acetylcholine receptor antibodies

> > ► Remission in some cases diagnosed early

Prevention

► None known

SEIZURE DISORDERS

▶ Transient disturbance of cerebral function secondary to an abnormal paroxysmal neuronal discharge in the brain.

▶ Epilepsy is common, affecting approximately 0.5 percent of the population in the United States.

▶ Types

▷ · Generalized

▶ Absence (petit mal) seizures

▷ Atypical absences

▷ · Tonic-clonic (grand mal) seizures

▷ An aura may precede a generalized seizure by a few seconds or minutes.

▷ It is part of the attack and arises locally from a restricted region of brain.

▷ · Partial

▶ One cerebral hemisphere

▷ · Simple seizures

▶ Consciousness preserved

▷ · Complex

▶ Consciousness impaired, accompanied or followed by dysphasia, dysmnesic symptoms, deja vu illusions, affective disturbances, or structured hallucinations

▷ · Tonic-clonic seizures

▶ Tonic phase

▷ Extension of extremities lasting 5–30 seconds

▶ Clonic phase

▷ Rhythmic jerky contraction and relaxation, incontinence

▷ · Postictal phase

▶ Lethargic, stuporous, confused

Risk Factors

▶ Epilepsy

▶ Congenital abnormalities and perinatal injuries

▶ Metabolic disorders

▶ Trauma

▶ Tumors and space-occupying lesions

▶ Vascular disorders

▶ Degenerative disorders

▶ Infectious diseases

Signs and Symptoms

▶ Nonspecific changes

▷ ' Headache, lethargy, mood alterations.

▷ 'Myoclonic jerking may precede impending seizure by hours.

Diagnostic Tests

▶ Detailed history and physical to determine underlying cause

▷ Neurological exam usually normal

▶ Focal deficits seen with underlying lesion.

▶ 'Motor events, typically tonic muscle contractions to clonic jerking.

▶ Mental or focal neurologic symptoms may persist postictally for hours.

▶ Recurrent seizures

▷ ' Electroencephalogram (EEG)

▶ Identifies abnormal brainwaves and changes

▶ Normal in 50 percent

▷ ' MRI, CT scan

▶ Identify causes and treatment

▷ ' Positron emission tomography (PET) scan

▶ Locate origin

▷ ' Spinal tap

▶ If infection suspected

Differential Diagnoses

▶ Head trauma

▶ Abnormal vessels in brain

▶ Brain tumor or lesions

▶ Brain abscess, meningitis, or encephalitis

▶ Cerebrovascular accident

▶ Cerebral palsy

▶ Fever

▶ Heredity

▶ Drug use

Management

- ▶ Educate patients about
  - ▷ Medication adherence and side effects,
  - ▷ Driving safety,
  - ▷ Effects of alcohol and medication,
  - ▷ Accessing psychological counseling, support groups,
  - ▷ Signs of impending seizure, and
  - ▷ Sleep hygiene.
- ▶ ♥ Individual seizures of <5 minutes' duration generally require no medications.
- ▶ Anticonvulsants are first-line treatment for tonic-clonic seizures.
  - ▷ ● Carbamazepine (Tegretol) 200 mg p.o. q12h
    - ▶ Increase weekly by 200 mg/day divided p.o. q6–8h
  - ▷ ● Phenytoin (Dilantin) 100 mg p.o. b.i.d.–q.i.d.
    - ▶ Titrate up to up to 200 mg t.i.d.
    - ▶ Therapeutic range: 10–20 mcg/L
  - ▷ ♦ Valproic acid (Depakote) 10–15 mg/kg/day p.o.
    - ▶ Increase by 5–10 mg/kg/day weekly up to 60 mg/kg/day
  - ▷ ● Fosphenytoin (Cerebyx)
    - ▶ Loading dose: 10–20 mg PE/kg phenytoin sodium equivalent) IV or intramuscularly (IM).
    - ▶ Maintenance: 4–6 mg PE/kg/day IV or IM in divided doses.
    - ▶ Infuse slowly over 30 minutes, not to exceed 150 mg PE/min.
    - ▶ Primarily used for status epilepticus and preventing and treating seizures during neurosurgical procedures.
    - ▶ Indicated for short-term, parenteral use.
    - ▶ Has not been effectively evaluated for more than 5 days of therapy.
  - ▷ ● Phenobarbital 1–3 mg/kg/day p.o. or IV in 1–2 divided doses
    - ▶ Therapeutic range 10–40 mcg/L (43–172 micromoles/L)
  - ▷ ● Primidone (Mysoline)
    - ▶ Initially 100–125 mg p.o. h.s. for 3 days, then
    - ▶ 100–125 mg b.i.d. for 3 days, then
    - ▶ 100–125 mg t.i.d.for 3 days, then
    - ▶ 250 mg t.i.d.–qid
    - ▶ Not to exceed 2 g/day
  - ▷ Gabapentin (Neurontin) 300 mg p.o. q8hr up to 600 mg q8hr
  - ▷ Levetiracetam (Keppra) 500–3000 mg in divided doses

▶ Titrate 1000 mg in divided doses daily q 2 weeks to maximum dose
▶ Surgical intervention

Prevention

▶ Patient education to include

▷ Avoid flashing lights and video games;

▷ Do not use illicit drugs;

▷ Limit alcohol use;

▷ Minimize stress; and

▷ Obtain adequate sleep.

PARKINSON'S DISEASE

▶ Neurological motor disorder from loss of dopamine-producing brain cells leading to dopamine and acetylcholine imbalance.

▶ Occurs in all ethnic groups.

▶ Dopamine depletion is due to degeneration of dopaminergic nigrostriatal system that leads to dopamine and acetylcholine (neurotransmitters in corpus striatum) imbalance.

Risk Factors

▶ ˈ Onset at between 45 and 65 years old

▶ ˈ Male:female ratio 3:2

▶ Heredity

▶ Environmental factors

Signs and Symptoms

▶ Cardinal signs

▷ ˋ Tremor

▶ Hands, arms, legs, jaw, and face

▶ Tremor of 4–6 cycles per second, most noticeable at rest

▷ Enhanced by emotional stress

▷ Less severe during voluntary activity

▷ ˋ Rigidity

▶ Cogwheel type

▷ Tension in muscles that responds with small jerks when muscles are passively stretched

▶ Flexed posture because of rigidity

▷ • Bradykinesia

▶ Slowness of voluntary movement

▶ Reduced automatic movements

▷ Arm swing lost while walking, slow movements

▷ • Posture

▶ Progressive instability

▷ Difficulty rising from sitting position and beginning walking

▷ Unsteadiness turning, difficulty in stopping, and tendency to fall

▶ Gait

▷ Small, shuffling steps

▶ • Seborrhea

▶ • Hypersalivation

▶ • Orthostatic hypotension

▶ Mild intellectual decline

▶ • Soft, poorly modulated voice

▶ • Impaired fine or rapidly alternating movements

▶ Tendon and plantar reflexes intact

Differential Diagnoses

▶ Benign essential tumor

▶ Depression or dementia

▶ Cardiovascular disease

▶ Medications

▶ Anticholinergics, antipsychotics

▶ Drug-induced Parkinson's

▶ Carbon monoxide poisoning

▶ Normal pressure hydrocephalus (NPH)

▶ Huntington's disease

▶ Creutzfeldt-Jakob disease

Management

▶ Education and emotional support related to disease and progressive nature

▶ • Nutritional counseling for low-protein diet

▶ • Physical, occupational, and speech therapy

▶ Fall precautions

▶ Considerations in treatment of older adults:

▷ Prescribe medications cautiously because of heart, renal, liver disease

▷ Increased side effects from anticholinergics

▶ Confusion, agitation, arrhythmias, urinary retention

▷ Differentiate Parkinson's tremors from benign essential tremor

▶ Pharmacological intervention:

▷ Monoamine oxidase-B inhibitors

▶ Selegiline (Eldepryl) 5 mg p.o. b.i.d.

▷ At low dose, is an MAO inhibitor and can be taken with levodopa

▷ Catechol-o-methyltransferase inhibitors

▶ Tolcapone (Tasmar) 100–200 mg p.o. t.i.d.

▶ Entacapone (Comtan) 200 mg p.o. daily with levodopa or carbidopa

▷ Not to exceed 1,600 mg per day

▷ Dopaminergics

▶ Levodopa/carbidopa (Sinemet, Sinemet CR) 100/25 mg t.i.d.–q.i.d. or 100/10 mg t.i.d.–q.i.d.

▷ Titrate up by 1 tablet q 2–7 days as tolerated and needed.

▷ Do not exceed 800 mg levodopa or 200 mg carbidopa daily.

▶ Levodopa (Larodopa, Dopar) 0.5–1 g daily

▷ Take in 2 or more divided doses with food.

▷ Titrate up by 0.75 g q 3–7 days to 8 g.

▷ Dopaminergic agonists

▶ Pergolide (Permax) 0.05 mg p.o. × 2 days

▷ Titrate by 0.1 or 0.15 mg/day q 3 days over 12 days, then

▷ Increase 0.25 mg/day q 3 days to therapeutic dose.

▶ Bromocriptine (Parlodel) 1.25 mg p.o. q12h

▷ Increase 2.5 mg/day q 2–4 weeks

▷ Safety at >100 mg/day not established

▶ Pramipexole (Mirapex) 0.125 mg p.o. t.i.d.

▷ Titrate up to 1.5 mg t.i.d. over 7 weeks.

▶ Ropinirole (Requip) 0.25 mg t.i.d.

▷ Titrate weekly up by 1.5 mg daily to dose of 24 mg daily.

▷ Maintenance dose is 3–24 mg daily.

▶ Amantadine (Symmetrel) 100 mg per day p.o.

▷ May increase to 100 mg q12h after 1 week

▷ Up to 400 mg/day only in special circumstances

    ▷ Anticholinergic drugs

        ► Benztropine (Cogentin) 1–2 mg daily

    ▷ Thalamotomy or pallidotomy

Prevention

► None known

MULTIPLE SCLEROSIS (MS)

► MS is a chronic autoimmune demyelinating disease of the central nervous system in which damage to myelin sheath slows or blocks messages between brain and body.

► Strong association between multiple sclerosis and specific human lymphocyte antigens (HLA-DR2) supports the theory of genetic predisposition.

► More common in western European lineage in temperate zones; no high-risk population exists between latitudes 40°N and 40°S.

► Types:

    ▷ Relapsing remitting (RRMS): Relapse followed by near or complete recovery

    ▷ Secondary progressive (SPMS): Progression of disability with few or no relapses

    ▷ Primary progressive (PPMS): Progressive disease from the beginning

Risk Factors

► Between the ages of 20 and 50 years

► Female:male ratio 1:5

► Heredity

► More common in people of Western European descent

► Temperate zones

► Environmental factors

Signs and Symptoms

► Episodic sensory abnormalities.

► Blurred vision

► Sphincter disturbance

► Weakness, numbness, tingling, or unsteadiness in a limb.

► Spastic paraparesis.

► Retrobulbar neuritis.

► Diplopia.

► Disequilibrium.

▶ Symptoms progress to include optic atrophy, nystagmus, dysarthria, internuclear ophthalmoplegia and pyramidal, sensory, or cerebellar deficits in some or all limbs.

▶ Infection, trauma, pregnancy, heat, or stress may trigger exacerbations. (Ferri 2016)

Diagnostic Tests

▶ • Lumbar puncture

   ▷ Elevated immunoglobulin G (IgG) in cerebrospinal fluid with discrete bands of IgG oligoclonal bands

▶ • Brain and cervical spine MRI

   ▷ Single pathologic lesion cannot explain clinical findings.

   ▷ Multiple foci best visualized by MRI.

   ▷ Focal, often perivenular demyelination with reactive white matter gliosis in brain, spinal cord, and optic nerves.

Management

▶ Refer to neurologist

▶ Refer to urologist

▶ Physical and occupational therapy

▶ • Corticosteroids

   ▷ Methylprednisolone 1g IV daily × 3–5 days, then

   ▷ 7–10 day course of prednisone tapering dose

▶ Immunosuppressive therapy

▶ • Cyclophosphamide-azathioprine

▶ • Beta interferons: Avonex, Betaseron, Extavia, Rebif, and Peginterferon beta-1a (Plegridy)

   ▷ Need CBC, liver function, and thyroid-stimulating hormone tests during therapy

▶ Cop 1 (random polymer-simulation myelin basic protein)

▶ • Pain

   ▷ Carbamazepine, gabapentin, amitriptyline

▶ • Spasticity

   ▷ Baclofen, tizanidine, diazepam, lorazepam

▶ • Spastic bladder

   ▷ Oxybutynin, tolterodine, propantheline

Prevention

▶ None known

DEMENTIA

▶ Decline in mental function, severe enough to interfere with activities of daily living (ADLs).

▶ Memory loss by itself is not indicative of dementia. Two or more brain functions, such as memory and language, are affected.

▶ Many different diseases can cause dementia, including Alzheimer's disease and stroke. (National Institute on Aging [NIA] 2017d)

Lewy Body Dementia (LBD)

▶ A "disease associated with abnormal deposits of a protein called alpha-synuclein in the brain" (NIA 2017e)

▶ There are two types of LBD (NIA 2017e):

▷ Dementia with Lewy bodies and

▷ Parkinson's disease dementia.

Risk Factors

▶ Increasing age (50 or over)

▶ Male

▶ Having a family member with Lewy body dementia or Parkinson's disease

▶ • Parkinson's disease

▶ REM sleep behavior disorder

▶ Lack of healthy lifestyle (regular exercise, mental stimulation, healthy diet)

▶ Anxiety and depression
(NIA 2017c; Boot et al. 2013; Lewy Body Dementia Association 2017)

Signs and Symptoms

▶ • Like Alzheimer's dementia (AD; see below), but includes hallucinations, shuffling gait, flexed posture

▶ See Lewy Body Dementia Association Common Symptoms Checklist: http://www.lbda.org/sites/default/files/2013_comprehensive_lbd_symptom_checklist.pdf

Diagnostic Tests

▶ CT scan and MRI can be used to rule out other disorders.

▶ Neuropsychological tests

▷ There are no brain scans or medical tests that can *definitively* diagnose LBD. Currently, LBD can be diagnosed with certainty only by a brain autopsy after death. (NIA 2017a)

Differential Diagnoses

▶ Alzheimer's dementia

▶ Parkinson's disease

▶ Hydrocephalus

Management

▶ ● "The FDA has approved one Alzheimer's drug, rivastigmine (Exelon), to treat cognitive symptoms in Parkinson's disease dementia" (NIA 2017b)

▶ ● "LBD-related movement symptoms may be treated with a Parkinson's medication called carbidopa-levodopa (Sinemet, Parcopa, Stalevo)" (NIA 2017b)

▶ Physical, speech, music or expressive art, and occupational therapy

▶ Mental health counselors for patients and families

▶ Palliative care specialists (NIA 2017b)

Prevention

▶ Researchers have not yet identified any specific causes of LBD.

Vascular Dementia

▶ Second most common dementia

▶ ● Brain damage from inhibited vascular function

▷ ●Cerebrovascular, cardiovascular issues

Risk Factors

▶ ● HTN

Signs and Symptoms

▶ Similar to AD

▶ Personality and emotions affected in late stages

Diagnostic Tests

▶ MRI

▶ Neurocognitive testing

▶ CT scan

Differential Diagnoses

▶ Alzheimer's disease

▶ Neurosyphilis

▶ Malignancy

▶ Lewy body dementia

Management

▶ No drugs have been approved to treat vascular dementia.

▶ • Certain medications such as cholinesterase inhibitors and memantine (Namenda) approved by the FDA to treat Alzheimer's disease may also help people with vascular dementia.

▶ ⁹ Risk factor control: Blood pressure, blood glucose, and cholesterol control. (Alzheimer's Association 2017b)

Prevention

▶ Control blood pressure, blood glucose, and cholesterol.

▶ Healthy living: Healthy diet, regular exercise, maintain healthy weight.

▶ Avoid smoking and excessive alcohol consumption. (Alzheimer's Association 2017b)

Frontotemporal Dementia (FTD)

▶ Frontal and temporal lobe nerve cell degeneration

Risk Factors

▶ "Frontotemporal degenerations are inherited in about a third of all cases.... There are no known risk factors for any frontotemporal degenerations except for a family history or a similar disorder" (Alzheimer's Association 2017a).

▶ Most diagnoses are made between 40 and 60 years of age (Alzheimer's Association 2017a).

Signs and Symptoms

▶ • Judgment and social behavior issues

▶ ₀ Compulsive behaviors

▶ ◦ Eventual motor skill and memory loss

Diagnostic Tests

▶ Made by clinical evaluation

▶ Cognitive and neuropsychological tests

▶ CBC, glucose, liver function, kidney function, thyroid-stimulating hormone tests, toxicology screen, urinalysis

　▷ Help rule out treatable causes

▶ Spinal tap

　▷ Normal

　▷ May be helpful in identifying causes in rapidly progressive cases

▶ CT, MRI

　▷ Identify stroke

Differential Diagnoses

▶ Parkinson's dementia or syndromes

▶ Vascular dementia, AD

▶ Pick's disease

▶ Creutzfeldt-Jakob disease

▶ Metabolic or pharmacologic delirium

Management

▶ Educate regarding disease progression and care.

▶ Treat underlying conditions.

▶ • Stop or change medicines that are causing memory loss or confusion.

▶ ◉ Cholinesterase inhibitors

▷ Treat cognitive impairment, hallucinations, sleep disorders, anxiety.

▶ ◉ Antidepressants for depression and irritability.

▶ ◉ Antipsychotics

▷ Treat hallucinations (relatively uncommon in FTD).

Prevention

▶ None known

ALZHEIMER'S DISEASE (AD)

▶ AD is characterized by progressive loss of cognitive skills, memory, language, insight, and judgment.

▶ • Most common cause of dementia over the age of 65 years, and accounts for 50–75 percent of all dementias.

▶ ◉ AD results from amyloid plaques and neurofibrillary tangles in the brain.

Risk Factors

▶ ◉ Advanced age

▶ ◉ Family history (genetic)

▶ ◉ Possible risk factors

▷ Female

▷ Low educational level

▷ Head injury

Signs and Symptoms

▶ ◦ Memory loss

▶ ◦ Aphasia, apraxia, agnosia

▶ ▫ Difficulty performing complex tasks

  ▷ Balancing checkbook

  ▷ Later: Abstract thinking affected

▶ ▫ Impaired reasoning, judgment

  ▷ Getting lost, driving difficulties

▶ • Behavioral changes

  ▷ Moody, apathetic

  ▷ Later: Agitation, psychosis

Diagnostic Tests

▶ Criteria to diagnose

  ▷ ▫ Documented Mini–Mental Status Exam (MMSE)

  ▷ ▫ Deficits occurring in two or more cognitive areas

    ▶ Memory, calculation, judgment

  ▷ Progressive worsening of memory and cognitive functions

  ▷ ▫ No disturbance of consciousness

  ▷ ▫ Onset between ages 40 and 90 years

  ▷ Lack of systemic disorders or other brain diseases that may result in progressive deficits

  ▷ Progressive deterioration of specific cognitive functions

  ▷ ▫ Impaired ADLs and altered patterns of behavior

  ▷ Family history of similar disorder

▶ History and physical exam

▶ ▫ Depression screening

  ▷ ▫ Neuropsychological testing, which might provide more direction and support for the patient and the caregivers

    ▶ Normal (age-related) nonspecific changes in EEG: increased slow-wave activity

    ▶ Evidence of cerebral atrophy on CT; progression documented on serial studies

    ▶ Normal lumbar puncture

▶ Cognitive state evaluation

  ▷ ▫ Folstein's MMSE

  ▷ ▫ Clock-drawing test

    ▶ Correlates with executive functions

  ▷ ▫ Mini-Cog

    ▶ Combination of clock-drawing test and three-word recall

> ▶ Montreal Cognitive Assessment (MoCA)

▶ Functional assessment

   ▷ Detect dementia and monitor cognitive decline based on declining ADLs and instrumental activities of daily living (IADLs).

Differential Diagnoses

▶ Cancer

   ▷ Brain tumor or neoplasm

▶ Infection

   ▷ HIV or neurosyphilis

▶ Organ failure

   ▷ Vascular disorders

▶ Cerebrovascular accident, vasculitis, subdural hematoma

   ▷ Depression

Management

▶ • Identify and address safety risks.

   ▷ Driving, wandering, cooking

▶ • Behavioral therapy.

   ▷ Social inappropriateness, withdrawal, compulsive behaviors, wandering

▶ • Pharmacological interventions.

   ▷ Mild-to-moderate Alzheimer's:

      ▶ Cholinesterase inhibitors

        ▷ May delay or slow worsening of symptoms

      ▶ Razadyne or Reminyl (galantamine) 4 mg p.o. b.i.d. with food

        ▷ Increase by 4 mg b.i.d. q 4 weeks

        ▷ Target dose 8–12 mg b.i.d.

      ▶ Exelon (rivastigmine) 1.5 mg p.o. b.i.d. with food

        ▷ Increase by 1.5 mg b.i.d. weekly

        ▷ Target dose 3–6 mg b.i.d.

      ▶ Aricept (donepezil) 5 mg p.o. daily for 4–6 weeks

        ▷ Target dose 10 mg daily

   ▷ Moderate-to-severe Alzheimer's:

      ▶ N-methyl D-aspartate (NMDA) antagonist

        ▷ Delays progression of symptoms and improves memory

> ▶ Namenda (memantine) 5 mg p.o. daily
>> ▷ Increase by 5 mg weekly
>> ▷ Target dose 10 mg b.i.d.

Prevention

▶ None known

DELIRIUM

▶ Acute, transient, usually reversible cause of cerebral dysfunction commonly caused by physical or mental illness, oxygen deprivation, substance abuse, infections, or fluid and electrolyte disturbances

Risk Factors

▶ Age

▶ Dementia

▶ Frailty

▶ Visual or hearing impairments

▶ Chronic diseases

▶ Infection

Signs and Symptoms

▶ Quick mental status change

▶ Difficulty maintaining attention

▶ Disorientation, illusions

▶ Hallucinations

▶ Motor abnormalities

Diagnostic Tests

▶ Screening tools
>> ▷ Confusion Assessment Method (CAM)
>> ▷ Depression scales
>>> ▶ Beck Depression Inventory, Hamilton Depression Rating Scale, Geriatric Depression Scale
>> ▷ Delirium Symptom Interview (DSI)
>> ▷ Confusion Assessment Method for the Intensive Care Unit (CAM-ICU)
>> ▷ Intensive Care Delirium Screening Checklist (ICDSC)

Differential Diagnoses

► Dementia, depression

► Infections

   ▷ Urinary tract infection (UTI), pneumonia, meningitis

   ▷ Syphilis or HIV

► Hypoxemia

► Trauma

► Drug toxicity

► Fecal impaction, constipation

Management

► Find and treat cause.

► Provide supportive care.

   ▷ Minimize environmental stimuli.

   ▷ Provide glasses or hearing aids.

   ▷ Orientation aids.

   ▷ Clock, watch, calendar.

► Haloperidol (Haldol) 0.5 mg IM or p.o. q2–6h for agitation.

Prevention

► Good sleep patterns.

► Orientation to surroundings if changed.

► Minimize medications.

► Treat comorbid conditions.

► Avoid narcotics.

REFERENCES

Alzheimer's Association. 2017a. "Frontotemporal Dementia." Alzheimer's and Dementia. https://www.alz.org/dementia/fronto-temporal-dementia-ftd-symptoms.asp#causes.

———. 2017b. "Vascular Dementia." Alzheimer's and Dementia. http://www.alz.org/dementia/vascular-dementia-symptoms.asp#treatments.

American Migraine Foundation. 2016. "What Type of Headache Do You Have?" https://cdn2.hubspot.net/hubfs/2611652/AMF%20-%20PC-%20What%20Type%20of%20Headache%20do%20You%20Have-.pdf?t=1501120140417.

Boot, B. P., C.F. Orr, J.E. Ahlskog, T.J. Ferman, R. Roberts, V.S. Pankratz, …, B.F. Boeve. 2013. "Risk factors for dementia with Lewy bodies: A case-control study." Neurology. http://www.ncbi.nlm.nih.gov/pubmed/23892702.

Dunphy, L., J. Winland-Brown, B. Porter, and D. Thomas, eds. 2015. *Primary Care: The Art and Science of Advanced Practice Nursing*. 4th ed. Philadelphia: F. A. Davis.

Ferri, F. F. 2016. *Ferri's Clinical Advisor 2016*. Philadelphia: Elsevier Health Sciences.

Lewy Body Dementia Association. 2017. "The Basics of Lewy Body Dementia: Causes and Risk Factors". http://lbda.org/content/lbd-booklet/lbd-causes-risk-factors.

National Institute on Aging. 2017a. "Diagnosing Lewy Body Dementia." https://www.nia.nih.gov/health/diagnosing-lewy-body-dementia.

———. 2017b. "Treatment and Management of Lewy Body Dementia." https://www.nia.nih.gov/health/treatment-and-management-lewy-body-dementia.

———. 2017c. "What Causes Lewy Body Dementia?" https://www.nia.nih.gov/health/what-causes-lewy-body-dementia.

———. 2017d. "What Is Dementia?" https://www.nia.nih.gov/health/what-dementia.

———. 2017e. "What Is Lewy Body Dementia?" https://www.nia.nih.gov/health/what-lewy-body-dementia#lewy%20bodies.

Prescribers' Digital Reference. 2017. "Mycophenolate Mofetil – Drug Summary." http://www.pdr.net/drug-summary/cellcept?druglabelid=988.

CHAPTER 15

ENDOCRINE DISORDERS

LEARNING OBJECTIVES

▶ Recognize common endocrine disorders and analyze processes to make differential diagnoses among them.

▷ Risk factors

▷ Signs and symptoms

▷ Diagnostic tests

▷ Differential diagnoses

▶ Describe treatment and management of endocrine disorders.

▷ Management

▷ Prevention

AGE-RELATED CONCERNS

TABLE 15–1.
AGE-RELATED CHANGES THAT AFFECT PHARMACOTHERAPY

PHARMACOKINETICS	IMPLICATION
Absorption Increased gastric pH; decreased motility, absorptive surface area, first-pass effect	Slower absorption and delayed onset, greater bioavailability of drugs with high hepatic extraction
Distribution Decreased total body fluid, increased body fat, decreased lean muscle mass and albumin	Small older adults more sensitive to dose, lipophilic drugs have increased half-life, hydrophilic drugs have increased peak concentrations
Metabolism Decreased liver and renal blood flow, glomerular filtration rate (GFR), altered cytochrome P450 metabolism	Increased or decreased effect and toxicity of drugs metabolized
Excretion Decreased liver and renal blood flow and renal tubule secretory function	Increased effect and toxicity of renally eliminated drugs and those metabolized in liver

HYPOTHERMIA

▶ Condition in which the body cannot adequately regulate body temperature because of overwhelming cold conditions in the environment.

▶ Hypothermia is diagnosed when core body temperature is ≤95°F (32°C; Dunphy et al. 2015).

▷ Mild hypothermia

▶ A core temperature of 89.6°F–95°F (32°C–35°C)

▷ Moderate hypothermia

▶ A core temperature of 82.4°F–89.6°F (28°C–32°C)

▷ Severe hypothermia

▶ A core temperature of <82.4°F (28°C)

Risk Factors

▶ Thyroid disease

▶ Cardiovascular disease

▶ Exposure to cold

▶ Age: >75 years

▶ Alcohol use

▶ Antidepressants

▶ Electrolyte imbalance

▶ Inactivity

▶ Extended periods in cold environment

▶ Homelessness and mental illness

Signs and Symptoms

▶ Shivering

▷ Indicates heat regulation still active

▷ May stop as hypothermia progresses

▶ Slow and shallow breathing, weak pulse

▶ Altered level of consciousness

▶ Confusion, memory loss

▶ Drowsiness, exhaustion

▶ Slurred or mumbled speech

▶ Loss of coordination

Diagnostic Tests

- ▶ Arterial blood gases
    - ▷ Altered if body temperature is <98.6°F (37°C)
    - ▷ ●May show higher oxygen or carbon dioxide or low pH
- ▶ Electrolytes
    - ▷ ● Potassium > 10 mmol/L associated with poor prognosis
    - ▷ Serum glucose levels
        - ▶ ● Hyperglycemia may be seen in acute hypothermia.
        - ▶ ● Hypoglycemia may be seen in chronic hypothermia.
- ▶ ● Elevated hematocrit

Differential Diagnoses

- ▶ Alcohol or drug toxicity
- ▶ Carbon monoxide poisoning
- ▶ Stroke
- ▶ Ventricular fibrillation or tachycardia
- ▶ Therapeutic hypothermia
- ▶ Myocardial infarction,
- ▶ Diabetic hypoglycemia or hyperglycemia
- ▶ Sepsis
- ▶ Hypothyroidism
  (Dunphy et al. 2015)

Management

- ▶ Remove any wet clothing.
- ▶ Protect from further heat loss with warm, dry clothes and blankets.
- ▶ ● Warm blankets (electric blanket, hot packs, heating pad) to torso, axilla, neck, groin.
- ▶ Move to a warm, dry area.
- ▶ ● Warm liquids intravenously and orally, lavage, humidified oxygen.
- ▶ ● Bretylium (5 mg/kg initially) for ventricular ectopy.
- ▶ ● Observe for signs of rhabdomyolysis.
- ▶ Warmed IV saline, rewarm body temp 1–2°C per hour. (Dunphy et al. 2015)

Prevention

- ▶ ● Avoid alcohol and caffeine when in cold environments for extended periods.
- ▶ Wear warm clothes in layers.

▶ Know the signs of cold weather illnesses and injuries.

▶ Take breaks in warm shelters when in cold for extended time.

HYPERTHERMIA

▶ Condition in which the body cannot adequately regulate body temperature because of being overwhelmed by hot conditions in the environment.

▶ Hyperthermia is diagnosed when core body temperature is ≥99°F (37.2°C).

Risk Factors

▶ Thyroid disease

▶ Cardiovascular disease

▶ • Sustained muscle activity

▶ • Dehydration

▶ No air conditioning

▶ • Lack of mobility

▶ Overdressing

▶ Overcrowding

▶ Chronic medical conditions

▶ Environmental exposure to heat

▶ • Drug toxicity

Signs and Symptoms

▶ • Heat exhaustion

▷ Occurs when there is a prolonged period of fluid loss (e.g., from perspiration, diarrhea, or use of diuretics) and exposure to warm ambient temperatures without adequate fluid and electrolyte replacement (Dunphy et al. 2015, 1139)

▷ Normal to slightly elevated core temperature

▷ • Mental status intact

▷ • Fatigue or malaise

▷ • Orthostatic hypotension, tachycardia

▷ • Dehydration

▷ • Nausea, vomiting, diarrhea

▶ Due to splanchnic vasoconstriction

▶ • Heatstroke

▷ Occurs when core body temperature reaches >105°F (40.6°C; Dunphy et al. 2015)

▷ • Confusion, ataxia, coma, seizures, delirium

▷   Hot, dry skin

▷ ● Vague weakness, nausea, vomiting, headache

▷ ● High central venous pressure, low systemic vascular resistance

▷ ● Elevated transaminase

▷ ● Coagulopathy

▷ ● Rhabdomyolysis

▷ ● Renal failure

Diagnostic Tests

▶ ● Complete blood count (CBC)

▶ ● Thyroid panel

Differential Diagnoses

▶   Thyroid storm

▶   Meningitis

Management

▶   Reduce temperature

▶   Aggressive temperature reduction if hemodynamically unstable

▶   Responsive to cool environment, fluid and electrolyte replacement

▶   Heatstroke management

▷ ● Rapid cooling; if ice packs are used, place them in groin and axillary region.

▷ ● Monitor rectal temperature.

▷ ● Supplemental oxygen, including possible intubation, may be necessary.

▷ ● IV fluids (usually 0.9 percent normal saline; Dunphy et al. 2015, 1139)

▶ ● Neuroleptic malignant syndrome and malignant hyperthermia

▷ ● Dantrolene 2.5 mg/kg repeated q5min.

▷   Until reaction occurs or total dose of 10—20 mg/kg reached.

▷   Discontinue offending drug.

Prevention

▶   Dress appropriately for weather, dress in layers.

▶ ● Drink extra fluids.

▶ ● Avoid caffeine and alcohol.

▶ Stay indoors on hot, humid days.

▶ Keep air conditioner on or use a fan to circulate air.

▶ If no air conditioning, go to community cooling center.

DIABETES MELLITUS

▶ Twenty-nine million Americans are living with diabetes and 86 million are living with prediabetes, a serious health condition that increases a person's risk of type 2 diabetes and other chronic diseases.

▶ Type 2 diabetes accounts for about 90–95 percent of all diagnosed cases of diabetes, and type 1 diabetes accounts for about 5 percent. The health and economic costs for both are enormous:

▷ Diabetes was the seventh leading cause of death in the United States in 2013 (and may be underreported).

▷ Diabetes is the leading cause of kidney failure, lower-limb amputations, and adult-onset blindness.

▷ More than 20 percent of healthcare spending is for people with diagnosed diabetes (Centers for Disease Control and Prevention [CDC] 2016).

▷ Costs for diabetic care exceed $245 billion annually; one in five healthcare dollars is spent on diabetes each year.

Types

▶ Type 1 diabetes, caused by beta-cell destruction, usually leading to absolute insulin deficiency

▶ Type 2 diabetes, caused by progressive loss of insulin secretion on the background of insulin resistance

▶ Gestational diabetes mellitus (GDM), diagnosed in the second or third trimester of pregnancy and not clearly overt diabetes

▶ Specific types of diabetes attributable to other causes (American Diabetes Association [ADA] 2015)

Complications

▶ Retinopathy, blindness, cataracts, glaucoma

▶ Nephropathy, renal failure

▶ Cardiovascular disease, atherosclerosis, myocardial infarction (MI)

▶ Cerebrovascular disease, stroke

▶ Peripheral neuropathy

▶ Infection

▶ Foot ulcers, bacterial and fungal skin infections

- ▶ Hyperosmolar nonketotic coma
- ▶ • Diabetic ketoacidosis (DKA)

Screening

- ▶ Screening for prediabetes and risk for future diabetes with an informal assessment of risk factors or validated tools should be considered in asymptomatic adults.
- ▶ • For all people, testing should begin at age 45 years.
- ▶ • Testing for prediabetes and risk for future diabetes in asymptomatic people should be considered in adults of any age who are overweight or obese (body mass index [BMI] >25 kg/m² or >23 kg/m² in Asian Americans) and who have one or more additional risk factors for diabetes:
  - ▷ A1C > 5.7 percent (39 mmol/mol), IGT, or IFG on previous testing
  - ▷ First-degree relative with diabetes
  - ▷ High-risk race/ethnicity (e.g., African American, Latino, Native American, Asian American, Pacific Islander)
  - ▷ Women who were diagnosed with GDM
  - ▷ History of cardiovascular disease (CVD)
  - ▷ Hypertension (HTN; >140/90 mmHg or on therapy for HTN)
  - ▷ HDL cholesterol level < 35 mg/dL (0.90 mmol/L) and/or a triglyceride level 250 mg/dL (2.82 mmol/L)
  - ▷ Women with polycystic ovary syndrome
  - ▷ Physical inactivity
  - ▷ Other clinical conditions associated with insulin resistance (e.g., severe obesity, acanthosis nigricans)
- ▶ If tests are normal, repeat testing carried out at a minimum of 3-year intervals is reasonable (ADA 2017).

TYPE 1 DIABETES MELLITUS (FORMERLY CALLED INSULIN-DEPENDENT DIABETES OR IDDM)

- ▶ Beta-cell destructive autoimmune disease that develops in response to an environmental trigger. It is a syndrome produced by disorders in metabolism of carbohydrates, proteins, and fats caused by an absolute absence of insulin that then results in hyperglycemia. Without insulin, ketoacidosis rapidly develops.

Risk Factors

- ▶ Exposure to viruses, toxic chemicals, or cytotoxins
- ▶ Genetic predisposition

▶ • First-degree relative with type 1 diabetes

▶ ⁹ Autoimmune disorders

Signs and Symptoms

▶ ⁹ Acute onset

▶ ⁸ Polyuria, polydipsia

▶ ○ Polyphagia, weight loss

▶ • Blurred vision

▶ ⁹ Fatigue

▶ ◦ Abdominal pain, nausea and vomiting

▶ ▲ Vaginal itching and infections

▶ ⁹ Unhealed wounds, skin infections, rashes

▶ ⁹ Dehydration

▶ ⁹ Hypoglycemia or ketotic episodes

▶   See table 15–2

TABLE 15–2.
COMMON FINDINGS IN DIABETES MELLITUS

BODY SYSTEM	EXAM FINDINGS
Skin	Cellulitis; lower leg ulcers; candidiasis
Eyes	Ptosis; glaucoma; abnormal retinal exam
Mouth	Oral *Candida* infections
Heart	Resting tachycardia; silent MI
Abdomen	Gastroparesis; residual urine
Peripheral vasculature	Decreased circulation; edema
Central nervous system	Decreased proprioception, vibration, and light touch; ataxia

Diagnostic Tests

▶ ▲ Fasting plasma glucose (FPG) *or*

▶ • Oral glucose tolerance test (OGTT): Plasma glucose value 2 hours after a 75-gram oral glucose challenge *or*

▶ ○ Glycosylated hemoglobin (A1C)

▶ ⁹ Diagnostic criteria for diabetes:

    ▷   A1C > 6.5 percent *or*

    ▷   FPG > 126 mg/dL *or*

    ▷   OGTT plasma glucose > 200 mg/dL 2 hours after 75-gram anhydrous glucose load following an 8-hour fast *or*

▷ Random plasma glucose > 200 mg/dL with classic symptoms of hyperglycemia or hyperglycemic crisis

▶ •Diagnostic criteria for prediabetes:

▷ A1C 5.7–6.4 percent *or*

▷ FPG 100 mg/dL to 125 mg/dL *or*

▷ OGTT plasma glucose 140–199 mg/dL 2 hours after 75-gram anhydrous glucose load following an 8-hour fast

▶ •Decreased C-reactive protein (CRP)

▶ •Glucose and ketones in urine

▶ •Blood urea nitrogen (BUN), creatinine elevated if patient dehydrated

▶ •Urinalysis, urine microalbumin

▶ •Fasting lipids

▷ Triglycerides > 150 mg/dL

▶ •Thyroid-stimulating hormone level

Differential Diagnoses

▶ Type 2 diabetes, diabetes insipidus

▶ Pancreatic disease

▶ Pheochromocytoma

▶ Cushing's syndrome or acromegaly

▶ Liver disease

▶ Salicylate poisoning

▶ Renal disease with glucosuria

▶ Secondary effects of oral contraceptives, corticosteroids, thiazides, phenytoin, nicotinic acid

Management

▶ Replace lost endogenous insulin.

▶ •Most people with type 1 diabetes should be treated with multiple-dose insulin injections (three to four injections per day of basal and prandial insulin) or continuous subcutaneous insulin infusion (see table 15–3).

▶ •Match prandial insulin to carbohydrate intake, premeal blood glucose, and anticipated physical activity.

▶ •For most patients (especially those at elevated risk of hypoglycemia), use insulin analogs.

▶ •For patients with frequent nocturnal hypoglycemia, recurrent severe hypoglycemia, or hypoglycemia unawareness, a sensor-augmented low glucose threshold suspend pump may be considered (ADA 2016a).

- ▶ A1C goals
  - ▷ • A reasonable A1C goal for many nonpregnant adults is <7 percent (53mmol/mol).
  - ▷ More stringent A1C goals (such as <6.5 percent [48 mmol/mol]) for selected individual patient if this can be achieved without significant hypoglycemia or other adverse effects of treatment (e.g.., polypharmacy). Appropriate patients might include those with short duration of diabetes, type 2 diabetes treated with lifestyle or metformin only, long life expectancy, or no significant cardiovascular disease.
  - ▷ • Less stringent A1C goals (such as <8 percent [64 mmol/mol]) may be appropriate for patients with a history of severe hypoglycemia, limited life expectancy, advanced microvascular or macrovascular complications, extensive comorbid conditions, or long-standing diabetes for whom the goal is difficult to achieve despite diabetes self-management education, appropriate glucose monitoring, and effective doses of multiple glucose-lowering agents including insulin (ADA 2017).
  - ▷ • Treat HTN, proteinuria, nephropathy, dyslipidemia with angiotensin-converting enzyme inhibitors (ACEI) unless contraindicated (renal protective).
- ▶ Goal blood pressure (BP) < 140 mm Hg
  - ▷ BP < 130 mm Hg may be appropriate for some patients with diabetes, such as younger patients, those with albuminuria, and those with HTN and one or more additional atherosclerotic cardiovascular disease risk factors (ADA 2016b).
  - ▷ • Aspirin 81–325 mg daily (unless contraindicated)
  - ▷ Reduces risk of diabetic atherosclerosis
  - ▷ Treat dyslipidemia

Prevention
- ▶ None known

TYPE 2 DIABETES MELLITUS (FORMERLY CALLED NON-INSULIN-DEPENDENT DIABETES)

- ▶ Elevated blood glucose levels caused by reduced pancreatic production of insulin and inability to use insulin efficiently, including insulin resistance

Risk Factors
- ▶ • Obesity, inactivity
- ▶ More than 20 percent over ideal body weight or BMI (BMI > 25 kg/m^2 or > 23 kg/m^2 in Asian Americans)
- ▶ • High refined carbohydrate, high-fat, low-fiber diet
- ▶ Family history

TABLE 15–3.
INSULIN PRODUCTS

PREPARATION	BRANDS	ONSET	PEAK	DURATION	ROUTE
Rapid-Acting Insulin analogs	NovoLog Humalog	15 min	60 min	3 hr	SC before meals
Rapid-Acting	AFREZZA (insulin human)	12–15 min	60 min	2.5–3 hr	Inhalation; administer at the beginning of a meal
Rapid-Acting	APIDRA (insulin glulisine [rDNA origin] injection)	15 min	60 min	2–4 hr	SC 15 minutes before or within 20 minutes after starting a meal
Short-Acting Regular	Novolin R Humulin R	30 min	2–4 hr	6–8 hr	SC, IM, IV before meals
Intermediate-Acting NPH	Novolin N Humulin N	1–2 hr	6–12 hr	18–24 hr	SC b.i.d.
Long-Acting Ultralente	Humulin L	1–3 hr	6–12 hr	18–24 hr	SC q12h
Long-Acting Insulin glargine	Lantus	1 hr	None	24 hr	SC at h.s.
Long-Acting Insulin detemir	Levemir Levemir FlexPen	1–3 hr	8–10 hr	18–26 hr	
Long-Acting Insulin glargine	Toujeo	1–1½ hr	No peak	20–24 hr	SC once a day
Ultra Long-Acting Insulin	Degludec Tresiba	30–90 min	No peak	42 hr	SC once daily at any time of day

Note: SC = subcutaneous; IV = intravenous; IM = intramuscular

▶ ● People of African American, Asian American, Hispanic, Native American, Pacific Island descent at higher risk

▶ ● Advanced age; as age increases, the risk of diabetes increases.

▷ Generally, type 2 diabetes occurs in middle-aged adults, most frequently after age 45 (American Heart Association [AHA] 2017)

▶ ● Previous impaired glucose tolerance

▶ ● Metabolic syndrome

▶ ● Lipid abnormalities

▷ High-density lipoprotein (HDL) < 35 mg/dL or triglycerides > 250 mg/dL

Signs and Symptoms

▶ · Polyuria and polydipsia

▶ Increased appetite

▶ · Extreme fatigue, blurred vision

▶ · Slow wound healing

▶ · Tingling, pain, numbness in hands or feet

Diagnostic Tests

▶ · Urinalysis

▷ For protein, glucose, ketones, and microalbuminuria

▶ · BUN and creatinine

▷ Serum and urine

▶ · Serum cholesterol, lipid profile

▶ · A1C

▶ · Fasting blood glucose (FBG)

Differential Diagnoses

▶ Type 1 diabetes

▶ Diabetes insipidus

Management

▶ • If FBG < 250 mg/dL:

▷ Nutrition counseling and exercise for 3 months

▷ Lifestyle modifications

▷ Dietary changes

▷ Weight reduction

▷ Daily exercise

▷ Glycemic control

▶ A1C goals:

▷ A reasonable A1C goal for many nonpregnant adults is <7 percent (53mmol/mol).

▷ More stringent A1C goals (such as <6.5 percent [48 mmol/mol]) for selected individual patient if this can be achieved without significant hypoglycemia or other adverse effects of treatment (e.g., polypharmacy). Appropriate patients might include those with short duration of diabetes, type 2 diabetes treated with lifestyle or metformin only, long life expectancy, or no significant cardiovascular disease.

▷ Less stringent A1C goals (such as <8 percent [64 mmol/mol]) may be appropriate for patients with a history of severe hypoglycemia, limited life expectancy, advanced microvascular or macrovascular complications, extensive comorbid conditions, or long-standing diabetes for whom the goal is difficult to achieve despite diabetes self-management education, appropriate glucose monitoring, and effective doses of multiple glucose-lowering agents including insulin (ADA 2017).

▶ Pharmacologic treatment (see table 15–4)

    ▷ • Metformin, if not contraindicated and if tolerated, is the preferred initial pharmacologic agent for the treatment of type 2 diabetes.

        ▶ Metformin monotherapy should be started at diagnosis of type 2 diabetes.

TABLE 15–4.
ORAL AND NONINSULIN INJECTABLE HYPOGLYCEMIC AGENTS

GENERIC AND CLASS	BRAND NAME
Second-Generation Sulfonylureas	
Glipizide	Glucotrol, Glucotrol XL
Glyburide	DiaBeta, Micronase
Glyburide, micronized	Glynase, Press Tab
Meglitinides	
Repaglinide	Prandin
Nateglinide	Starlix
Biguanides	
Metformin	Glucophage XR
	(Calculate creatinine clearance. Do not give to older patients if clearance is <50 cc/min. Use in ages >80 years is not FDA-approved.)
Thiazolidinediones	
Pioglitazone	Actos
Rosiglitazone	Avandia
Alpha-Glucosidase Inhibitors	
Acarbose	Precose
Miglitol	Glyset
Incretin Mimetics	
GLP-1 Agonists	
Exenatide	Byetta
Liraglutide	Victoza
Albiglutide	Tanzeum
Dulaglutide	Trulicity
Amylin Analog	
Pramlintide	Symlin
DPP-4 Inhibitors	
Sitagliptin	Januvia
Saxagliptin	Onglyza
Linagliptin	Tradjenta

▷ • When A1C is >9 (75 mmol/mol), consider initiating dual combination therapy.

▷ • Consider initiating insulin therapy (with or without additional agents) in patients with newly diagnosed type 2 diabetes who are symptomatic and/or have A1C ≥ 10 percent (86mmol/mol) and/or blood glucose levels >300 mg/dL (16.7 mmol/L).

▷ • If noninsulin monotherapy at maximum tolerated dose does not achieve or maintain the A1C target after 3 months, add a second oral agent, a glucagon-like peptide-1 receptor agonist, or basal insulin.

▷ Lifestyle therapy plus antihyperglycemic therapy is recommended.

    ► • Treat HTN, proteinuria, nephropathy, dyslipidemia with ACEIs unless contraindicated (renal protective).

► • Goal: BP < 140 mm Hg

► • BP < 130 mm Hg may be appropriate for some patients with diabetes, such as younger patients, those with albuminuria, and those with HTN and one or more additional atherosclerotic cardiovascular disease risk factors (ADA 2016b)

▷ • Aspirin 81–325 mg daily (unless contraindicated).

► Reduces risk of diabetic atherosclerosis

▷ Treat dyslipidemia.

Prevention

► Maintain optimal weight.

► Exercise.

► Healthy balanced diet, avoiding simple carbohydrates.

HYPOTHYROIDISM

► Endocrine disorder caused by inadequate thyroid hormone secretion; constitutes 90 percent of cases of primary hypothyroidism (gland cannot produce hormone).

► • Hashimoto's thyroiditis is an autoimmune disorder resulting in hypothyroidism and is the most common cause of hypothyroid after age 8.

Risk Factors

► • Hypothyroidism two to three times more common in women (Dunphy et al. 2015, 856)

► • Presence of thyroid antibodies

► • Treatment of hyperthyroidism

► • Family history of thyroid or autoimmune disease

► • Pituitary or hypothalamus disease

► • Type 1 diabetes

▶ ▸ Postpartum

   ▷   Maternal thyroid-stimulating hormone-binding antibodies

▶ Surgery

▶ ▪ Previous radiation to head or neck area

▶ ▪ Iodine deficiency or excess

▶ ▪ Medications

   ▷   Lithium, sulfonamides, phenylbutazone, amiodarone, prolonged treatment with iodides

Signs and Symptoms

▶ Affects all systems (see table 5–5).

▶ ▪ Thyroid gland may or may not be palpable.

   ▷   If palpable, may be enlarged or atrophied, tender, nodules

▶ ▪ Fatigue, lethargy.

▶ ▪ Muscle weakness, stiffness.

▶ ▪ Memory loss, depression.

▶ ▪ Slowed speech, hoarseness.

▶ ▪ Periorbital edema.

▶ ▪ Dry skin, coarse hair, hair loss.

▶ ▪ Temporal thinning of brows, brittle nails.

▶ ▪ Weight gain.

▶ ▪ Constipation.

▶ ▪ Cold intolerance.

TABLE 15–5.
HYPOTHYROID PHYSICAL CHANGES

SYSTEM AFFECTED	SIGNS
Face	Facial periorbital edema, swollen tongue, outer eyebrow loss
Skin	Dryness, coarse hair, nail loss
Ears	Decreased acuity
Thyroid	Goiter or atrophy, tender, nodules
Respiratory	Dyspnea, pleural effusion
Cardiac	Bradycardia, low-voltage electrocardiogram (ECG)
Abdominal	Hypoactive bowel sounds, ascites
Extremities	Edema in hands, legs, feet; weight gain
Neurological	Dementia, paranoia, slow or delayed reflexes, cerebellar ataxia, carpal tunnel syndrome

Diagnostic Tests

▶ Thyroid-stimulating hormone (TSH) assay

▷ Elevated

▷ Low if due to pituitary insufficiency

▶ Free T4

▷ Elevated TSH or low free T4

▶ Confirms hypothyroidism

▷ Subclinical hypothyroidism

▶ Elevated TSH with normal free T4

▷ Pituitary or hypothalamic failure

▶ TSH normal or low or mildly elevated free T4

▷ If secondary hypothyroid suspected

▶ Serum prolactin, neuroradiological studies, pituitary and adrenal, pituitary gonadal function studies

▷ CBC, electrolytes, BUN, creatinine, glucose, calcium, phosphates, albumin, pregnancy test, urine protein, lipids as indicated

Differential Diagnoses

▶ Depression, dementia

▶ Obesity

▶ Ischemic heart disease, chronic heart failure

▶ Kidney failure, nephrotic syndrome

▶ Cirrhosis

▶ Congenital or transient hypothyroidism

▶ Thyroid hormone resistance

▶ Hypopituitarism

Management

▶ Thyroid hormone replacement.

▷ Lifelong thyroid hormone replacement is necessary.

▶ First-line therapy for primary hypothyroidism.

▷ Levothyroxine (T4) 25–50 mcg p.o. daily in healthy persons

▷ Start at the lowest dose in frail older adults.

▷ Overreplacement can trigger cardiovascular problems, and atrial fibrillation.

▶ Repeat TSH in 6–8 weeks after initiating therapy.

▶ • Increase every 6–8 weeks until TSH is in normal limits, then repeat TSH every 6 months when regulated.

▶ • Monitor for signs and symptoms of hyperthyroidism.

▶ • Improvement seen within 1 month of starting medication.

▶ • Symptom resolution within 3–6 months.

▶ • Check lipids annually.

Prevention

▶ Monitor thyroid levels closely when taking replacement or medications known to decrease thyroid hormones.

HYPERTHYROIDISM AND THYROTOXICOSIS

▶ Endocrine disorder caused by overproduction of thyroid hormone T4 (thyroxine) and T3 (triiodothyronine)

Risk Factors

▶ Family history of thyroid and autoimmune disorders

▶ • Thyroid replacement hormone

▶ • Graves's disease

▶ • Multinodular goiter or solitary nodule

▶ • Transient thyroiditis

▶ • Drug-induced

  ▷ Iodide-containing drugs

   ▶ Amiodarone, contrast media

Signs and Symptoms

▶ • Weight loss, increased appetite

▶ • Insomnia, nightmares

▶ • Palpitations

▶ • Fatigue, weakness

▶ • Sensitivity to heat

▶ • Irritability, anxiety

▶ • Severe depression in older adults

▶ • Increased frequency of bowel movements

▶ • Diarrhea, pernicious vomiting

▶ See table 15–6 for physical changes

TABLE 15–6.
HYPERTHYROID PHYSICAL CHANGES

SYSTEM	SIGNS
Adrenergic	Tachycardia, sweating, palpitations, tremor, lid lag
Skin	Warm, moist, diaphoresis, thin or fine hair, spider angiomas
Eyes (Graves's disease only)	Periorbital edema, exophthalmos, blurred vision, photophobia, diplopia
Cardiac	Atrial fibrillation, angina, congestive heart failure, systolic flow murmurs, widened pulse pressure

Diagnostic Tests

▶ TSH, free T4

▷ TSH low or undetectable; T4 elevated

▷ If free T4 normal, order T3

▶ T3 elevated

▶ Other labs

▷ •Hypercalcemia, elevated alkaline phosphatase, low hemoglobin or hematocrit

▷ Perform urine pregnancy test if abnormal menses

▶ Thyroid autoantibodies

▷ ⁹ Elevated serum antinuclear antibody

▷ ⁴ Elevated TSH receptor antibody

▶ ₐ Radioactive uptake

▷ Normal values:

▶ In 6 hours: 3–16 percent

▶ In 24 hours: 8–25 percent

▷ High radioactive iodine uptake

▶ Graves's disease, goiter

▷ Low radioactive iodine uptake

▶ Thyroiditis

▶ ₐThyroid uptake scan or ultrasound for palpable nodules to rule out cold nodule

▶ ⁹Thyroid biopsy

▶ • CT scan for eye findings to rule out tumor

▶ ○ ECG in older adults

Differential Diagnoses

▶ Thyrotoxic phase of Hashimoto's thyroiditis

▶ Psychological disorders

▷   Anxiety, panic, psychosis

►   Infection

►   Hormone ingestion

►   Plummer's disease

►   Toxic multinodular goiter

►   Acromegaly

►   Malignancy

►   Congestive heart failure (CHF), new onset or worsening angina

►   Orbital tumors

►   Myasthenia gravis

Management

► ⇒ Radioactive iodine

   ▷   Treatment of choice for Graves's disease, symptomatic multinodular goiter, single hyperfunctioning adenoma, and older adults

   ▷   1–2 doses orally

      ► ⇒ Euthyroid in 2–6 months.

      ► ⇒ Hypothyroidism may result.

►   Antithyroid medications

   ▷ • Propylthiouracil (PTU) 100–150 mg p.o. q8h initially

      ►   50–100 mg b.i.d. maintenance

   ▷ • Methimazole (Tapazole) 20–30 mg p.o. q12 h initially

      ►   5–10 mg daily maintenance

      ►   Euthroid in 4–6 weeks

   ▷ • Usually on medication for 1–2 years, then gradually weaned

►   Symptom management

   ▷ • Beta blocker

      ►   For catecholamine symptoms

      ►   Propranolol 10–60 mg p.o. q6h for catecholamine symptoms

      ►   Atenolol 50–100 mg p.o. daily

   ▷ • Multivitamin

   ▷ • Calcium with vitamin D, bisphosphonate

      ►   Replenish bone

   ▷ • Diltiazem

      ►   If unable to take beta blockers

▷ • Check bone density (dual-energy X-ray absorption [DXA]); if indicated, give bisphosphonate

▷ Eye lubricants for ophthalmopathy

Prevention

▶ Monitor thyroid levels closely when taking replacement or medications known to increase thyroid hormones.

THYROID NODULE AND THYROID CANCER

▶ Abnormal growth in thyroid gland.

▶ May function independent of hypothalamic and pituitary feedback.

▶ More than one nodule is called multinodular goiter.

▶ A fluid- or blood-filled nodule is a thyroid cyst.

▶ • A nodule that produces thyroid hormone is autonomous.

▷ • Autonomous nodules (hot nodule on thyroid scan) are usually benign and may cause symptoms of hyperthyroidism.

▶ • A nonfunctioning nodule (cold nodule on thyroid scan) may be malignant.

▷ Most thyroid cancers are found between ages 20 and 50.

▷ • A solitary nodule is more likely to be cancerous than multiple nodules.

▷ The majority of nodules are benign.

▷ 90 percent of women older than age 60 years have a nodular thyroid gland.

▷ 60 percent of men older than age 80 years have a nodular thyroid gland.

Risk Factors for Thyroid Nodule

▶ • Iodine deficiency

▶ • Female

▶ • Increasing age

▶ • Residing in area of endemic iodine deficiency

Risk Factors for Thyroid Cancer

▶ Family history of thyroid cancer or multiple endocrine metaplastic type II carcinoma

▶ • Male

▶ • Age < 15 years or > 70 years

▶ • Head, neck, chest radiation exposure

▶ • Single nodule

Signs and Symptoms

▶ • History of hypothyroidism or hyperthyroidism

   ▷ Hyperthyroid symptoms if nodule is producing thyroid hormone

▶ • Hoarseness, cough, dysphagia, obstruction, shortness of breath

   ▷ Hoarseness may be caused by nodule location and causing pressure

▶ • Ear, jaw, throat pain; neck tenderness, swelling, or enlargement

▶ • Malignant

   ▷ Hoarseness, enlarged cervical nodes

   ▷ Dyspnea; palpable fixed, painless, hard, irregular mass (tumor)

▶ • Benign

   ▷ Multiple nodules palpable

      ▶ Nodular Hashimoto's thyroiditis or multinodular goiter

Diagnostic Tests

▶ Fine-needle biopsy aspiration

   ▷ • If palpable nodules > 1.5 cm

▶ • Thyroid-stimulating hormone

   ▷ If low, do free T4

▶ • Radionuclide scans to determine cytologic results

   ▷ Hot

      ▶ 98 percent benign

   ▷ Cold

      ▶ 5–10 percent malignant

▶ • Ultrasound

   ▷ Determines if cystic

▶ • Antithyroperoxidase and antithyroglobulin antibodies

   ▷ Rule out thyroiditis

▶ • Serum calcitonin for family history of medullary thyroid carcinoma

Differential Diagnoses

▶ Malignant versus benign nodules

▶ Cysts

▶ Thyroiditis

Management

▶ ◦ Refer all persons with thyroid nodules for biopsy (Dunphy et al. 2015).

▶ ◦ Adequate iodine intake.

▶ Surgical resection for malignant or disfiguring tumors.

▶ • Monitor benign nodules.

▶ ◦ Suppressive thyroid hormone to shrink nodule.

▶ Education

▶ Follow up for changes.

▷ Lymphadenopathy, dysphagia, hoarseness, new or worsening symptoms of hypothyroidism or hyperthyroidism

Prevention

▶ None known

REFERENCES

American Diabetes Association. 2002. "Diabetes Mellitus and Exercise." *Diabetes Care* 25 (S1): S64–S68. http://care.diabetesjournals.org/content/25/suppl_1/s64.full.

———. 2012. "Clinical Practice Recommendations," supplement, *Diabetes Care* 35 (S1).

———. 2015. "Standards of Medical Care in Diabetes—2015," supplement, *Diabetes Care* 38 (S1). http://dx.doi.org/10.2337/dc15-s001.

———. 2016a. "Approaches to Glycemic Treatment." In "Standards of Medical Care in Diabetes–2016," supplement, *Diabetes Care* 39 (S1): S52–S59. http://dx.doi.org/10.2337/dc16-s010.

———. 2016b. "Cardiovascular Disease and Risk Management." In "Standards of Medical Care in Diabetes–2016," supplement, *Diabetes Care* 39 (S1): S60–S71. http://dx.doi.org/10.2337/dc16-s011.

———. 2016c. "Classification and Diagnosis of Diabetes." In "Standards of Medical Care in Diabetes–2016," supplement, *Diabetes Care* 39 (S1): S13–S22. http://dx.doi.org/10.2337/dc16-s005.

———. 2016d. "Glycemic Targets." In "Standards of Medical Care in Diabetes–2016," supplement, *Diabetes Care* 39 (S1): S39–S46. http://dx.doi.org/10.2337/dc16-s008.

———. 2017. "Classification and Diagnosis of Diabetes." *Diabetes Care* 40 (S1): S11–S24. http://dx.doi.org/10.2337/dc17-s005.

American Heart Association. 2017. "Understand Your Risk for Diabetes." http://www.heart.org/HEARTORG/Conditions/More/Diabetes/UnderstandYourRiskforDiabetes/Understand-Your-Risk-for-Diabetes_UCM_002034_Article.jsp.

Centers for Disease Control and Prevention. 2013. "Surveillance Reports." Diabetes Reports and Publications. https://www.cdc.gov/diabetes/library/reports/surveillance.html.

———. 2016. "Diabetes." Chronic Disease Prevention and Health Promotion. http://www.cdc.gov/chronicdisease/resources/publications/aag/diabetes.htm.

Dunphy, L., J. Winland-Brown, B. Porter, and D. Thomas, eds. 2015. *Primary Care: The Art and Science of Advanced Practice Nursing*. 4th ed. Philadelphia: F. A. Davis.

CHAPTER 16

HEMATOLOGICAL DISORDERS

LEARNING OBJECTIVES

▶ Recognize common hematological disorders and then analyze processes useful to providing differential diagnosis among them.

  ▷ Risk factors

  ▷ Signs and symptoms

  ▷ Diagnostic tests

  ▷ Differential diagnoses

▶ Describe treatment and management of hematological disorders.

  ▷ Management

  ▷ Prevention

ANEMIA

TABLE 16–1.
NORMAL RANGES FOR RED BLOOD COUNT (RBC) STUDIES

TEST	WOMEN	MEN
Hematocrit (HCT; calculated from mean corpuscular volume [MCV] and RBC)	36–48 percent	40–52 percent
Hemoglobin (Hgb)	12–16 g/dL	13.5–17.7 g/dL
RBC (×106/uL)	4.0–5.4	4.5–6.0
MCV	80–100 fL	80–100 fL
Mean corpuscular hemoglobin concentration (MCHC)	31–37 percent Hgb/cell	31–37 percent Hgb/cell
Serum iron	50–170 mcg/dL	65–175 mcg/dL
Total iron-binding capacity (TIBC)	250–450 mcg/dL	250–450 mcg/dL

(continued)

TABLE 16–1. (CONTINUED)

TEST	WOMEN	MEN
Ferritin	10–120 ng/mL (average 55)	20–250 ng/mL (average 125)
Reticulocyte count	0.5–1.5 percent of RBC	0.5–1.5 percent of RBC
Lactate dehydrogenase (LDH)	208–378 U/L	208–378 U/L
Haptoglobin	26–185 mg/dL	26–285 mg/dL

TABLE 16–2.
BLOOD VALUES TO DIFFERENTIATE ANEMIAS

ANEMIA	MCV	ADDITIONAL VALUES	APPEARANCE OF RBC
Iron deficiency	<80 fL	TIBC elevated; iron (Fe) or ferritin low	Normocytic or microcytic, hypochromic
Thalassemia	<80 fL	**Minor:** MCV and HCT low; Fe normal; reticulocytes normal or high; Hgb defects	Microcytic
		Major: HCT low; reticulocyte high; Heinz bodies; Hgb H 10–40 percent of Hgb	
Sideroblastic	<80 fL	Hgb low; sideroblasts ringed; Fe high	Hypochromic
Sickle cell	<80 fL	Hgb low; target cells; reticulocytes high	Sickle cells, normochromic
Folate deficiency	>100 fL	Folate decreased	Macrocytic, hyperchromic
Vitamin B12	>100 fL	Vitamin B12 decreased	Macrocytic, hyperchromic
Chronic disease	Normal		Normochromic, normocytic or microcytic
Glucose-6-phosphate dehydrogenase (G6PD)	Normal		Heinz bodies, bite cells, blister cells
Drug-induced	Normal		Normocytic, normochromic
Aplastic	Normal		Normocytic, normochromic
Posthemorrhagic	Normal		Normocytic, normochromic

Sources: Maakaron, Taher, and Conrad 2016; Braunstein 2017

Microcytic Anemia

▶ Microcytic anemia is characterized by a low MCV and the presence of small, often hypochromic red blood cells in a peripheral blood smear. (See table 16–3)

Iron-Deficiency Anemia

▶ Decreased iron in red cells or hemoglobin in blood unable to support normal red blood cell production.

▶ Iron deficiency anemia is the most common blood condition in United States, affecting 3.5 million Americans.

▶ Women, young children, older adults, and people with chronic diseases are at higher risk.

TABLE 16–3.
MICROCYTIC ANEMIAS

	THALASSEMIA MAJOR	THALASSEMIA MINOR
Cause	Both parents transmit gene	One parent transmits gene
Genetically transmitted defect in alpha or beta Hgb	Excess iron deposits in myocardium, liver, and pancreas result in organ damage. If untreated, leads to heart and liver failure.	**Alpha Major** if both genes are altered **Alpha Minor** if missing one gene, "silent" carrier; no signs of illness If missing two genes, alpha thalassemia **Beta Minor** if one a carrier (National Heart, Lung, and Blood Institute [NHLBI] 2012)
Risk Factors	**Beta Major** Cooley's anemia, beta genes affected Primarily affects Mediterranean ethnicities Lead poisoning, chronic illness or inflammation, and sideroblastic anemia	**Alpha Major** Asian (especially Chinese), Mediterranean, African American ethnicities
Signs and Symptoms	Fatigue, shortness of breath, facial deformities, bronze skin, stunted growth	Usually asymptomatic; diagnosis of exclusion
Diagnostic Tests	CBC, Fe, reticulocyte count, peripheral smear; electrophoresis	CBC, Fe, reticulocyte count, peripheral smear; electrophoresis
Management	Blood transfusions, folate supplements, bone marrow transplant, splenectomy *No iron supplements*	No treatment
Prevention	None	None

Note: CBC = complete blood count

Risk Factors
- ▶ · Heavy menstrual bleeding
- ▶ · Gastrointestinal (GI) ulcers, gastritis, hemorrhoids
- ▶ · Cancer, menstruation
- ▶ · Childbirth
- ▶ · Female
- ▶ · Inability to absorb iron (celiac disease)
- ▶ · Iron intake < 2 mg/day
- ▶· Slow, persistent blood loss

Signs and Symptoms
- ▶ · Pale, dry skin and mucus membranes
- ▶ ·Fatigue, weakness, dizziness

▶ ' Headache, irritability

▶ ' Dyspnea on exertion, palpitations

▶ ' Trouble concentrating

▶ ' Pica

Diagnostic Tests

▶ Complete blood count (CBC) with differential and smear

▷ Men: Hgb < 13.5 gram/100 ml

▷ Women: Hgb < 12.0 gram/100 ml.

▷ MCV or mean corpuscular hemoglobin (MCH)

▷ Decreased

▶ MCV <80 mcg/dL

▷ Red cell distribution width (RDW) >15

▷ ' Platelets increased >400,000

▷ Reticulocytes

▶ Elevated in blood loss

▶ ' Decreased in iron deficiency

▶ Serum Fe, TIBC, ferritin, transferrin

▷ Fe < 30 mcg/dL

▷ TIBC > 400 mcg/dL

▷ Ferritin

▶ <10 ng/dL women

▶ <20 ng/dL in men

▷ Transferrin saturation <15 percent

▶ Consult hematologist if

▷ ' HCT < 24 percent,

▷ ' Unexplained bleeding, or

▷ ' Hgb does not increase over 4 weeks.

Differential Diagnoses

▶ Thalassemia

▶ G6PD deficiency

▶ Infection

▶ Cancer

▶ Chronic illness

▶ Lead poisoning

▶ Hypothyroidism

▶ Renal failure

Management

▶ Treat underlying cause.

▶ • Iron 325 mg p.o. t.i.d.

▶ ` May see nonadherence because of constipation, diarrhea, nausea

▶ ` Vitamin C supplement.

▶ • Iron-rich foods: Meats, vegetables, whole grains, iron-fortified cereals.

▶ Consult physician if unexplained bleeding occurs or Hgb does not increase over 4 weeks.

Prevention

▶ Eating a well-balanced diet that includes iron-rich foods may help prevent iron-deficiency anemia.

▶ Taking iron supplements also may lower the risk for the condition if patient is unable to get enough iron from food (NHLBI 2017).

Macrocytic Anemias

See table 16–4.

TABLE 16–4.
OTHER MACROCYTIC ANEMIAS

	PERNICIOUS ANEMIA	B12 DEFICIENCY
Cause	• Failure of gastric parietal cells to produce sufficient intrinsic factor to permit absorption of adequate dietary vitamin B12	• A lack of vitamin B12 because of poor nutrition
Risk Factors	• Poor nutrition lacking B12 • Alcoholism • Digestive problems: Crohn's disease, celiac disease, tapeworm	• Older adults • Caucasians, especially northern Europeans • Intestinal flora overgrowth • Gastrectomy • Atrophic gastritis • Autoimmune response to gastric parietal cells • Addison's or thyroid disease, hypoparathyroidism • Hypopituitarism • Myasthenia gravis • Type 1 diabetes

(continued)

TABLE 16–4. (CONTINUED)

	PERNICIOUS ANEMIA	B12 DEFICIENCY
Signs and Symptoms	• Constipation or diarrhea • Lack of energy, fatigue • Light-headedness on standing or exertion, shortness of breath with exertion • Pallor • Appetite loss • Problems concentrating • Smooth, beefy red tongue; bleeding gums	
Neurological Symptoms	• Confusion • Depression • Loss of balance • Numbness and tingling in hands and feet	
Diagnostic Tests	• CBC, reticulocyte count • Serum cobalamin, folic acid, methylmalonic acid, LDH, homocysteine assays • Peripheral smear • Indirect bilirubin • Intrinsic factor antibody • Gastric secretions evaluation • Schilling test (not available in most centers) • Bone marrow aspiration if diagnosis is unclear	• CBC, reticulocyte count • Vitamin B12 level, LDH level • Esophagogastroduodenoscopy (EGD) to examine stomach • Enteroscopy to examine small bowel • Bone marrow biopsy if the diagnosis is not clear
Management	• Vitamin B12 injections monthly or p.o. daily. • Injections may be required more frequently in beginning.	
Prevention	• Eating foods high in vitamin B12 can help prevent low vitamin B12 levels. • Limit alcohol consumption. • Early detection and treatment can help reduce complications.	• Eating foods high in vitamin B12 can help prevent low vitamin B12 levels

Source: NHLBI 2012

Folate Deficiency

▶ Macrocytic anemia in which inadequate folic acid is present in DNA synthesis and RBC maturation

Risk Factors
- ▶ ▸ Malnourishment
- ▶ ▸ Hemolytic anemia
- ▶ ▸ Alcoholism
- ▶ ▸ Illicit drug use
- ▶ ▸ Drugs
  - ▷ Oral contraceptives, phenytoin, phenobarbital, antimalarials, methotrexate, sulfasalazine, triamterene, pyrimethamine, trimethoprim-sulfamethoxazole, barbiturates

Signs and Symptoms
- ▶ ▸ Fatigue
- ▶ ▸ Headache
- ▶ ▸ Pallor
- ▶ ▸ Sore mouth and tongue

Diagnostic Tests
- ▶ ▸ Low CBC, serum folate
- ▶ ▸ Normal B12 and Schilling test
- ▶ Rarely, bone marrow aspiration

Differential Diagnoses
- ▶ Pernicious anemia

Management
- ▶ ▸ Folate 1 mg daily.
- ▶ Correct underlying cause(s).
- ▶ ▸ Include green leafy vegetables and citrus fruits in diet.

Anemia of Chronic Disease

- ▶ Mildly hypoproliferative reticulocyte count is decreased by decreased bone marrow production.
- ▶ ▸ Its cause is unknown, but red blood cell life span and production are decreased, and it is associated with chronic disease, infections, and malignancies that have persisted for 1–2 months.

Risk Factors

- ▶ Chronic disease
- ▶ Liver, renal, endocrine disease, rheumatoid arthritis, some cancers
- ▶ Infections

Signs and Symptoms

▶ All signs of iron deficiency

▷ Pale, dry skin and mucus membranes

▷ Fatigue, weakness, dizziness

▷ Headache, irritability

▷ Dyspnea on exertion, palpitations

▷ Trouble concentrating

▷ Pica

▶ Underlying chronic disease symptoms

Diagnostic Tests

▶ CBC, reticulocytes

▷ Hgb < 10

▶ Serum iron and TIBC: Low

▶ Serum ferritin: Normal

Differential Diagnoses

▶ Iron deficiency anemia, aplastic anemia

▶ Chronic liver, endocrine diseases

▶ Chronic renal insufficiency

▶ Posthemorrhagic anemia

▶ AIDS (acquired immune deficiency syndrome)

Management

▶ No specific therapy.

▶ Look for underlying etiology, occult malignancy.

▶ Treat underlying disorder.

▶ Transfuse blood when needed.

▶ Considerations for anemia in older adults:

▷ Most anemias present as normocytic anemia.

▷ MCV increases slightly with age.

▷ Elevated reticulocytes, indirect bilirubin, elevated LDH indicate hemolytic anemia.

▷ Low reticulocytes, elevated indirect bilirubin; elevated LDH suggest ineffective erythropoiesis.

▷ Macrocytosis suggests B12 or folate deficiency.

▷ Evaluate if Hgb falls >1 g/dL in year.

▷ Evaluate if >65 years and Hgb < 13.

▷ Check white blood count (WBC) and peripheral blood smear.

▷ • Do not exclude infection with normal or low WBC (neutrophil response blunted).

▷ Do not assume anemia with chronic inflammatory disease is "anemia of chronic disease."

▷ Nutritional deficiencies are major causes of anemia.

   ▶ • Assess and treat B12 deficiency before treating folate deficiency.

▷ • Do not treat iron-deficiency anemia without finding site of blood loss.

▷ Mixed anemias are common; check for multiple causes.

Prevention

▶ Treat underlying cause.

▶ Proper nutrition.

Hemolytic Anemias

See table 16–5.

TABLE 16–5.
HEMOLYTIC ANEMIAS

	SICKLE CELL TRAIT (HG AS)	SICKLE CELL ANEMIA (HG SS)
Causes	• Autosomal recessive genetic disorder in which HgS develops instead of HgA, causing sickle-shaped red blood cells.	• Autosomal recessive genetic disorder in which HgS develops instead of HgA, causing sickle-shaped red blood cells
	• Sickle cell gene from one parent causes sickle cell trait.	• If both parents have gene, one in four chance child will have disease
Risk Factors	• African descent	
Signs and Symptoms	• Usually no symptoms; considered a carrier	• Sudden pain
		• Low-grade fever
	• May experience painful symptoms under extreme altitudes or hypoxia	• Jaundice
		• Delayed puberty
		• Shortened life span
		• Sickle cell crisis
		• Severe pain in bones, abdomen, other organs
		• Increased chest pain, dyspnea
		• Fever

(continued)

TABLE 16–5. (CONTINUED)

	SICKLE CELL TRAIT (HG AS)	SICKLE CELL ANEMIA (HG SS)
Diagnostic Tests	• CBC • Peripheral smear • Hgb electrophoresis	
Differential Diagnoses (Maakaron and Taher 2017)	• Acute anemia • Carotid cavernous fistula • Hemoglobin C disease • Hemolytic anemia • Legg-Calvé-Perthes disease imaging • Ophthalmologic manifestations of leukemias • Osteomyelitis in emergency medicine • Pulmonary embolism • Rheumatoid arthritis hand imaging • Septic arthritis	
Management	• No treatment • Genetic counseling	• • Hydroxyurea prevents painful episodes • • Nonsteroidal anti-inflammatory drugs (NSAIDs) • Genetic counseling • • Stem cell transplant • Crisis • • Pain control with opioids, NSAIDs • • Blood transfusions, oxygen • • Intravenous (IV) or oral fluids • Antibiotics
Prevention	• None known	

Sickle Cell Anemia

▶ Autosomal recessive disorder in which hemoglobin S (HgS) develops instead of hemoglobin A (HgA).

▶ One of the most common inherited anemias.

▶ Mutated hemoglobin leads to chronic hemolytic anemia and results in a variety of severe clinical consequences.

▶ Primarily affects people of African descent.

▶ There are approximately 90,000–100,000 with sickle cell anemia in the United States.

G6PD Deficiency

▶ • Genetic disorder in enzyme G6PD that causes red blood cells to break down prematurely, resulting in hemolysis.

▶ • Mainly affects red blood cells, which carry oxygen from lungs to tissues in body.

▶ • Occurs most often in males of African American and Middle Eastern decent.

Risk Factors

▶ • Infection

▶ • Ingestion of fava beans

▶   Oxidant drugs

▶ • Antibiotics

  ▷   Dapsone, nalidixic acid, nitrofurantoin, sulfonamides

▶ • Antimalarials

  ▷   Primaquine, quinine

▶ • Phenazopyridine, doxorubicin, quinidine

▶   Triggers

  ▷ • Bacterial or viral infections

  ▷ • Antibiotics

  ▷ • Antimalarials

  ▷ • Ingesting fava beans or inhaling fava plant pollen

Signs and Symptoms

▶ • Pallor

▶ - Jaundice

▶ • Dark urine

▶ • Fatigue

▶ • Shortness of breath

▶ • Tachycardia

▶ • Enlarged spleen

Differential Diagnoses

▶   Suspect Mediterranean variant if anemia severe

▶   Iron-deficiency anemia

▶   Combined anemias

  ▷   Sickle cell and G6PD deficiency

▶   Acute hemolytic transfusion reaction

  ▷   Positive Coombs test

Management

▶ ꞏ Avoid triggers

▶ ꞏ Antibiotics

▶ ꞏ Stop drugs causing RBC lysis

▶ ꞏ Transfusions

▶ Genetic counseling

Prevention

▶ Genetic disorder, not preventable

LEUKEMIAS

▶ Abnormal white blood cell production in bone marrow that crowds out healthy blood cells

▶ ꞏ Chronic lymphocytic leukemia (CLL) most common in older adults

▶ Etiology unknown, but may be caused by exposure to chemical or ionizing radiation, genetic factors, or viral agents

Risk Factors

▶ ꞏ Immunodeficiency

▶ ꞏ Chemical and radiation exposures

▶ ꞏ Chromosomal abnormalities

▶ ꞏ Cigarette smoking

▶ Likelihood of some types increases with age

Signs and Symptoms

▶ ꞏ Fever, malaise

▶ ꞏ Bruising, bleeding

▶ ꞏ Joint pain

▶ ꞏ Weight loss, anorexia

▶ ꞏ Hepatosplenomegaly

▶ ꞏ Lymphadenopathy

▶ ꞏ Lymphocytosis on CBC

▶ ꞏ People with chronic lymphocytic leukemia (CLL) may have no symptoms.

Diagnostic Tests

- ▶ Physical assessment:
  - ▷ ˙ Acute lymphocytic leukemia (ALL)
    - ▶ Joint pain, limping, anorexia, infection
    - ▶ Generalized lymphadenopathy, hepatosplenomegaly, petechiae
  - ▷ ˙ Acute myelogenous leukemia (AML)
    - ▶ Sternal tenderness, mouth sores, occasional lymphadenopathy
  - ▷ ˙ Chronic lymphocytic leukemia (CLL)
    - ▶ Might be asymptomatic; dyspnea on exertion, hepatosplenomegaly, lymphadenopathy, sustained absolute lymphocytosis, bone marrow positive for lymphocytes
  - ▷ ˙ Chronic myelogenous leukemia (CML)
    - ▶ Might be asymptomatic; night sweats, blurred vision, anorexia, respiratory distress, sternal tenderness, splenomegaly, priapism, Philadelphia chromosome in bone marrow
- ▶ ˙ CBC with differential, platelets, coagulation profile, peripheral smear, reticulocytes, complete metabolic panel
- ▶ ˙ Bone marrow aspiration
- ▶ ˙ Consider X-ray or computed tomography (CT) scan of chest

Differential Diagnoses

- ▶ Aplastic anemia
- ▶ Viral diseases
- ▶ Mononucleosis
- ▶ Pertussis
- ▶ Paroxysmal nocturnal hemoglobinuria
- ▶ Gaucher's disease
- ▶ Myelodysplastic syndromes

Management

- ▶ ˙ Refer to oncologist.
- ▶ ˙ Chemotherapy.
- ▶ ˙ Radiation therapy.
- ▶ ˙ Stem cell transplant.

Prevention

- ▶ None known

MULTIPLE MYELOMA

▶ Malignant disease of plasma cells characterized by replacement of bone marrow, bone destruction, and paraprotein formation

Risk Factors

▶ Incidence peaks in the seventies.

▶ Exposure to radiation, asbestos, benzenes, herbicides, insecticides.

▶ Antigenic exposure of reticuloendothelial system.

▶ Family history.

Signs and Symptoms

▶ Pain in back, chest, or extremities

▶ Weakness, fatigue

▶ Abnormal bleeding

▶ Pathological fractures

▶ Pallor, radiculopathy

▶ Hepatosplenomegaly

Diagnostic Tests

▶ Palpable liver and spleen

▷ CBC with differential

▶ Normochromic; normo- or microcytic anemia

▷ Erythrocyte sedimentation rate (ESR) increased

▷ Creatinine or calcium elevated

▷ Bone marrow aspiration

▶ Infiltrated with plasma cells

▷ Chest X-ray (CXR)

▷ Immunoelectrophoresis

▶ Monoclonal spike (M spike) in >90 percent

▷ Urine immunoelectrophoresis

▶ Bence-Jones proteins, hypercalcemia, proteinuria, high serum protein

▶ International staging for multiple myeloma

▷ Stage I

▶ Serum beta-2 microglobulin <3.5 (mg/L) and albumin levels are ≥ 3.5 (g/dL).

    ▷ Stage II

        ► Neither stage I nor III, meaning that either

           ▷ The beta-2 microglobulin level is 3.5–5.5 (with any albumin level), *or*

           ▷ Albumin and beta-2 microglobulin levels are both <3.5.

    ▷ Stage III

        ► Serum beta-2 microglobulin is ≥5.5.

Differential Diagnoses

- ► Leukemias
- ► Malignant lymphoma
- ► Bone disease
- ► Waldenstrom's
- ► Monoclonal gammopathy

Management

- ► According to stage
- ► Chemotherapy
  - ▷ Side effects: Hair loss, mouth sores, loss of appetite, nausea and vomiting, low blood counts
- ► Plasmapheresis
- ► Radiation therapy
- ► Stem cell transplant
- ► Biphosphates to maintain bone health during treatment
- ► Interferon
- ► Surgery

Prevention

- ► None known

NON-HODGKIN LYMPHOMA

- ► Malignant disease of the lymphoreticular system without Reed-Sternberg giant cells
- ► Sixth most common neoplasm

Risk Factors

- ► Median age of diagnosis: 50 years
- ► HIV (human immunodeficiency virus)

Signs and Symptoms

▶ · Cough

▶ · Fever, night sweats

▶ · Weight loss

▶ · Painless peripheral lymphadenopathy

Diagnostic Tests

▶ · CBC with differential

▷ Mild anemia

▶ · LDH

▷ Elevated

▶ Chemistry profile

▶ Urinalysis

▶ CXR

▶ · Lymph node biopsy

▷ No Reed-Sternberg giant cells

Differential Diagnoses

▶ Hodgkin disease

▶ Viral infections

▶ Metastatic carcinoma

Management

▶ · If lymphoma suspected, refer to hematology

Prevention

▶ None known

HODGKIN LYMPHOMA

▶ · Cancer of the lymph tissue of unknown origin (but past infection with the Epstein-Barr virus may contribute to its development).

▶ · Most common among people ages 15–35 and 50–70 years.

▶ · HIV infection increases risk.

Risk Factors

- ▶ HIV infection
- ▶ Epstein-Barr infection
  - ▷ Mononucleosis
- ▶ Age: 15– 40 and after age 55 years
- ▶ Family history
- ▶ Higher socioeconomic status

Signs and Symptoms

- ▶ Fever and chills, night sweats
- ▶ Urticaria, diaphoresis
- ▶ Loss of appetite
- ▶ Painless adenopathy in neck, axilla, or groin
- ▶ Unexplained weight loss
- ▶ Coughing, chest pain, dyspnea
- ▶ Skin flushing

Diagnostic Tests

- ▶ CBC, chemistry profile, liver, kidney, protein, uric acid levels
- ▶ CT, positron emission tomography (PET) scan
- ▶ Bone marrow biopsy
- ▶ Lymph node biopsy
  - ▷ Reed-Sternberg giant cells

Differential Diagnoses

- ▶ Non-Hodgkin lymphoma
- ▶ Viral infections
- ▶ Metastatic carcinoma

Management

- ▶ Consider type of Hodgkin lymphoma
  - ▷ Most people have classic Hodgkin lymphoma.
  - ▷ Stage (where the disease has spread); tumor size >4 inches (10 cm) wide.
  - ▷ Age and medical issues.

▶ – Referral to oncologist

▶ ˙ Chemotherapy

▶ ˙˙ Radiation

▶ ⋅⋅ Stem cell transplant

▶ ˜ Complications

⊳ Bone marrow diseases (such as leukemia)

⊳ Heart disease

⊳ Infertility

⊳ Lung disease

⊳ Other cancers

⊳ Thyroid problems

Prevention

▶ None known

DRUG-INDUCED THROMBOCYTOPENIA

▶ – Disorder in which platelet count is <150,000

▶ ⋅⋅ May be immune globulin G–mediated response to drug or its metabolites, or idiopathic

Risk Factors

▶ New or continued use of a variety of drugs

⊳ – Quinine and quinine-like drugs, valproic acid, heparin, antibiotics (cephalosporins, penicillin, sulfa), anti-inflammatory drugs, digoxin, procainamide, amiodarone, diuretics, H2 antagonists, antihistamines, antineoplastic drugs

Signs and Symptoms

▶ – Easy bruising, purpura

▶ – Petechiae, usually lower legs

▶ – Prolonged bleeding from cuts

▶ – Bleeding from gums or nose

▶ – Blood in urine or stools

Diagnostic Tests

▶ Platelet count

  ▷ • Low normal platelet count

▶ ‹ Prothrombin time (PT) and bleeding times: Normal

▶ • Partial thromboplastin time (PTT): Greatly prolonged

▶ Clotting factors VIII and IX: Normal, unless patient has hemophilia

Differential Diagnoses

▶ Von Willebrand's disease

▶ Vitamin K deficiency

▶ Disseminated intravascular coagulation (DIC)

▶ Other platelet disorders

Management

▶ Education and supportive therapy.

▶ ‹ Refer to hematologist upon diagnosis.

▶ Promptly treat any trauma or injury.

▶ Avoid aspirin and other NSAIDs.

▶ Stop offending agent if possible.

▶ Lifespan considerations:

▶ ‹ Malignancies and anemia are *not* a consequence of age.

▶ There is controversy regarding cancer screening in older adults.

  ▷ •American Geriatrics Society states screening should be reserved for people younger than 70 years.

  ▷ ‹ Many older than 70 years request screening; functional status should be considered.

  ▷ If patient is too ill or frail to undergo treatment of a malignancy, screening should not be done.

▶ Anemic older adults should be treated to ensure quality of life.

  ▷ *However*, how aggressively to search for cause should depend on functional status, patient desire, and patient risk involved in work-up.

Prevention

▶ Avoid exposure to the medication again.

REFERENCES

Braunstein, E. M. 2017. "Evaluation of Anemia." Approach to the Patient with Anemia. http://www.merckmanuals.com/professional/hematology-and-oncology/approach-to-the-patient-with-anemia/evaluation-of-anemia.

Maakaron, J. E., and A. T. Taher. 2017. "Sickle Cell Anemia Differential Diagnoses." Medscape. http://emedicine.medscape.com/article/205926-differential.

Maakaron, J. E., A. T. Taher, and M. E. Conrad. 2016. "Anemia." Medscape. http://emedicine.medscape.com/article/198475-overview.

National Heart, Lung, and Blood Institute. 2012. "What Causes Thalassemias?" https://www.nhlbi.nih.gov/health/health-topics/topics/thalassemia/causes.

———. 2014. "How Can Iron-Deficiency Anemia Be Prevented?" https://www.nhlbi.nih.gov/health/health-topics/topics/ida/prevention.

World Health Organization. 2006. "Chronic Diseases and Their Risk Factors." Facing the Facts No. 1. http://www.who.int/chp/chronic_disease_report/media/Factsheet1.pdf.

CHAPTER 17

PSYCHIATRIC AND MENTAL HEALTH

LEARNING OBJECTIVES

▶ Recognize and differentiate among different common psychiatric and mental health disorders.

▷ Risk factors

▷ Signs and symptoms

▷ Diagnostic tests

▷ Differential diagnoses

▶ Describe treatment and management of psychiatric and mental health disorders.

▷ Management

GENERAL APPROACH TO PSYCHIATRIC ISSUES

▶ Dementia and depression

▷ ꜱ Can present similarly in older adults and

▷ ꜱ Often coexist, especially with early dementia.

▷ ꜱ If depression or dementia cannot be differentiated, treat for depression and observe for improvement.

▶ Mental disorders are underdiagnosed and undertreated in older adults.

▶ Recognition and treatment are not stressed in primary care.

▶ Social stigma prevents mental illness discussion.

PSYCHOSOCIAL CHANGES OF AGING

▶ Personality

▷ Consistent with earlier years in healthy aging

▷ • Change caused by pathology or response to events or things affecting self-image

▶ Memory

▷ Long-term intact

▷ Short-term diminished (benign senescence)

▶ Changes in learning

▷ Spatial awareness and intuitive creative thought decline

▷ Verbal and abstract abilities remain

▷ Basic intelligence not changed

▷ Material must be relevant

▷ Use simple association rather than analysis

▶ Relationships

▷ Close relationships have positive effect

▶ Less stress

▶ Better mental health

▶ Improved life satisfaction

▷ Social network of friends shrinks

▶ Loss

▷ Can result in social change

▶ May need to learn new roles and how to manage tasks of daily living

▷ Spiritual

▶ Search for meaning

▶ May have crisis of faith and meaning

DEPRESSION

▶ Clinical syndrome of depressed mood with a wide variety of causes, types, and treatment modalities.

▶ Affects 9 to 16 million Americans.

▶ Adolescents and older adults at highest risk.

▶ May be family history.

▶ Depression is the most common mental illness seen in primary care practices.

▶ Recurrence rate greater than 50 percent.

Risk Factors

▶ ' Recent stressful events

▶ ' Death, divorce, finances, job loss, trauma, abuse

▶ Prior episodes of depression

▶ ॰ Lack of close relationships

▶ › Losing a parent before age 11 years

▶ Family history of depression

▶ Chronic illness

MAJOR DEPRESSIVE DISORDER (MDD)

Risk Factors

▶ Family history

▶ ' Major negative life events

▶ Illness

Signs and Symptoms

▶ A variety of symptoms are possible; see "Diagnostic Tests" below

▶ One of the following *must* be present:

▷ • Depressed mood

▷ ⸀Anhedonia

Diagnostic Tests

▶ Rule out physical problems.

▶ A variety of depression screening tools are available.

▶ *Diagnostic and Statistical Manual of Mental Disorders* (DSM-5; American Psychiatric Association [APA] 2013) symptom criteria for major depression: Five or more of the following symptoms have been present during the same 2-week period and represent a change from previous functioning

▷ • One of the symptoms *must be* either depressed mood or anhedonia, meaning loss of interest or pleasure.

▶ Depressed mood expressed as feelings of sadness or hopelessness

▷ • Irritability may be the primary symptom in adolescents.

▷ • Apathy: Markedly diminished interest in most activities.

▷ › Change in appetite.

▷ ' Insomnia or hypersomnia.

▷ • Behavioral agitation or retardation.

> ▷ . Loss of energy.
>
> ▷ • Feelings of worthlessness or guilt.
>
> ▷ ، Loss of concentration.
>
> ▷ ، Recurrent thoughts of death or suicide.
>
> ▷ ، These symptoms cause significant functional impairment and are not caused by a medical illness or substance use.

Differential Diagnoses

- ▶ Electrolyte imbalance
- ▶ Chronic fatigue syndrome
- ▶ Chronic obstructive pulmonary disease
- ▶ Bereavement
- ▶ Bipolar or psychotic disorders, schizophrenia
- ▶ Substance abuse
- ▶ Mononucleosis
- ▶ Chronic illnesses
- ▶ Medications
  - ▷ Opioids, steroids, estrogen, antihypertensives, digoxin, anti-Parkinson's medications, beta blockers, sedatives and hypnotics, antimicrobials, antineoplastics, psychotropics, analgesics, anti-inflammatories including nonsteroidal anti-inflammatory drugs (NSAIDS)

Management

- ▶ ˉ Psychotherapy
- ▶ ، Cognitive behavioral therapy (CBT)
- ▶ ، Evaluation for suicide ideation
- ▶ ، Electroconvulsive therapy for severe depression or if not responsive to medications
  - ▷ Memory loss may occur for up to 2 weeks after treatment.
- ▶ Medication therapy
  - ▷ Most useful in otherwise healthy persons
  - ▷ Selective serotonin reuptake inhibitors (SSRIs) and serotonin-norepinephrine reuptake inhibitors (SNRIs): First-line drug choice (table 17–1)
    - ▶ ·، No effect on cardiac conduction
    - ▶ • No anticholinergic effects
    - ▶ • May cause loss of libido
    - ▶ ˉ Side effects related to central nervous system (CNS) agitation
    - ▶ ˮ Lowers seizure threshold
    - ▶ ، Need several weeks of therapy before results seen

▷ Tricyclic antidepressants (TCAs): require careful monitoring (table 17–2)

▶ Less costly than newer drugs

▶ ˙ Need several weeks of therapy before results seen

▶ ˙ Cardiac effects: Hypotension, prolonged QT interval—get baseline electrocardiogram (ECG)

▶ Anticholinergic effects significant

▷ ˙ Dry mouth, tachycardia, blurred vision, urinary retention, constipation, sedation, delirium

▶ Sedative effects more prevalent

TABLE 17–1.
SSRI AND SNRI MEDICATIONS FOR DEPRESSION IN ADULTS

MEDICATION	INITIAL DOSE	TARGET DOSE
Fluoxetine (Prozac)	20 mg in a.m. daily	20–80 mg daily
Sertraline (Zoloft)	50 mg daily	50–100 mg daily
Paroxetine (Paxil)	20 mg in a.m. daily	20–50 mg daily
Citalopram (Celexa)	20 mg daily	40–60 mg daily
Escitalopram (Lexapro)	10 mg daily	10–20 mg daily
Duloxetine (Cymbalta)	40 mg daily	40–60 mg daily

TABLE 17–2.
TRICYCLIC ANTIDEPRESSANTS

MEDICATION	INITIAL DOSE	TARGET DOSE
Amitriptyline (Elavil)	25 mg h.s. daily	50–100 mg, divided doses
Desipramine (Norpramin)	25 mg daily	75–300 mg daily
Imipramine (Tofranil)	25 mg h.s. daily	75–300 mg daily
Nortriptyline (Pamelor)	10–25 mg h.s. daily	75–150 mg daily or divided doses

BIPOLAR DISORDER

Risk Factors

▶ ˙ Family history

▶ ˙ Substance abuse

▶ ˙ Increased stress

Signs and Symptoms

▶ ˙ Psychological disorder characterized by periods of acute mania, hypomania, and depression

▷ Mania

▶ ' Distinct period of abnormally, persistently elevated, expansive, or irritable mood

▶ ' May last at least 1 week; significant functional decline

▷ Hypomania

▶ Distinct period of persistently elevated, expansive, or irritable mood

▶ May last 4 days; no functional decline

▶ . Hypomania has same symptoms as mania *but*

▷ Never severe enough to cause problems working or socializing, and

▷ There are never any psychotic features present in a hypomanic episode.

▷ ' Depression

▶ Distinct period of feeling sad or hopeless

▶ Thoughts of death or suicide, or attempting suicide

▷ : Mixed episode

▶ Criteria met for a manic episode and for a major depressive episode

▷ , Cyclothymia

▶ Alternating mood states for at least 2 years that do not meet full criteria for depressive, manic, or mixed episodes

▷ Bipolar not otherwise specified (NOS)

▶ A mood episode that does not meet specific criteria for any specific bipolar disorder

Diagnostic Tests

▶ ' Diagnosis made on the basis of symptoms

▶ ' Psychiatric assessment

Differential Diagnoses

▶ Bipolar I

▶ Bipolar II
(Dunphy et al. 2015)

Management

▶ ' Referral for psychotherapy

▶ ' Atypical antipsychotics

▶ . Mood stabilizers:

▷ Lithium

▷ ▸ Divalproex (Depakote)

▷ ▸ Carbamazepine (Tegretol)

▶ Medications to treat individual symptoms (see table 17–3)

TABLE 17–3.
MEDICATIONS FOR TARGET SYMPTOMS

SYMPTOMS	EFFECTIVE MEDICATIONS
Psychomotor retardation	SSRI, venlafaxine, bupropion
Anxiety	SSRI (especially Paxil)
Insomnia	Mirtazapine, trazodone
Weight loss	Mirtazapine
Weight gain	SSRI, bupropion

GRIEF AND BEREAVEMENT

▶ Etiology is loss.

▷ ▸ Emotional and physiological reaction to death or loss of a loved one.

▷ ▸ Grief and bereavement are normal reactions to death or loss.

▷ ▸ Uncomplicated grief presents as situational and time-limited depressed mood.

▶ ▸ Grief that lasts longer than 2 months should be evaluated for mood disorder.

Risk Factors

▶ ▸ History of MDD, other mental illness, or prior suicide attempts

Signs and Symptoms

▶ ▸ Patient verbalizes suicidal ideation, plan, or desire to join deceased loved one.

▶ ▸ Suicide attempts or suicidal ideation with plan are psychiatric emergencies. Immediately refer to mental health specialist or emergency department for evaluation and treatment.

▶ ▸ Symptoms last 2 months.

▶ ▸ Symptoms intensify and severely impair daily function.

Differential Diagnosis

▶ Depression

Management

▶ ▸ Weekly during acute phase.

▶ ▸ Consult psychiatrist or mental health specialist for symptoms lasting longer than 2 months.

- ▶ ᾽ Depression risk continues through second year of bereavement.
- ▶ ᾽ Older adults without adequate social and familial support at high risk for MDD and suicidal ideation.
- ▶ Expected course:
  - ▷ ᾽ Uncomplicated grief or bereavement for 2 months, but can last longer.
  - ▷ ᾽ Brief, limited symptoms close to date of loss are common.
  - ▷ • Cognitive behavioral therapy and social supports associated with improved prognosis.

ANXIETY DISORDERS

Risk Factors

- ▶ ᾽ Family history
- ▶ ، Increased stress
- ▶ ᾽ Shyness

Signs and Symptoms

- ▶ ᾽ Unpleasant feeling of dread, apprehension, or tension
- ▶ • Multiple categories of anxiety disorders
- ▶ Generalized anxiety disorder (GAD)
  - ▷ Excessive anxiety or worry most days for more than 6 months; difficulty controlling worry
  - ▷ Associated with more than three of the following symptoms:
    - ▶ ᾽ Restlessness
    - ▶ ᾽ Muscle tension
    - ▶ ، Fatigue
    - ▶ ᾽ Sleep disturbance
    - ▶ ، Irritability
    - ▶ ، Difficulty concentrating
- ▶ Panic disorders
  - ▷ Excessive dread of a harmless object or situation
- ▶ Obsessive-compulsive disorder (OCD)
  - ▷ Repetitive thoughts or acts, or both
- ▶ Post-traumatic stress disorder (PTSD)
  - ▷ Delayed anxiety related to a severe trauma

▶ Panic attack

   ▷ Discrete period of intense fear or discomfort with more than four of the following symptoms (DSM-5 criteria; APA 2013):

      ▶ Palpitations, tachycardia, chest pain or discomfort

      ▶ Sweating, chills, or hot flashes

      ▶ Feeling dizzy, unsteady, or faint

      ▶ Trembling or shaking

      ▶ Feeling short of breath or smothered, fear of dying

      ▶ Choking feeling

      ▶ Nausea or abdominal distress

Diagnostic Tests

▶ Thorough history and physical exam

▶ Complete blood count (CBC), basic metabolic panel, thyroid function

▶ ECG, Holter monitor

▶ Mini–Mental Status Exam (MMSE)

▶ Hamilton Anxiety Rating Scale

Differential Diagnoses

▶ Panic disorder

▶ Social anxiety disorder (SAD)

▶ Substance abuse

▶ Hyperthyroidism

▶ Arrhythmias

Management

▶ CBT

▶ Exercise

▶ Stress reduction programs

▶ Counseling

▶ Lifestyle modification

▶ Medication reduction or adjustment

▶ Antidepressants: First-line drug of choice

   ▷ Dosage usually higher than needed to treat depression

   ▷ Numerous antianxiety medications available

▶ Food and Drug Administration (FDA)–approved antidepressants for anxiety disorders:
  ▷ OCD
    ▶ ˙ Fluoxetine (Prozac)
  ▷ OCD, panic, PTSD
    ▶ ˙ Sertraline (Zoloft)
  ▷ OCD, panic, SAD
    ▶ ˙ Paroxetine (Paxil)
  ▷ GAD
    ▶ ˙ Venlafaxine (Effexor)
    ▶ ˙ Duloxetine (Cymbalta)
    ▶ ˙ Buspirone (BuSpar)
▶ Serotonin 1A partial agonist
  ▷ ˙ Not effective for acute anxiety
  ▷ Takes 2–4 weeks for therapeutic effect
  ▷ No dependence, tolerance, withdrawal, CNS depression, or significant drug interactions
  ▷ Adverse reactions are seen in 2030 percent of anxious older adults.
  ▷ GAD, PTSD
    ▶ ˙ Mirtazapine (Remeron)
▶ Medications for panic attack
  ▷ SSRIs, beta blockers, and antipsychotics
  ▷ Benzodiazepines (table 17–4)
    ▶ ˙ For acute anxiety only.
    ▶ Use with great caution in older adults.
    ▶ ˙ Can be used short-term until other medication has reached therapeutic level.
    ▶ Avoid those with long half-lives (flurazepam, diazepam).
    ▶ ˙ Linked with falls, dependence.
    ▶ Can be fatal if combined with alcohol.

TABLE 17–4.
BENZODIAZEPINE THERAPY FOR ANXIETY ATTACKS

BENZODIAZEPINE	STARTING DOSE	USUAL DOSE
Alprazolam (Xanax)	0.25 mg daily or b.i.d.	0.5–3 mg/day
Lorazepam (Ativan)	0.25 mg q h.s.	0.5–1.5 mg/day (in divided doses)
Clonazepam (Klonopin)	0.25 mg daily or b.i.d.	1–2 mg/day

ALCOHOL AND SUBSTANCE ABUSE

► Harmful overuse of alcohol, drugs, or both

► DSM-5 criteria (APA 2013):

▷ Substance-use disorders: Pathological behaviors associated with substance-seeking activities

▷ Substance-induced disorders: Intoxication, withdrawal, and mental disorders caused by a medication or a substance

▷ The severity of substance-use disorders is identified as

► Mild: Two or three symptoms,

► Moderate: Four or five symptoms, or

► Severe: Six or more symptoms.

▷ Major symptom criteria need to occur within the previous 12 months with at least two of the following symptoms:

► Impaired control

▷ Use of a substance in greater amounts than intended or for more prolonged periods of time

▷ Persistent desire to use a substance or unsuccessful efforts aimed at decreasing or controlling substance use

▷ Extensive amounts of time spent obtaining, using, or recovering from the substance

▷ Intense desire or craving for the substance

► Social impairment

▷ Recurrent substance use results in work, school, or home obligation failures

▷ Continued substance use despite persistent interpersonal or social problems

▷ Continued substance use resulting in social isolation or withdrawal from recreational and family activities

► Risky use

▷ Recurrent substance use in physically hazardous situations

▷ Continued use despite physical or psychological problems

► Tolerance

▷ Marked increase in the amount needed to achieve the desired effect or intoxication, or a marked decrease in the effect achieved with the same amount of substance

► Withdrawal

▷ Symptoms that occur when a substance has not been used, or the substance is used to relieve the symptoms of withdrawal (Dunphy et al. 2015, 1085)

Risk Factors

▶ · Family history

▶ · Abuse of other substances

▶ Cultural conditioning

▶ · Domestic violence or abuse

▶ Psychiatric disorder

▶ Stressful events

Signs and Symptoms

▶ · Decline in grooming, physical appearance

▶ · Bloodshot eyes, dilated or constricted pupils

▶ · Appetite or sleep changes

▶ · Sudden weight loss or gain

▶ · Tremors, slurred speech, or impaired coordination

▶ · Erectile dysfunction

Diagnostic Tests

▶ Toxicology

▷ · Older adults experience higher blood alcohol concentration (BAC) levels per amount consumed because of decreased lean body mass and total body water depletion.

▶ Liver function tests

▷ · Liver less efficient in older adults

▶ · Thyroid function tests

▶ · B12, folate

▶ · Prothrombin time, partial thromboplastin time (PT, PTT)

▶ · Lipid panel

▶ · Complete blood count (CBC) if anemia or infection suspected

▶ · Metabolic panel if pancreatitis suspected

▶ · **CAGE** questionnaire

C – Have you ever felt you should **C**ut down on your drinking?

A – Does others' criticism of your drinking **A**nnoy you?

G – Have you ever felt **G**uilty about your drinking?

E – Have you ever had an "**E**ye opener" to steady your nerves or get rid of a hangover?

Differential Diagnoses

▶ Anxiety disorder

▶ Bipolar disorder

Management

▶ Alcohol abuse

▷ Alcohol counseling

▷ Hospitalization for detoxification for acute withdrawal

▷ • Many medications interact with alcohol (NSAIDs, acetaminophen, statins)

▷ Control seizures with benzodiazepines and antipsychotics

▷ • Disulfiram (Antabuse); naltrexone

▷ Thiamine, folic acid, and B complex supplements

▶ Drug abuse

▷ • Usually placed in a controlled setting, like long-term care

▷ Gradually wean medication; small decrease in dose every 2–4 weeks

▶ Maintenance therapy

▷ • Naltrexone; methadone (Dolophine)

▷ Drug counseling

▷ Alcohol and substance abuse counseling

TOBACCO USE AND CESSATION

▶ Repetitive use of tobacco or nicotine despite recurrent and significant adverse medical consequences.

▶ Tobacco- and nicotine-seeking behaviors have accompanying physical dependence, tolerance, and withdrawal.

▶ Links between smoking and poor health are well known.

▶ Fire hazards

▷ Particularly with use of oxygen

▶ Smoking behavior linked to other behaviors.

Management

▶ • Make a plan: Identify

▷ Health beliefs to enhance success.

▷ Smoking-related serious disease.

▷ Strength or will to make an honest attempt.

▷ How benefits of quitting outweigh risks of smoking.

▷ Someone who suffered health problems from smoking.

▷ Set a date to stop within next month.

▷ Decide whether to use nicotine replacement.

▷ Refer to community support groups, smoking cessation classes, or both.

▷ Get rid of cigarettes and smoking items on quit day.

▷ Pick buddy or friend to provide support.

▶ Managing withdrawal

▷ Pharmacological aids

▶ Bupropion (Zyban) 150 mg b.i.d. × 12 weeks

▶ Combined with nicotine replacement, doubles quit rate to 30 percent at 12 months

▶ Contraindicated in seizure disorders

▷ Nicotine replacement

▶ Nicorette gum: 9–12 pieces per day

▷ Nicotine transdermal patches up to 12 weeks

▶ Nicotine spray or inhalers: 6–16 per day

▶ Do not use pharmacological interventions when

▷ Smoker is very motivated,

▷ Smokes <10 cigarettes daily, or

▷ Recent myocardial infarction, uncontrolled hypertension, arrhythmias, severe angina, gastric ulcers; cognitively impaired.

ELDER ABUSE AND NEGLECT

▶ Two-part definition: "(a) Intentional actions that cause harm or create serious risk of harm (whether or not harm is intended) to a vulnerable elder by a caregiver or other person who is in a trust relationship to the elder or (b) failure by a caregiver to satisfy the elder's basic needs or to protect the elder from harm" (Bonnie and Wallace 2003, 40).

Risk Factors

▶ Dementia, mental illness

▶ Dependence

▶ Substance abuse

▶ Inadequate coping

▶ Abused as a child

Signs and Symptoms

- ▶ Anxiety
- ▶ Unexplained bruising, fractures, lacerations
- ▶ Frequent emergency department visits
- ▶ Repeated falls
- ▶ Signs of sexual abuse
- ▶ Older adult states they are being abused

Diagnostic Tests

- ▶ Identify signs and symptoms of abuse
- ▶ Evaluate plausibility of explanations for injuries and conditions
- ▶ Assess cognitive status and health
- ▶ Perform abuse screenings ("Detection of Elder Mistreatment"; Caceres and Fulmer 2012).

Differential Diagnoses

- ▶ Mechanical falls
- ▶ Self-inflicted injuries

Management

- ▶ Ensure safety of abuse victim first.
- ▶ Nurses are mandated by law to report all suspected abuse and neglect of older and disabled adults to adult protective services.
- ▶ Manage medical conditions.
- ▶ A major consideration: Abuse may escalate unless intervention is undertaken.
- ▶ Provide expert testimony.
- ▶ Counseling services.

REFERENCES

American Psychiatric Association. 2013. *Diagnostic and Statistical Manual of Mental Disorders: DSM-5*. 5th ed. Arlington: American Psychiatric Publishing.

American Psychological Association Practice Central. 2015. "Reaching Out to Diverse Populations: Opportunities and Challenges." http://www.apapracticecentral.org/good-practice/secure/Summer07-Populations.pdf.

Bonnie, R. J., and R. B. Wallace, eds. 2003. *Elder Mistreatment: Abuse, Neglect, and Exploitation in an Aging America*. Washington, DC: National Academies Press. https://www.nap.edu/read/10406/chapter/4.

Caceres, B., and T. Fulmer. 2012. "Mistreatment Detection." In *Evidence-Based Geriatric Nursing Protocols for Best Practice*, edited by M. Boltz, E. Capezuti, T. Fulmer, and D. Zwicker, 544–61. 4th ed. New York: Springer.

Dunphy, L., J. Winland-Brown, B. Porter, and D. Thomas, eds. 2015. *Primary Care: The Art and Science of Advanced Practice Nursing*. 4th ed. Philadelphia: F. A. Davis.

APPENDIX A

REVIEW QUESTIONS

1. Which of the following patients may fall outside of the scope of practice of the Adult-Gerontology Primary Care Nurse Practitioner (AGPCNP)?

    a. An 80-year-old woman with advanced cognitive impairments

    b. A 65-year-old man with hypertension

    c. A 10-year-old boy with otitis media

    d. A 70-year-old woman with osteoporosis.

2. Which is true about prescriptive privileges for advanced-practice nurses (APNs)?

    a. Prescriptive privileges require one pharmacy affiliation.

    b. Prescriptive privileges are mandated by state Boards of Nursing.

    c. Prescriptive privileges are contracted through a physician's credentials.

    d. Prescriptive privileges vary from state to state in the United States.

3. The family of a terminally ill, homebound patient who has less than 6 months to live wants to be involved in her end-of-life care. What action is most appropriate?

    a. Admit her into a hospital and take turns being with her 24 hours a day.

    b. Place her in a nursing home with private duty nurses.

    c. Access respite care.

    d. Enroll her in hospice care.

4. A group of nurses want to form a journal club to discuss evidence-based practice studies published in a research-based journal. The director discourages them stating, "Oh that stuff will never help you improve patient outcomes. We've tried that before." The best reply is:

    a. It may be a good time again. This journal has evidenced-based articles for practice.

    b. You're right, why change what we have always done?

    c. Let's ask Dr. Jones, our head of cardiology, to see what he says.

    d. Negativity never solved any problem.

5. A nurse practitioner is teaching a class to a group of younger and older adults. What is important for the NP to remember when preparing educational handouts?

    a. Make most of the information written.

    b. Use a variety of colors to catch attention.

    c. Provide information in several languages.

    d. Maintain a 5th- to 6th-grade reading level.

6. An AGPCNP instructs an older patient about his use of an inhaler. The patient appears puzzled but when asked if he has questions, he says "No, I have no questions." What is the most appropriate action by the AGPCNP?

    a. Ask if he would like written instructions.

    b. Ask a family member to come into the room.

    c. Ask another nurse to help instruct the patient.

    d. Ask the patient to demonstrate how he uses his inhaler to assess his knowledge.

7. An older adult patient who lives alone and has no family has been admitted to the hospital three times in the past 3 months for dehydration, falls, and failure to thrive. What principle is the NP exercising by encouraging the patient to move to a nursing home?

    a. Beneficence
    b. Justice
    c. Autonomy
    d. Fidelity

8. Mrs. L. is an 80-year-old woman with end-stage Alzheimer's disease. She is aphasic, unaware of her surroundings, dependent for all activities of daily living (ADLs), and is progressively failing. She is newly admitted to the nursing home. The facility's AGPCNP has been unsuccessful in obtaining information regarding a living will or advance directive, so there is no do-not-resuscitate (DNR) order documented in her chart. Family members have had little contact with her for several years, and do not have an opinion about whether she should be resuscitated in the event of cardiac arrest. Members of the nursing staff express their discomfort regarding performing cardiopulmonary resuscitation, given Mrs. L.'s condition. What is the AGPCNP's best option?

    a. Contact the physician and request a DNR order.
    b. Convene a multidisciplinary conference to consider alternatives.
    c. Contact the family and tell them CPR will not be performed.
    d. Arrange a meeting with the facility's Ethics Committee.

9. Mrs. Jones is an 80-year-old woman who presents for a physical examination. She recently moved to be closer to her daughter and lives in her own home with her 86-year-old husband. She states she has no restrictions in her ability to perform activities of daily living (ADLs), and she delivers for Meals-on-Wheels twice a week. She wears glasses for reading, smokes 1–2 packs of cigarettes weekly, and drinks a glass of wine with her supper. She takes a daily baby aspirin, a multivitamin, and medication for her high blood pressure. Currently her vital signs are blood pressure (BP) 130/78 mm Hg, heart rate 72 beats per minute, respiration 14 per minute, temperature 97.6° F. Her weight is 210 pounds, and height is 5 feet 5 inches. What preventative health counseling will the NP provide?

    a. BP control, low-fat diet, birth control
    b. Breast exam, alcohol moderation, PSA testing
    c. BP control, tobacco cessation, diet & exercise
    d. Alcohol moderation, tobacco cessation, low-fat diet

10. When taking a nutritional history on an older adult patient, what issue raises a red flag that requires immediate intervention?

    a. A patient with diabetes not eating at regular intervals
    b. Drinking soft drinks, coffee, and tea but no water
    c. A weight loss of more than 10 percent in the last 6 months without trying
    d. Eating only canned vegetables

11. Which of the following fall prevention interventions is most effective in a senior residential facility?

    a. Resident-centered interventions

    b. Environmental interventions

    c. Protective hip pads

    d. Structured, multidisciplinary interventions to reduce residents' risk factors

12. While performing a skin assessment, the NP discovers a suspicious mole. Which of the following characteristics of a mole necessitates immediate intervention?

    a. A symmetrical, uniform brown mole larger than 6 mm on the thigh, unchanged for 5 years

    b. Multiple small, round, flat, smooth-edged dark brown moles across the upper back

    c. A 3-cm waxy facial papule with a "stuck on" appearance

    d. A new 2-cm (20 mm) brown mole with red, irregular border that is occasionally pruritic

13. A 22-year-old complains of a painful, red eye after he got hit in the eye while biking. What is most appropriate in his care?

    a. Ophthalmic antibiotic and cortisone ointment q.i.d.

    b. Normal saline irrigation

    c. Topical anesthetic drops for comfort

    d. Refer to an ophthalmologist

14. When a patient is being treated with Timolol eye drops for glaucoma, what medication would cause concern?

    a. Aspirin prophylaxis for myocardial infarction (MI)

    b. Ranitidine for gastroesophageal reflux disease (GERD)

    c. Inderal for hypertension

    d. Alprazolam for anxiety

15. Routine screening of a 38-year-old man with no risk factors for CAD reveals a total cholesterol of 236. The next step in his plan of care is:

    a. Provide dietary information and recheck cholesterol in 1 year.

    b. Check his low density lipoprotein (LDL) and suggest an exercise program.

    c. Refer to a cardiologist and cardiac rehabilitation.

    d. Check lipid panel and provide information for low-fat diet.

16. How long is the average therapy for tuberculosis (TB)?

    a. 6 weeks to 2 months

    b. 4–6 months

    c. 6 months to a year

    d. 1 year

17. Ms. Piccard is a 38-year-old who reveals that she has smoked a pack of cigarettes daily for over 20 years. She states that for the past year, she has had an intermittent, productive cough. Today, she states that she has had a persistent productive cough for 2 months. What physical finding is the most consistent with Ms. Piccard's history?

    a. Pneumothorax

    b. Pneumonia

    c. Pleural effusion

    d. Increased anterior–posterior chest diameter

18. Which is true of peptic ulcer disease (PUD) in the older adult?

    a. Smoking does not increase the risk.

    b. Ulcers are uncommon in older adults.

    c. Perforation is rare.

    d. Symptoms are often vague.

19. A careful history reveals that a patient has abdominal pain with diarrhea alternating with constipation. What is the most likely diagnosis?

    a. Drug-induced diarrhea

    b. Cholelithiasis

    c. Irritable bowel syndrome (IBS)

    d. Giardiasis

20. A 75-year-old patient is complaining of constipation. Which of the following medications is most likely the cause?

    a. Selective serotonin reuptake inhibitors (SSRIs)

    b. Angiotensin II receptor blockers (ARBs)

    c. Magnesium-based antacids

    d. Anticholinergics

21. A 36-year-old female patient complains of lower abdominal and low back pain, dyspareunia, dysuria, and cramps. What does the NP suspect?

    a. Endometriosis

    b. Vaginitis

    c. Pelvic inflammatory disease (PID)

    d. Urinary tract infection (UTI)

22. Tom is a 24-year-old who came to the clinic with complaints of nausea, fever, malaise, and anorexia for the past 2 days. He drinks 1–2 drinks a month and does not use drugs. He is single and dates weekly. He vacationed in Central America about a month ago, traveled much of the time, stayed at a variety of hotels, and sampled food from retail and local eateries. The NP ordered a hepatitis panel and received the following results:

Total anti-HAV: Positive

IgM anti-HAV: Positive

Total anti-HBc: Positive

IgM antihepatitis B core antigen: Negative

HBsAg: Negative

anti-HBs: Positive

anti-HCV: Negative

What is the diagnosis?

   a.   Acute hepatitis A
   b.   Chronic hepatitis A
   c.   Acute hepatitis B
   d.   Neither hepatitis A nor B

23. What management is appropriate for a patient with acute hepatitis A?

   a.   Bed rest for 6 weeks
   b.   Education
   c.   Quarantine of 15 days
   d.   Hospitalization

24. What is the most sensitive screening test for an active infection with hepatitis C?

   a.   Recombinant immunoblot assay (RIBA)
   b.   Anti-HCV
   c.   Anti-HCV IgG
   d.   HCV RNA

25. What risk factor is associated with breast cancer?

   a.   Being underweight
   b.   Socially drinking alcohol
   c.   Smoking
   d.   High-sodium diet

26. What bacterium is the most common cause of UTIs?

   a. *Escherichia coli*

   b. *Staphylococcus aureus*

   c. *Proteus mirabilis*

   d. *Staphylococcus epidermidis*

27. While assessing a patient's understanding of benign prostatic hypertrophy (BPH), he relates the following information. Which is correct?

   a. Bladder infections are normal because of my enlarged prostate.

   b. I need to be examined twice a year for cancer.

   c. If I need surgery, I will become impotent.

   d. Enlarged prostate is common in older men.

28. What antibiotic is most appropriate for outpatient treatment of mild pyelonephritis?

   a. Ciprofloxacin 500 mg orally twice daily for 7–10 days

   b. Flagyl 500 mg every 6 hours for 7–10 days

   c. Vancomycin 1 g intravenously every 12 hours for 10 days

   d. Tetracycline 250 mg orally four times a day for 14 days

29. After starting outpatient antibiotic therapy for mild pyelonephritis, what important intervention will the NP stress with a patient?

   a. Limit fluid intake

   b. Void less frequently

   c. Kegel exercises

   d. Screen urine routinely

30. If a patient treated as an outpatient for mild pyelonephritis has recurrent symptoms of frequency, urgency, hesitancy, and nocturia, what is the NP's next recommendation?

   a. Refer to a specialist

   b. A kidney biopsy

   c. Another course of antibiotics

   d. A cystoscopy

31. A 17-year-old presents with pain and swelling in his left testis. Pain began suddenly and is rated 8/10. He denies dysuria, frequency, urgency, urethral discharge, fever, chills. He has no significant PMH. He denies sexual activity. Physical exam reveals very painful testis significantly higher in the scrotum than the right, and the cremasteric reflex is negative. The NP has to work quickly. What does the NP think the most likely diagnosis is?

   a. Gonorrhea

   b. Testicular torsion

   c. Prostatitis

   d. Epididymitis

32. An HIV-positive patient presents with several raised, painless, purple, persistent facial lesions. The most likely cause is:

    a. Seborrheic dermatitis

    b. Molluscum contagiosum

    c. Kaposi's sarcoma

    d. Fungal infection

33. In a discussion of treatment with a young woman who has been diagnosed with genital herpes, what information is important for the nurse practitioner to include?

    a. She can be treated and cured with antibiotic therapy for 2 weeks.

    b. The lesions become worse with each subsequent outbreak.

    c. If she ever becomes pregnant she will have to have a cesarean section.

    d. She can spread herpes even if the lesions are not visible.

34. What circumstances most often cause a meniscal tear?

    a. The knee is almost completely extended and the tibia externally rotated.

    b. A strong external force causes external rotation or hyperextension of the knee.

    c. Valgus or varus pressure on the knee occurs at full extension and at 30 degree flexion.

    d. The knee is jammed

35. A frail, petite, 85-year-old Asian woman complains of a sudden onset of thoracic back pain. An X-ray shows a compression fracture. What is the most likely diagnosis?

    a. Osteoarthritis

    b. Herniated disk

    c. Osteoporosis

    d. Rheumatoid arthritis

36. Mrs. T. is a 54-year-old woman who complains of aching in her right knee that worsens with walking and improves with rest. She reports no morning stiffness. What does the NP suspect?

    a. Osteoarthritis

    b. Rheumatoid arthritis

    c. Gout

    d. Osteoporosis

37. What initial intervention should an NP consider for a middle-aged patient with osteoarthritis in the knee?

    a. Acupuncture

    b. Surgery

    c. Allopurinol

    d. Physical therapy

38. What is a good exercise program for a patient newly diagnosed with knee osteoarthritis to start with?

    a. Badminton
    b. Yoga
    c. Cycling
    d. Jogging

39. A patient is about to begin taking Levothyroxine for hypothyroidism. What dietary consideration does she need to be made aware?

    a. Vitamin B supplements should be added.
    b. Levothyroxine should be taken 30 minutes to 1 hour before eating.
    c. Low-salt diet diminishes the effectiveness of Levothyroxine.
    d. Foods high in calcium are contraindicated.

40. Mr. James is a 45-year-old man with diabetes treated with insulin. His blood glucose average ranges from 55 to 60 mg/dL in the morning, around 140 mg/dL at lunch, about 120 mg/dL at dinner, and 100 mg/dL at bedtime. He takes NPH 30 units a day. Before dinner he takes NPH 18 units. What instructions will be most effective?

    a. Decrease evening NPH by 1 unit.
    b. Check blood glucose between 2 a.m. and 4 a.m. for the next few days.
    c. Increase morning regular insulin by 2 units.
    d. Order a fasting blood sugar.

41. Mr. James is a 45-year-old man with diabetes treated with insulin. His blood glucose average ranges from 55 to 60 mg/dL in the morning, around 140 mg/dL at lunch, about 120 mg/dL at dinner, and 100 mg/dL at bedtime. He takes NPH 30 units a day. Before dinner he takes NPH 18 units. Decreasing the evening NPH insulin has not helped to elevate the morning blood sugars significantly. What does the NP believe may be happening?

    a. Mr. James may be exhibiting the dawn phenomenon.
    b. Mr. James has developed insulin resistance.
    c. Mr. James is not eating a substantial bedtime snack.
    d. Mr. James may be experiencing Somogyi effect.

42. A 38-year-old patient with type 1 diabetes continues to have elevated morning blood sugars above 200 mg/dL despite increasing her bedtime insulin. What does the NP suspect is happening?

    a. The patient is not adhering to a diabetic diet.
    b. The patient may be experiencing Somogyi effect.
    c. The patient is not taking her insulin correctly.
    d. The patient is not testing her blood sugar correctly.

43. The NP knows that the Somogyi effect and dawn phenomenon are diagnosed by doing what?

    a. Limiting glucose monitoring to 2 hours postprandial testing.

    b. Increasing glucose monitoring to before and after meals.

    c. Having morning glucose testing done in a lab for a week.

    d. Checking blood sugar at 3 a.m.

44. A 63-year-old African-American woman who presents for her first visit tells the AGPCNP that her finger-stick blood sugar was 243 and her BP was 140/90. What does the AGPCNP recommend?

    a. Antihypertensive medication

    b. Lipid panel

    c. Stress management intervention

    d. Fasting blood sugar

45. Mrs. Warren presents with weight loss, anorexia, weakness, diarrhea, and frequent stools. The nurse practitioner reviews the lab work and discovers that Mrs. Warren's TSH is decreased, and free T4 is elevated. What does she suspect?

    a. Hypothyroidism

    b. Graves' disease

    c. Hyperthyroidism

    d. Thyroid storm

46. The AGPCNP suspects that an anemic 82-year-old patient has pernicious anemia. What is the most likely cause?

    a. Decreased gastric acid secretion

    b. Iron deficiency

    c. Calcium malabsorption

    d. Anemia of chronic disease

47. Which of the following is most likely to cause folic acid (folate) deficiency anemia?

    a. Alcoholism

    b. Coronary artery disease

    c. Diabetes

    d. COPD

48. A 60-year-old woman presents with new-onset headaches and temporal and scalp tenderness on palpation. Her complete blood count (CBC) is normal, but she has an elevated erythrocyte sedimentation rate (ESR). What does the NP suspect?

    a. Prodromal stage of shingles

    b. Temporal arteritis

    c. Rheumatoid arthritis

    d. Hypothyroidism

49. A patient complains of daily, severe, unilateral headaches that involve one eye with increased lacrimation, edema of the eyelid, runny nose, and nasal congestion, lasts from 1 to 4 hours with each episode over a period of weeks and then not occuring again for months. What type of headache does the NP know presents with such signs and symptoms?

    a. Arteritis

    b. Migraine headache

    c. Cluster headache

    d. Sinus headache

50. When Mr. Bart gets up from his chair to walk to the examination room, the NP notices that his movements are rigid and bradykinesic, his gait is shuffling, his posture is stooped and leans forward, and he barely swings his arms. What disease will the NP suspect?

    a. Depression

    b. COPD

    c. Spinal stenosis

    d. Parkinson's disease

51. While a patient with suspected Parkinson's disease is sitting, his right thumb and fingers exhibit alternating tremors (pill-rolling). What does the NP know about the tremors of Parkinson's disease?

    a. Tremors subside with intentional movement.

    b. Emotional distress does not affect tremors of Parkinson's disease.

    c. Tremors remain constant.

    d. Tremors are symmetrical and are more common in lower extremities.

52. What changes associated with Parkinson's disease are most associated with risk for falls?

    a. Increased weight

    b. Mental affect and memory

    c. Gait changes and gait velocity

    d. Stooped posture and vision

53. Which of the following patients has the greatest risk of suicide?

    a. An 85-year-old white man who recently lost his wife of 65 years

    b. A 65-year-old black woman with arthritis

    c. A mildly demented man with decreased impulse control

    d. An 86-year-old white woman who needs assistance and is moving in with her daughter.

54. Mrs. B. is a 67-year-old woman who presents with complaints of fatigue, difficulty sleeping, and vague muscle aches and pains. In conversation, she reveals that a year ago she retired as executive director of a large organization. Her daughter is getting divorced and recently moved in with Mrs. B. with her two school-age children. Mrs. B.'s husband is pressuring her to move to Florida to relax and enjoy her retirement. Mrs. B.'s exam is normal. The NP comments that she is approximately 25 pounds overweight. Mrs. B. begins to cry, and states that her clothes no longer fit, and she feels "so old." What additional information does the NP need to make a diagnosis?

    a. How long has she been feeling this way?
    b. Has she ever had psychiatric treatment before?
    c. What is the quality of her relationship with her husband?
    d. How has she coped with similar events in the past?

55. When treating a person with antidepressants, what must the NP remember?

    a. Initially, high doses of antidepressant are given to alleviate symptoms.
    b. Psychotherapy and drugs together are more effective than either in isolation.
    c. Antidepressants are expensive and potential side effects may not be worth it.
    d. Antidepressants will not be effective for sleep difficulties.

56. Mrs. B. is a 67-year-old woman who presents with complaints of fatigue, difficulty sleeping, and vague muscle aches and pains. In conversation, she reveals that a year ago she retired as executive director of a large organization. Her daughter is getting divorced and recently moved in with Mrs. B. with her two school-age children. Mrs. B.'s husband is pressuring her to move to Florida to relax and enjoy her retirement. Mrs. B.'s exam is normal. The NP comments that she is approximately 25 pounds overweight. Mrs. B. begins to cry, and states that her clothes no longer fit, and she feels "so old." The NP is considering an antidepressant for Mrs. B. Which would be the best choice?

    a. Lithium
    b. Alprazolam (Xanax)
    c. Citalopram (Celexa)
    d. Quetiapine (Seroquel)

57. What is known about depression?

    a. It rarely responds well to treatment.
    b. It is precipitated by shame and self-accusations.
    c. It is rare without a history of depression.
    d. It may be exhibited as inappropriate guilt or low self-esteem.

58. A patient has been diagnosed with generalized anxiety disorder (GAD). Which of the following medications may be used to treat it?

    a. Alprazolam (Xanax) or diazepam (Valium)
    b. Venlafaxine (Effexor) or duloxetine (Cymbalta)
    c. Trazodone (Desyrel) or sertraline (Zoloft)
    d. Venlafaxine (Effexor) or hydroxyzine pamoate (Vistaril)

59. A patient is scheduled for a series of tests to determine whether his dementia is treatable. What forms of dementia can be arrested or reversed?

    a. Dehydration

    b. Multiple sclerosis

    c. Alzheimer's disease

    d. None

60. Mr. Taft is a 76-year-old recently widowed man who presents to the office with complaints of weakness, insomnia, and health concerns. He appears agitated and is having difficulty focusing on any one aspect of his physical complaints. He previously was in excellent health except for an enlarged prostate for which he had surgery. Four weeks after surgery he started complaining of burning in his bladder. The urologist's repeated examinations revealed no abnormalities. Before this visit he was calling the office daily with updates on his complaints and newly developed health issues. He mentions that he was arrested over the weekend for firing a gun in his yard because he wanted to see if it still worked. He denies any thoughts of self-harm or suicide. What does the NP need to consider?

    a. He is responding normally to his stress.

    b. He is moderately depressed.

    c. He has antisocial tendencies

    d. He is at risk for suicide.

61. What is the next step for the NP to take in treating an older adult patient suspected to be at risk for suicide?

    a. Immediately commit him for in-patient psychiatric treatment.

    b. Counsel him about worrying making his symptoms worse.

    c. Remind him that he is in better shape than many of his peers.

    d. Refer him for a psychiatric evaluation today.

62. What should NPs know about electroconvulsive shock therapy (ECT) in the treatment of depression?

    a. ECT usually requires 2 weeks to improve depressive symptoms.

    b. ECT treatment does not cause memory problems.

    c. ECT is used for severe depression not responding to antidepressants.

    d. ECT is effective in 30–40 percent of patients who receive it.

63. The AGPCNP is examining an older adult patient for nursing home placement and notices bruising across the patient's back and upper arms in varying stages of healing. The patient states, "Oh, I am always tripping and falling." Her daughter asks to come into the examination room and the patient immediately becomes very quiet and withdrawn. What is the best action for the AGPCNP to take?

   a. Ask the daughter to go to the receptionist to fill out paperwork before coming into the exam room so you can ask the patient questions regarding possible abuse.

   b. Allow the daughter to come into the examination room so that she can provide more concrete explanations about the falling habits of her mother.

   c. Immediately call Adult Protective Services to investigate whether there has been abuse if the patient returns to another appointment with more bruises.

   d. Do not get involveThe patient is going into nursing home anyway.

64. Which of the following statements is true regarding breast cancer?

   a. Edema of breast is usually not indicative of cancer.

   b. All newly developed breast masses in older woman are cancer.

   c. Nipple retraction is not usually a sign of cancer

   d. Change in size or shape of the breast is an important sign of cancer

APPENDIX B

REVIEW QUESTION ANSWERS

1. **Correct Answer**: **C**. AGPCNP scope of practice preparation is population-focused and ensures competencies in adult-gerontology primary care advanced nursing practice. Other Nurse Practitioner (NP) practice preparation that requires population-focused education are in family, neonates, pediatrics, psychiatric–mental health, and women's health areas. Additional preparation in specialized areas of practice (e.g., palliative care, orthopedics, cardiology) are beyond role and population foci and require additional education.

2. **Correct Answer: D.** APN prescriptive privileges, just like APN credentialing, vary from state to state and are mandated through legislation.

3. **Correct Answer: D.** Hospice and palliative care provide medical care, pain management, and emotional and spiritual support for life-limiting illness or injury. Both support the right to die pain-free, with dignity, with support for patients and family. Hospice care is limited to those who are terminally ill or within 6 months of death. Palliative care is available at any stage of illness whether terminal or not. Respite care provides short-term care to the ill outside the home to provide relief to family caregivers.

4. **Correct Answer: A.** In change theory, this is an example of letting go of counterproductive ideations (unfreezing) to embrace productive change (moving to a new level) and embracing change (refreezing).

5. **Correct Answer: D.** Reading ability of the average U.S. citizen is about at the 8th-grade level. Educational reading materials should be between 5th- and 6th-grade levels to maximize comprehension.

6. **Correct Answer: D.** As a component of interactive communication to summarize knowledge, the patient relays or demonstrates what he or she knows to enable the nurse to evaluate the patient's understanding and learning needs.

7. **Correct Answer: A.** *Beneficence* is action that is done for the benefit of another to help prevent harm or to improve a bad situation of another ("Do no harm").

8. **Correct Answer: D.** The facility's Ethic Committee assists in clarifying the ethical principles and the facility's policies as they relate to the rights of the patient and laws of the state, so that action can be taken to move forward in decisions regarding resuscitation. Often such cases are taken to court so that a state-appointed guardian can be assigned to make decisions regarding care.

9. **Correct Answer: C.** Based on Mrs. Jones' risk factors for coronary artery disease (CAD)—being a smoker, overweight, and currently treated for hypertension—controlling BP, tobacco cessation guidance, changes to diet, and exercise are most appropriate to lower her risk for CAD.

10. **Correct Answer: C.** Unintentional weight loss of 5 percent in 30 days or 10 percent in 6 months is an indicator of poor nutrition.

11. **Correct Answer: D.** Multidisciplinary interventions are most effective for identifying and planning safety precautions and fall prevention measures in care settings for all patients, and especially older adults.

12. **Correct Answer: D.** Skin lesions that are > 6 mm with irregular borders, varying color, and itching are indicators that require follow-up.

13. **Correct Answer: D.** Acute corneal abrasion can occur when something gets into the eye and scratches the cornea. Symptoms include feeling as though something is in the eye, pain, tearing, redness, sensitivity to light, blurred vision, or vision loss. Refer to an ophthalmologist.

14. **Correct Answer: C.** Inderal is a beta blocker. Timolol is also a beta blocker. Beta blockers lower blood pressure. The combination of Timolol and Inderal can cause hypotension and should be monitored closely.

15. **Correct Answer: D.** A lipid panel should be done. The more elevated the LDL, the greater the risk for heart disease.

16. **Correct Answer: C.** Average TB treatment regimens are for 6 months to a year.

17. **Correct Answer: D.** In a 2-pack-a-day smoker, chronic obstructive pulmonary disease (COPD) is probable. The anterior–posterior chest diameter is often increased 2:1.

18. **Correct Answer: D.** Symptoms of PUD are blunted in older adults, who often do not present any signs until they begin to hemorrhage.

19. **Correct Answer: C.** In addition to cramping and bloating, IBS symptoms can include alternating episodes of diarrhea and constipation.

20. **Correct Answer: D.** Medications with anticholinergic effects (antiemetics, cold preparations, and psychotropics) may cause constipation.

21. **Correct Answer: C.** PID causes dyspareunia, lower abdominal or low back pain, dysuria, and cramps.

22. **Correct Answer: A.** Specific serologic studies distinguish the forms of viral hepatitis. Hepatitis A is confirmed with a positive IgM anti-HAV test. This test is widely available and results are usually available within 24 hours. The hepatitis B serologic tests indicate past, resolved infection with no chronic infection. Acute hepatitis C anti-HCV may be delayed for as long as 6 months after exposure. The most common signs and symptoms associated with acute hepatitis A include jaundice, fever, malaise, anorexia, and abdominal discomfort.

23. **Correct Answer: B.** There is no specific treatment for hepatitis A beyond treating the symptoms that occur. Bed rest does not hasten recovery. Quarantine is not necessary. Hepatitis A is spread by contaminated food and water via the fecal–oral root; therefore, education about disease spread, immunization, and safeguards to take when travelling outside the United States are important factors of hepatitis A management.

24. **Correct Answer: D.** Anti-HCV, RIBA, and anti-HCV IgG blood tests confirm the presence of antibodies that indicate either active or past infection. Testing for HCV RNA is necessary to confirm an active infection. If the HCV RNA test is positive, the genotype is determined and the viral load is measured.

25. **Correct Answer: C.** American Cancer Society's Cancer Prevention II study links smoking to breast cancer.

26. **Correct Answer: A.** *Escherichia coli* is the most common bacterium to cause UTIs (28 percent).

27. **Correct Answer: D.** Bladder infections may occur if incomplete emptying of the bladder is persistent, but they are not normal. Enlarged prostate is associated with aging and is common in men older than 50 years. BPH is unrelated to cancer. Though impotence may result from surgery, it is rare.

28. **Correct Answer: A.** Most commonly used antibiotics for outpatient treatment of pyelonephritis are oral fluoroquinolones (ciprofloxin [Cipro], levofloxin [Levoquin]), cephalosporins (ceftriaxone [Rocephin], ceftazidime [Fortaz]), penicillins (amoxicillin [Amox], ampicillin [Principen]), and sulfanimide (sulfamethoxazole and trimethoprim [*Bactrim DS*]). Outpatient treatment is appropriate for mild pyelonephritis.

29. **Correct Answer: D.** Urine should be screened routinely to identify recurrent infections. Fluids should be increased to 2–3 liters per day to decrease urine concentration. Voiding more frequently will avoid bladder distention.

30. **Correct Answer: A.** For recurrent infections, evaluation and treatment by a specialist is necessary to preserve kidney function.

31. **Correct Answer: B.** Sudden onset of testicular pain and a unilaterally elevated scrotum is highly suspicious for testicular torsion. It is a medical emergency. If torsion is corrected within 12 hours of onset, testicular salvage occurs in 80 percent of occurrences. After 24 hours, irreversible testicular infarction is expected.

32. **Correct Answer: C.** Kaposi's sarcoma is an AIDS-related vascular neoplasm that appears as dark, red-purple, plaques or nodules on cutaneous and mucosal surfaces. Most frequently affected are the face, trunk, oral cavity, and extremities. Seborrheic dermatitis is a severe inflammation of skin characterized by an erythemic, scaling rash where sebaceous glands are concentrated. Molluscum contagiosum is a viral infection that presents as small, hard, nodular, flesh-colored, grouped lesions that eventually become umbilicated in the center. In children, face, trunk, and extremities are involved but it presents most commonly in adults in the pubic and genital areas.

33. **Correct Answer: D.** It is important to know that even if there are no visible lesions, herpes can be spread through the skin and to sexual partners. Guidance for protected sex should be followed.

34. **Correct Answer: B.** Meniscus tears are usually the result of an injury from a sudden sharp force or blow to the knee that causes it to pivot and rotate. Sports such as hockey, basketball, or football are often involved.

35. **Correct Answer: C.** Fractures are sometimes the first indication of osteoporosis. Typical fracture sites are the vertebrae, wrist, femur, and ribs. Being older than 65 years, female, petite, and Asian or Caucasian increase risk for osteoporosis.

36. **Correct Answer: A.** Osteoarthritis occurs most often in weight-bearing joints. Symptoms are usually asymmetrical. Discomfort worsens with movement and is relieved with rest.

37. **Correct Answer: D.** One of the first and most beneficial interventions for osteoarthritis is to stay mobile to reduce pain and help maintain a healthy weight. Strengthening exercises build muscles around OA-affected joints, easing the burden on those joints and reducing pain. Range-of-motion exercise helps maintain and improve joint flexibility and reduce stiffness.

38. **Correct Answer: C.** High-impact exercise such as jogging, downhill skiing, and step aerobics place impact on knee, hips, and spine, and can worsen arthritis. Exercises and sports such as yoga, Pilates, gymnastics, volleyball, and basketball that tend to hyperextend the knee and lead to bone-on-bone contact can promote and aggravate osteoarthritis. Low-impact aerobic exercise such as swimming, walking, and cycling are generally safe and beneficial for osteoarthritis.

39. **Correct Answer: B.** The absorption of levothyroxine is decreased when taken with some foods, supplements, and drugs so, levothyroxine should be taken on an empty stomach 30 to 60 minutes before food intake to avoid erratic absorption of the hormone.

40. **Correct Answer: A.** Adjusting evening NPH may normalize glucose in the morning. One unit of insulin will drop glucose by 60 mg/dL for the duration of action of that particular insulin (short-acting insulin for 2–3 hours; intermediate-acting insulin for 12–24 hours; long-acting insulin for 24 hours).

41. **Correct Answer: C.** When using older insulins such as NPH and regular insulin, a high-protein and high-fat snack before bed will keep glucose levels higher as the insulin effects linger and help to decrease hypoglycemic episodes. Consider changing to newer long-acting insulin or using an insulin pump.

42. **Correct Answer: B.** Somogyi effect (rebound hyperglycemia) is a pattern of hypoglycemia episodes below 70 mg/dL followed by hyperglycemia above 200 mg/dL. Typically, this occurs with too much circulating insulin, and often occurs in the middle of the night. During the periods of hypoglycemia, stored glucose is released, causing hyperglycemia.

43. **Correct Answer: D.** Somogyi effect occurs as a result of too much circulating insulin, causing hypoglycemia that stimulates the release glucose resulting in hyperglycemia. Dawn phenomenon is the result of too little circulating insulin from early morning hormone release (growth hormone, cortisol, and catecholamines) resulting in hyperglycemia. Both occur in the middle of the night. Taking a 3 a.m. glucose level for a few nights will identify the cause. If the blood glucose is consistently low during this time, the Somogyi effect is the likely cause. If blood glucose is normal or high during this time, the dawn phenomenon is more likely the cause.

44. **Correct Answer: D.** In a patient who exhibits no symptoms of diabetes, a single fasting blood sugar at or above 126 mg/dL is diagnostic of diabetes. A second random blood sugar result of 200 mg/dL or higher, or an elevated A1C, would also confirm diabetes.

45. **Correct Answer: C.** A decreased TSH and elevated free T4 are diagnostic of hyperthyroidism. Conversely, an elevated TSH and decreased free T4 are diagnostic of hypothyroidism.

46. **Correct Answer: A.** Pernicious anemia is an autoimmune disorder that causes antibodies against intrinsic factor and gastric parietal cells, decreasing gastric acid secretion and thereby inhibiting absorption of vitamin B12.

47. **Correct Answer: A.** Along with overall malnutrition, alcoholism can cause folate deficiency. None of the other conditions are associated with folate deficiency.

48. **Correct Answer: B.** Being older than 50 years, having a new-onset headache, temporal and scalp tenderness, and an elevated ESR are suspect for temporal (giant-cell) arteritis. Vison may also be affected. If vision loss occurs, patients are immediately referred to an ophthalmologist.

49. **Correct Answer: C.** Cluster headaches cause daily, severe, unilateral, periorbital pain that may include ipsilateral rhinorrhea, nasal congestion, and eye redness. These headaches can last for weeks and then not occur again for months.

50. **Correct Answer: D.** Among other signs and symptoms, Parkinson's disease presents with bradykinesia; postural instability; slowed, shuffling gait; and rigidity.

51. **Correct Answer: A.** The tremors of Parkinson's often begin asymmetrically, affecting the arms more than the legs. They subside with intentional movement, and emotional distress and lack of sleep can aggravate them.

52. **Correct Answer: C.** Parkinsonian changes in gait are shuffling, bradykinesia, and rigidity, which increase the risk of falling.

53. **Correct Answer: A.** Older men who are socially isolated are at high risk for suicide.

54. **Correct Answer: A.** Establishing a timeline is important for developing a plan of care.

55. **Correct Answer: B.** Without psychotherapy to help deal with psychological issues, anti-depressants only relieve the depressive symptoms, and do not address the underlying problems.

56. **Correct Answer: C.** Selective serotonin reuptake inhibitors (SSRIs) and serotonin and norepinephrine reuptake inhibitors (SNRIs) are used in conjunction with counseling for the treatment of depression. They cause fewer effects than other antidepressants. Lithium is used to treat the manic episodes of manic depression. Alprazolam (xanax) is used to treat anxiety and panic disorders. Quetiapine (Seroquel) is an antipsychotic used to treat bipolar disorder (manic depression).

57. **Correct Answer: D.** Depression may exhibit as inappropriate guilt or low self-esteem, or poor sense of self-worth. It may be precipitated by the loss of friends, status, or abilities. *The Diagnostic and Statistical Manual of Mental Disorders,* Fifth Edition (DSM-5) requires depression or anhedonia plus four of the following to be present: 1) Appetite change with weight gain or loss of more than 5 percent of body weight in one month, 2) hypersomnia or insomnia, 3) psychomotor agitation or retardation, 4) fatigue, 5) decreased ability to concentrate, or 6) recurrent suicide or death thoughts.

58. **Correct Answer: B.** Selective serotonin reuptake inhibitors (SSRIs) and serotonin and norepinephrine reuptake inhibitors (SNRIs) are first-line treatment for GAD (especially with comorbid depression), and have lesser side effects than benzodiazepines or sedating antidepressants.

59. **Correct Answer: A.** Dementias that are reversible include those caused by dehydration, nutritional or metabolic disorders, vascular disease, space-occupying lesions, normal-pressure hydrocephalus, or depression. Irreversible dementias are Alzheimer's disease, multi-infarct dementia, Creutzfeldt-Jakob disease, Pick's disease, Parkinson's disease, Huntington's disease, cerebellar degenerations, amyotrophic lateral sclerosis (ALS), AIDS, Down syndrome, and Korsakoff's syndrome.

60. **Correct Answer: D.** Recently widowed and older men are four times more likely to commit suicide. Most male suicides are committed with firearms. His depression, agitation, and recent impulsive behavior place him at risk for suicide.

61. **Correct Answer: D.** Psychiatric evaluation is pertinent for identifying his risk for suicide, self-harm and need for in-patient treatment.

62. **Correct Answer: C.** ECT is mostly used when severe depression is unresponsive to other forms of therapy, and is one of the fastest ways to relieve symptoms in severely depressed or suicidal patients.. ECT begins to work quicker, often starting within the first week. Some people may experience memory problems, especially of memories around the time of the treatment. Sometimes the memory problems are more severe, but usually they improve over the days and weeks following the end of an ECT course. ECT response rates are typically in the 60–90% range.

63. **Correct Answer: A.** Anxiety, unexplained bruising, injuries, and claims of repeated falls in older adults are signs of elder abuse. Having time alone with a patient to ask questions regarding abuse without the presence of the possible abuser is pertinent to prevent further episodes and make sure the patient is safe.

64. **Correct Answer: D.** A change in breast size, nipple retraction or discharge, breast pain, itching, dimpling *peau d'orange* (warm, red, swollen breasts with or without a rash with dimpling of skin that resembles the skin of an orange) are all signs of breast cancer.